Building Resilient Healthcare Systems With ICTs

Patrick Ndayizigamiye
University of Johannesburg, South Africa

Macire Kante
University of Johannesburg, South Africa

A volume in the Advances in Healthcare Information Systems and Administration (AHISA) Book Series

IGI Global
PUBLISHER of TIMELY KNOWLEDGE

Published in the United States of America by
IGI Global
Medical Information Science Reference (an imprint of IGI Global)
701 E. Chocolate Avenue
Hershey PA, USA 17033
Tel: 717-533-8845
Fax: 717-533-8661
E-mail: cust@igi-global.com
Web site: http://www.igi-global.com

Library of Congress Cataloging-in-Publication Data

Names: Ndayizigamiye, Patrick, 1979- editor. | Kante, Macire, 1983- editor.

Title: Building resilient healthcare systems with ICTs / Patrick Ndayizigamiye and Macire Kante, editors.
Description: Hershey, PA : Medical Information Science Reference, [2022] | Includes bibliographical references and index. | Summary: "This book will highlight various ways ICTs could help build resilience within healthcare systems presenting multi-perspective stances within the book highlighting the various contexts in which resilience could be built within healthcare systems"-- Provided by publisher.
Identifiers: LCCN 2021050260 (print) | LCCN 2021050261 (ebook) | ISBN 9781799889151 (hardcover) | ISBN 9781799889168 (ebook)
Subjects: MESH: COVID-19--epidemiology | Pandemics--prevention & control | Information Technology | Delivery of Health Care | Africa
Classification: LCC RA644.C67 (print) | LCC RA644.C67 (ebook) | NLM WC 506.4 HA1 | DDC 614.5/92414--dc23/eng/20211207
LC record available at https://lccn.loc.gov/2021050260
LC ebook record available at https://lccn.loc.gov/2021050261

This book is published in the IGI Global book series Advances in Healthcare Information Systems and Administration (AHISA) (ISSN: 2328-1243; eISSN: 2328-126X)

British Cataloguing in Publication Data
A Cataloguing in Publication record for this book is available from the British Library.

Advances in Healthcare Information Systems and Administration (AHISA) Book Series

ISSN:2328-1243
EISSN:2328-126X

Editor-in-Chief: Anastasius Moumtzoglou, Hellenic Society for Quality & Safety in Healthcare and P. & A. Kyriakou Children's Hospital, Greece

MISSION

The **Advances in Healthcare Information Systems and Administration (AHISA) Book Series** aims to provide a channel for international researchers to progress the field of study on technology and its implications on healthcare and health information systems. With the growing focus on healthcare and the importance of enhancing this industry to tend to the expanding population, the book series seeks to accelerate the awareness of technological advancements of health information systems and expand awareness and implementation.

Driven by advancing technologies and their clinical applications, the emerging field of health information systems and informatics is still searching for coherent directing frameworks to advance health care and clinical practices and research. Conducting research in these areas is both promising and challenging due to a host of factors, including rapidly evolving technologies and their application complexity. At the same time, organizational issues, including technology adoption, diffusion and acceptance as well as cost benefits and cost effectiveness of advancing health information systems and informatics applications as innovative forms of investment in healthcare are gaining attention as well. **AHISA** addresses these concepts and critical issues.

COVERAGE

- Clinical Decision Support Design, Development and Implementation
- Management of Emerging Health Care Technologies
- Medical Informatics
- E-Health and M-Health
- Nursing Expert Systems
- IT security and privacy issues
- Measurements and Impact of HISA on Public and Social Policy
- Decision Support Systems
- Telemedicine
- Role of informatics specialists

IGI Global is currently accepting manuscripts for publication within this series. To submit a proposal for a volume in this series, please contact our Acquisition Editors at Acquisitions@igi-global.com or visit: http://www.igi-global.com/publish/.

The Advances in Healthcare Information Systems and Administration (AHISA) Book Series (ISSN 2328-1243) is published by IGI Global, 701 E. Chocolate Avenue, Hershey, PA 17033-1240, USA, www.igi-global.com. This series is composed of titles available for purchase individually; each title is edited to be contextually exclusive from any other title within the series. For pricing and ordering information please visit http://www.igi-global.com/book-series/advances-healthcare-information-systems-administration/37156. Postmaster: Send all address changes to above address.

Titles in this Series

For a list of additional titles in this series, please visit:
http://www.igi-global.com/book-series/advances-healthcare-information-systems-administration/37156

Prospects of Blockchain Technology for Accelerating Scientific Advancement in Healthcare
Malaya Dutta Borah (National Institute of Technology (NIT), India) Peng Zhang (Belmont University, USA) and Ganesh Chandra Deka (Ministry of Skill Development and Entrepreneurship, Government of India, India)
Medical Information Science Reference • © 2022 • 315pp • H/C (ISBN: 9781799896067) • US $285.00

Quality of Healthcare in the Aftermath of the COVID-19 Pandemic
Anastasius Moumtzoglou (P&A Kyriakou Children's Hospital, Greece)
Medical Information Science Reference • © 2022 • 403pp • H/C (ISBN: 9781799891987) • US $325.00

Handbook of Research on Applied Intelligence for Health and Clinical Informatics
Anuradha Dheeraj Thakare (Pimpri Chinchwad College of Engineering, Savitribai Phule Pune University, India) Sanjeev J. Wagh (Shivaji University, India) Manisha Sunil Bhende (Dr. D.Y. Patil Institute of Engineering, Management, and Research Akurdi, India & Savitribai Phule Pune University, India) Ahmed M. Anter (Beni-Suef University, Egypt) and Xiao-Zhi Gao (University of Eastern Finland, Finland)
Medical Information Science Reference • © 2022 • 470pp • H/C (ISBN: 9781799877097) • US $425.00

Developing Maternal Health Decision Support Systems in Developing Countries
Vincent Mzazi (University of South Africa, South Africa)
Medical Information Science Reference • © 2021 • 286pp • H/C (ISBN: 9781799839583) • US $265.00

For an entire list of titles in this series, please visit:
http://www.igi-global.com/book-series/advances-healthcare-information-systems-administration/37156

IGI Global
PUBLISHER of TIMELY KNOWLEDGE

701 East Chocolate Avenue, Hershey, PA 17033, USA
Tel: 717-533-8845 x100 • Fax: 717-533-8661
E-Mail: cust@igi-global.com • www.igi-global.com

Table of Contents

Detailed Table of Contents

Disease outbreaks do not only create health challenges; they also potentially affect public health communication. To complement the efforts of medical and health workers, health communication professionals often try to design semiotic resources to advance the goal of health and medical practice. This chapter, therefore, explores the various semiotic resources created with the aid of digital technologies and deployed by the Nigeria Center for Disease Control across digital platforms to combat the COVID-19 pandemic. Applying Kress and van Leeuwen's social semiotic theory to 12 NCDC images sourced online, the chapter demonstrates that the semiotic resources shared by the NCDC on hygiene practices to fight COVID-19 have the potential of broadening the scope of interpretation, meaning, and understanding of COVID-19, health problems, and medical practices on account of the texts' representational, interactional, and compositional structures, thereby helping in building a vibrant healthcare system in Nigeria.

In the current context of the COVID-19 pandemic, many healthcare institutions have resorted to eHealth to manage the disruption in healthcare brought by the pandemic. However, the extent to which eHealth has been used in the context of the COVID-19 pandemic has not been widely investigated. It is in this context that this study sought to systematically review research trends on the use of eHealth in the context of the COVID-19 pandemic era, the theoretical underpinnings of the studies on the use of eHealth in the context of the COVID-19 pandemic, and the contributions made by these studies. Findings revealed that most studies focused on the 'health in our hands' and 'interacting for health' components of eHealth while none of the studies focused on the 'data enabling health' component. In addition, none of the reviewed studies used a theoretical framework. Albeit with limitations, these studies shed light on the use of eHealth applications for patients' data management and the provision of telemedicine in the fight against COVID-19.

preliminary findings revealed that the derived model explains 32.9% of the user's self-disclosure intention on social network sites.

Preface

The Coronavirus (COVID-19) pandemic has imposed new challenges to healthcare systems as well as to the provision of healthcare services. These challenges have affected and continue to affect the healthcare systems' stakeholders. Consequently, these stakeholders are forced to adjust and manage new challenges related to healthcare services delivery arising from the pandemic. Thus, many healthcare institutions and other stakeholders have resorted to Information and Communication Technologies (ICTs), in their quest to build resilience in the face of the negative repercussions of the pandemic.

In broad terms, resilience can be defined as the capacity to cope with, adjust to, and potentially transform amid change and uncertainty (Heeks & Ospina, 2015). Healthcare Systems have three distinct components: structure (structural components and the relations amongst them), process (functions), and properties. Heeks & Ospina (2015) cautioned that resilience is neither a systemic structure nor a systemic process, but a systemic property. Thus, the adaptive capacity of healthcare systems should not be drawn simply from the structural elements but also from the properties of those elements in a systemic combination (Norris et al., 2008).

Information and Communication Technologies play an important role in building adaptive healthcare systems. Thus, the title of this book, "Building resilient healthcare systems with ICTs" implies the building of adaptive healthcare systems using ICTs. In this case, ICTs are seen as the enablers of such resilience. Information and Communication Technologies can help stakeholders in healthcare services delivery to swiftly respond to healthcare disasters and be adequately prepared for future adverse events. Furthermore, ICTs can also strengthen healthcare institutions to withstand external shocks. In the context of the Covid-19 pandemic, there has been many ICT-led interventions to monitor the spread of the disease, hospital admissions, and compliance with safety regulations, to name a few. The common denominator of all these interventions is that they enable stakeholders in the management of the disease to make informed decisions to curb the disease. Hence, there is evidence that ICTs can be one of the components of building resilient healthcare systems.

This book is intended for stakeholders who are involved in the design and implementation of healthcare systems. These include but are not limited to policymakers, researchers in healthcare, healthcare professionals, Information Technology (IT) professionals, and health care managers. This book will also be beneficial to anyone who may want to get insights into building resilience using ICTs.

The book is organized into ten chapters. A brief description of each of the chapters follows:

Chapter 1 investigated the implementation of a visual telerehabilitation protocol during the COVID-19 pandemic in Italy. In March 2020, the Italian Government declared the state of lockdown to curb the spread of COVID-19 pandemic. This led to many challenges in the provision of rehabilitation services to people with disabilities. Consequently, there was a transition to the telematic provision of healthcare as an adaptive approach to the constraints posed by the pandemic. In the visual rehabilitation field, the lack of international guidelines for telematic rehabilitation led to pioneering interventions which were challenged by difficulties in the use of technological devices by visually impaired individuals. The purpose of this chapter was to identify the peculiar features that could enable the provision of visual telerehabilitation during the pandemic by analyzing the procedures followed in the implementation of a visual telerehabilitation protocol in Italy and the outcomes thereof.

Chapter 2 explored the various semiotic resources created with the aid of digital technologies and deployed by the Nigerian Center for Disease Control (NCDC) across digital platforms to combat the COVID-19 pandemic. Applying the Kress and van Leeuwen's social semiotic theory to 12 NCDC's images sourced online, the chapter demonstrated that the semiotic resources shared by the NCDC on hygiene practices to fight COVID-19 have the potential of broadening the scope of interpretation, meaning and understanding of COVID-19, health problems, medical practices on accounts of the texts' representational, interactional, and compositional structures, thereby helping in building a vibrant healthcare system in Nigeria.

Chapter 3 posits that in the current context of the COVID-19 pandemic, many healthcare institutions have resorted to eHealth to manage the disruption in healthcare brought by the pandemic. However, the extent to which eHealth has been used in the context of the COVID-19 pandemic has not been widely investigated. Therefore, the study reported in this chapter sought to systematically review research trends on the use of eHealth in the context of the COVID-19 pandemic era, the theoretical underpinnings of the studies on the use of eHealth in the context of the COVID-19 pandemic, and the contributions made by these studies. Findings revealed that most studies focused on the 'health in our hands' and 'interacting for health' components of eHealth while none of the studies focused on the 'data enabling health' component. In addition, none of the reviewed studies used a theoretical framework. Albeit the limitations of these studies, they shed light on the use of eHealth applications for patients' data management and the provision of telemedicine in the fight against COVID-19.

Chapter 4 investigated the use of digital technologies as a response to the COVID-19 Pandemic in Sub-Saharan countries. The study explored possible ways towards building an open, inclusive, and secure digital ecosystem using digital technologies to create awareness of the Coronavirus pandemic. The qualitative approach and critical discourse analysis were adopted to critically analyze the effects of digital technologies in the healthcare sector of the Sub-Saharan African region while the technology determinism theory was used as the theoretical lens of the study. This study advocated the use of digital technologies as an effective tool to disseminate information about infectious diseases to the citizens of the Sub-Saharan African region.

Chapter 5 investigated factors that led to the successful implementation of mobile health interventions for public healthcare in the East African Community (EAC) and lessons learnt from these implementations that could assist in devising successful mHealth interventions. The findings of this study revealed that forging partnerships with key stakeholders, adapting mHealth interventions to the cultural context, leveraging local opportunities, involving users in the design phase of mHealth interventions, planning for sustainability of mHealth interventions from the design phase, having a policy framework, and a monitoring system to guide mHealth activities, are key factors that led to the success of these interventions.

Chapter 6 reported the results of a study which evaluated the impacts of an mHealth system named Cstock on the supply chain management of medical supplies in village clinics of Mangochi district in Malawi. The study found that Cstock mHealth was used for requesting health products, supply, and resupply from healthcare facilities. In terms of quality, it was reported that the Cstock system was fast, easy to learn, and rarely displayed error reports. Besides, Cstock mHealth yielded positive impacts through time and cost savings, improved communication, availability of essential medical stocks at all levels of the supply chain, and improved data visibility for decision-making. However, poor network coverage, lack of power source for charging phone batteries, absence of monetary incentives, and lack of technical support, compromised the effective utilisation of the Cstock system. The chapter offers insights to policy makers, implementers, and research practitioners on how to build resilience in the management medical supply chain in a primary healthcare setting through the use of innovative mHealth technology.

Chapter 7 investigated the reliability of performance factors for evaluating Electronic Health Information Systems (EHIS). The chapter posits that assessing Information System functions performance like EHIShas been an issue for Information Systems executives who continue to seek evidence for returns on information technology investments. Apparently, there is no fit-it-all standard performance evaluation approach designed for evaluating EHIS because choosing between indicators is dependent on values and objectives that informed the evaluation. In this chapter, different approaches for Information Systems performance evaluation and EHIS evaluation were assessed to establish factors that should be incorporated in performance evaluation. A questionnaire was used to collect data in 15 districts of Uganda based on the identified evaluation factors. Thus, this study established that Net Benefits, Quality of System, Quality of Information, System Use, Quality of Service, Organisational factors, Personnel factors, User Satisfaction, can be used as the measurements of the resilience of EHIS.

Chapter 8 investigated the impediments to mHealth adoption in Burundi. A survey was conducted with 212 healthcare professionals from 48 primary healthcare centres in Burundi. The findings reveal that although there is a high acceptance of mHealth capabilities from the primary healthcare workers, a host of factors mitigate against the implementation of mHealth interventions in Burundi. Amongst these are lack of skills to develop mHealth applications, high cost of mobile devices, low rate of cellphone and other mobile devices penetration, unreliable network coverage in rural areas, and a high cost of network connection. These factors have a low effect size on the acceptance of mHealth capabilities by primary healthcare workers in Burundi. Besides these impediments, the chapter also proposes partnerships between Burundi's Ministry of Health and mobile service providers, extensive consultation with potential users of mHealth systems, and a performance-based system, as the additional factors that need to be considered for the successful implementation of mHealth projects in Burundi.

Chapter 9 investigated the adoption of blockchain to support the National Health Insurance Implementation (NHI) in South Africa using the integrative literature review approach. The chapter highlighted that the South Africa's healthcare sector currently makes use of skewed healthcare financing systems, which makes it difficult to have a convergent healthcare scheme such as the NHI. Therefore, the chapter proposed that a new healthcare financing system is developed based on Artificial Intelligence (AI) and blockchain algorithms with embedded deep learning capabilities to facilitate the implementation of the NHI in South Africa. It is anticipated that the proposed healthcare financing system as depicted in this chapter will help build resilience in South Africa's healthcare financing system.

Chapter 10 depicted the nexus between social network security, healthcare systems, and resilience. Online platforms users including health systems' users (patients, doctors) are worried about their privacy being violated. While the users of social media enjoy the opportunity to learn, connect and share, their privacy on those platforms is at risk. A possible cause of this is the information privacy paradox, which describes a disconnection between users' stated concerns and actual behaviour. The chapter reported the results of a pilot study which sought to explain self-disclosure in Social Network Sites by determining the relationships between constructs of the Information Privacy paradox. Through Partial Least Squares structural equation modelling, the study revealed that the derived model explains 32.9% of the user's self-disclosure intention on Social Network Sites. The findings have implications that need to be considered when building resilience in the provision of online healthcare through social media.

Patrick Ndayizigamiye
University of Johannesburg, South Africa

Macire Kante
University of Johannesburg, South Africa

REFERENCES

Heeks, R., & Ospina, A. V. (2015). Analysing Urban Community Informatics from a Resilience Perspective. *The Journal of Community Informatics*, *11*(1), 1–18. doi:10.15353/joci.v11i1.2846

Norris, F. H., Stevens, S. P., Pfefferbaum, B., Wyche, K. F., & Pfefferbaum, R. L. (2008). Community resilience as a metaphor, theory, set of capacities, and strategy for disaster readiness. *American Journal of Community Psychology*, *41*(1), 127–150. doi:10.100710464-007-9156-6 PMID:18157631

Acknowledgment

The editors would like to acknowledge the help of all the people involved in this project. Without their support, this book would not have become a reality.

First, the editors would like to thank each one of the authors for their contributions. Our sincere gratitude goes to the chapter's authors who contributed their time and expertise to this book.

Second, the editors wish to acknowledge the valuable contributions of the reviewers regarding the improvement of quality, coherence, and content presentation of chapters.

Patrick Ndayizigamiye
University of Johannesburg, South Africa

Macire Kante
University of Johannesburg, South Africa

Chapter 1
Implementation of a Visual Telerehabilitation Protocol During the COVID-19 Pandemic:
Patient Outcomes in an Italian Case Study

Giulia Perasso
https://orcid.org/0000-0003-3265-3869
David Chiossone Institute, Italy

Chiara Baghino
David Chiossone Institute, Italy

Elisabetta Capris
David Chiossone Institute, Italy

Elena Cocchi
David Chiossone Institute, Italy

Silvia Dini
David Chiossone Institute, Italy

Valentina Facchini
David Chiossone Institute, Italy

Antonella Panizzi
David Chiossone Institute, Italy

Valentina Salvagno
David Chiossone Institute, Italy

ABSTRACT

In March 2020, the Italian Government declared a state of lockdown to curb the spread of the COVID-19 pandemic. This led to many challenges in the provision of rehabilitation services to people with disabilities. Consequently, there was a transition to the telematic provision of healthcare as an adaptive approach to the constraints posed by the pandemic. In the visual rehabilitation field, the lack of international

DOI: 10.4018/978-1-7998-8915-1.ch001

guidelines for telematic rehabilitation led to pioneering interventions, which were challenged by difficulties in the use of technological devices by visually impaired individuals. The purpose of this chapter is to identify the peculiar features that could enable the provision of visual telerehabilitation during the pandemic by analyzing the procedures followed in the implementation of a visual telerehabilitation protocol in Italy and the outcomes thereof.

INTRODUCTION

An international report on visual impairment prevalence (Bourne et al., 2020) shows that in 2020 49.1 million people all over the world were blind, 33.6 million people presented a severe visual impairment (VI), and 221.4 million people presented a moderate visual (VI) impairment. The prevalence of blind people increased by 42.8% from 1990 (34.4 million) to 2020 (49.1 million) (Bourne et al., 2020). Globally, the main causes for blindness and visual impairment are cataract, uncorrected refractive error, glaucoma, age-related macular degeneration, corneal opacity, trachoma, diabetic retinopathy (Ackland et al., 2017). Specifically, among the worldwide population, a significant increase in blindness percentage has risen between 2015 and 2020: 38.5 million individuals have acquired blindness from a previous cataract (from 13 million to 70 million), 13 million from uncorrected refractive error (2 million to 16 million), and 3 million from glaucoma (4 million to 11 million) (Flaxman et al., 2017).

In this field, rehabilitation protocols are addressed at preventing patients' vision loss and at supporting their autonomy and psychosocial wellbeing (Bittner et al., 2020). The spectrum of visual rehabilitation includes protocols to strengthening individual adaptive synaptic responses in terms of cortical plasticity (Karmarkar & Dan, 2006; Trauzettel-Klosinski, 2011) through training visual attention (Pilz et al., 2006), compensatory eye movements (White & Bedell, 1990), and eccentric fixation (Nilsson et al., 2003). Visual rehabilitation is a powerful tool to advocate for people with visual impairment social inclusion and autonomy (Shadrick, 2020), even during the Covid-19 pandemic and related socio-behavioral restrictions.

From March 2020, the healthcare system was globally challenged by the Covid-19 crisis to continue to provide rehabilitation for individuals with disabilities, notwithstanding lockdown and restrictive measures (Martinez et al., 2020). Professionals from many different rehabilitation areas and across different diagnoses needed to adapt their rehabilitation protocols to the telematic environment (Das & Christy, 2021; Salgueiro et al. 2021; Varela-Aldás et al., 2021). In the visual rehabilitation field, this was particularly challenging given the lack of international guidelines and the difficulties in the use of technology and digital devices by visually impaired or blind individuals (Murphy et al., 2008; Saltes, 2018; Senjam et al., 2021).

In that context, healthcare needed to find strategies to be resilient. Resilience is the capacity to bend without breaking, but also to gain hints for enrichment and growth from distressing events. In this sense, the chapter is focused on telemedicine and telehealth as tools to avoid breaking rehabilitation patterns. Firstly, it is targeted at understanding which peculiar features could enable the healthcare system to conduct visual telerehabilitation resiliently and successfully during the pandemic by analyzing the procedure and the outcomes of an Italian implementation experience. The chapter illustrates the procedure proposed for the visual telerehabilitation protocol developed during the first lockdown in Italy. During the first wave of the Covid-19 pandemic, Italian healthcare was not prepared to face the emergency and telematic rehabilitation of visually impaired people passed from being an utopistic project to be a necessary daily resource. The chapter offers a dual perspective on the intervention through two main methodologies: a quantitative and empirical study and a qualitative investigation. The chapter presents an empirical investigation to explore the protocol's successful outcomes among visually impaired children and adults, bringing knowledge about the application of ICTs in the telematic rehabilitation of visually impaired individuals. Subsequently, the chapter offers a qualitative perspective from orthoptists' point of view of the experience of visual telerehabilitation during the Covid-19 lockdown months in Italy (i.e., from March to May 2020).

BACKGROUND

Technology in Visual Disability Rehabilitation

Founded in 1869, David Chiossone Institute (Genoa, Italy) has a long tradition in visual impairment rehabilitation. With pandemic emergency, the orthoptists were required to implement their work in remote, experiencing for the first time the application of their well-known in-person protocols through the telematic environment. The telerehabilitation protocol implemented for patients with a visual disability has been proved ameliorating reaction time in training of attention, visual search, visual pursuit, spatial coordination, eye-hand coordination, and visual-aid use (Perasso et al., 2021). In this sense, Internet Communication Technology (ICT) constituted an essential basis to make the healthcare system resilient: it guaranteed that orthoptists could continue to work with patients from remote, overcoming Covid-19 socio-behavioral restrictions during the first lockdown through telemedicine. In this sense, the facilitating role of ICT was related to the capillary diffusion of the Internet and digital devices among families. The Internet became even more essential during the pandemic's spread as it guaranteed smart working, online shopping, information research, remote education, administrative services, and healthcare services (Yang et al., 2020). As regards this visual telerehabilitation experience, all the families presented smartphones and tablets and at least one personal computer per house.

It is worth noticing that individuals with a visual disability are capable of using ICTs and all the related devices (i.e., smartphones, tablets, personal computers) with specific settings or with the support of assistive technologies. Computer scientists describe with the label assistive technology (AT) all those technological tools, solutions, hardware, and software, that have been created to facilitate activities of daily living (ADLs) by individuals with disabilities or by elderly individuals (Parant et al., 2017). According to the conceptual and empirical model developed in the 1950s by Katz, ADLs include ambulation, dressing, grooming, bathing, device care, mobility and orientation, toileting, and also the use of technology (Wallace & Shelkey, 2007).

When it comes to the use of technology and ICTs by individuals with a disability, interfaces regulating human-machine interactions can simplify the input/output procedures (Beiling, 2009). Typically, ATs used to support human-machine interaction among people with visual disabilities are based on tactile and vocal tools to input and output information, like the following tools listed:

1. Settings and software allowing to enlarge the screen of computers and smartphones, personalize colors and pointer's dimension, enlarging icons, constitute a contribution similar to the video magnifier (Muranaka et al., 1985). In fact, this type of AT permits individuals with visual impairment to zoom texts and images according to their residual vision, providing them also with vocal support when combined with speech synthesis.
2. Speech synthesizers and screen readers help individuals with visual disabilities to understand textual information through vocal and/or tactile interfaces (Stent et al., 2011). In this way, web pages, textual files, and pop-ups appearing on the computer screen are accessible notwithstanding visual impairment. Tablets and smartphones present similar system settings. Plus, all devices can be linked to the electronic Braille pad, a tool translating the textual stimuli in the tactile language (Supriya & Senthilkumar, 2009).
3. Optical character recognition (OCR) tools scanner textual pages (i.e., books, printed documents, magazines) and translate them in vocal stimuli or enlarge the characters to allow reading (Pattillo et al., 2004).

AT allows people with visual disabilities to perform a wide range of activities that otherwise would not be accessible for them. Nevertheless, the formats in which such digital contents are realized arise usability and compatibility issues in the light of users' devices operative system. The proliferation of content in different formats may cause technical barriers to accessibility, risking hindering or limiting users' experience with AT. Beyond national guidelines, there are internationally recognized standards proposed by the World Wide Web Consortium (W3C) to get developers to create inclusive content across multifarious digital formats and disability levels (Chiang et al., 2005).

Visual Telerehabilitation Setting

To implement the visual telerehabilitation protocol with visually impaired children and adults, David Chiossone Institute's orthoptists had to know AT and related areas for application. Moreover, the orthoptists had to consider technical and pragmatic elements such as the home setting available for the patients. Firstly, orthoptists had to evaluate with the patient and her/his caregivers whether the devices and the environment constituted the best setting to practice the telerehabilitation sessions. Not all the patients presented devices and settings integrated with AT, others were provided with AT tools but had issues in using them. To create the best setting possible, the caregivers (i.e., parents for children, and family members for elders or adults with disabilities) were required to collaborate in the evaluation of the screen dimension, in positioning the patient at the right distance from the screen of her/his computer or tablet or smartphone. Parents of preschool children were engaged to place their sons and daughters at the right distance from the webcam, re-calibrating the positioning in case of movements altering the distance. The webcam, in fact, had to capture the patients' gaze to allow orthoptists to follow patients' eye movements.

The orthoptists guided the patients and the caregivers to make the setting comfortable and effective. For instance, parents were suggested to regulate the child's posture on a chair towards a desk. Children had to stay still at their desks during the procedure and should not be held by parents during the sessions. The presence of siblings was also discouraged, to prefer a quiet space for the child doing visual telerehabilitation.

On the other hand, the orthoptist conducted the sessions in a setting that was constituted of a desk-station with the personal computer, accessorized with a functioning webcam, a microphone, speakers, and Internet connection. Most of the orthoptists used devices with Windows operative system and different installed platforms for video-calling (e.g., zoom, Google Meet, Skype, WhatsApp). Video-calling platforms were chosen accordingly to devices availability of all patients and families to not leave out any patient. The use of various platforms for video-calling was related to the patients' needs: given Covid-19 emergency, patients' preferences and requirements were satisfied by orthoptists, who learned and adapted to conduct sessions on different virtual environments. In each virtual environment, the screen sharing function was fundamental to interact with the patient in different training activities and exercises, taking, or letting, or sharing the control of the screen.

Microsoft Office suite, PDF readers, antivirus, Google Docs, multimedia readers, and contents repository access were also required. Storing graphic, video, and interactive self-produced materials helped the orthoptist to cooperate by exchanging materials or accessing pre-existing web resources useful for telerehabilitation (e.g., cognitive training website: https://www.trainingcognitivo.it/). Google Documents was used by orthoptists with users with minor visual impairment and sufficient informatics knowledge to simultaneously edit textual material.

Some of the patients had no optical character recognition (OCR) tools at home. In those cases, the visual telerehabilitation experience was focused on training the residual vision through stimulation like reading, visual matching, visual discrimination, visual memory, visuospatial localization, and visual completion. Given the Covid-19 emergency, most of the contents were self-produced by orthoptists. In creating such exercises, graphical elements had been considered. For example, exercises were produced both in black on white background and white on black background, to encounter patients' contrast sensitivity. By the same token, reading exercises were aimed at avoiding visual overcrowding by presenting precise text characteristics in terms of dimension, used fonts, space between letters and between page rows, shape, page layout, contrast, and colors.

The Orthoptist's Role

Orthoptics was inaugurated by ophthalmologist Louis Emil Javal in the 19th century. Javal was the first scientist to document ocular exercises practice to counteract strabismus. In the 20th century, the ophthalmologist Ernest Maddox invented specific tools to test binocular vision. Subsequently, in 1928, his daughter, Mary Maddox, opened the first clinic for this practice at the Royal Westminster Hospital of London (Helveston, 2005). The word orthoptics is driven from ancient Greek words ὀρθός orthos, "straight" and ὀπτικός optikos, "sight". Orthoptists are professionals working to diagnose and treat eye movements problems and, in particular, binocular vision. Eye movement anomalies can be caused by eye-muscle issues or by nervous system problems (i.e., multiple sclerosis, stroke, brain tumors). Orthoptists work with adults or children. In all cases where surgery is not necessary, orthoptists can intervene to manage strabismus, eye movement disorders, and amblyopia (Fujita et al., 2000). Orthoptists are prepared to treat eye disorders with proper exercises, with the use of patches, and they train patients in the correct use of glasses and prisms. With a specific background, orthoptists also work to reduce and monitor the effect of eye diseases like cataract, diabetic retinopathy, and glaucoma (Vukicevic et al., 2013). In Italy the orthoptists acquire a bachelor's degree in the subject: the course is granted by the universities' departments of Medicine and Surgery. Moreover, orthoptic professionalism is regulated by the Ministerial Decree of September 14th,

1995, n. 74238 law n.251 August 10th, 2000 and it is officially encompassed in the sanitary professional's category since July 2018.

Orthoptists perform a wide range of activities (Iacobucci, 1991; Stanhope et al., 2014):

1. Diagnosis of ocular motility (McCarry, 1999), assessment of special needs (Fitzmaurice, 2000), rehabilitation in neurological disorders impacting the eye (1999), vision screening for preventing children's visual deficits (Jarvis et al., 1991; Tamura et al., 2020).
2. Assessment and management of low vision (Fitzmaurice, 1999), glaucoma (Scheetz et al., 2019), biometry (Edwards et al., 1999), visual electrodiagnosis (Trzepacz et al., 2019), fundus photography (Georgievski et al., 2007), retinoscopy and assessment of refractive errors with phoropter (Novis, 2020).
3. Participation in multidisciplinary teams for rehabilitation, assistance in surgical procedure, filter screening of patients waiting list for surgery (Banes et al., 2000; Horwood, 2018).

The Visual Telerehabilitation Protocol

The visual telerehabilitation protocol was administered to patients between March 2020 and May 2020. Weekly sessions were planned. Patients were required to be connected through a video call with the orthoptist using a tablet or a PC. In line with previous studies on the right choice-telerehabilitation apps (Panesi et al., 2018; Panesi et al., 2020), each participant followed a structured rehabilitation program according to her/his residual vision and diagnosis (i.e., visual impairment due to acquired brain injury, congenital brain injury, congenital pathologies of the eye). The rehabilitation exercises were stored in a Microsoft Teams archive to facilitate sharing and using them by orthoptists.

The visual telerehabilitation protocol encompassed various exercises that were conducted by the orthoptist screen-sharing the desktop with the patient. The exercises were structured on the different rehabilitation macro-areas:

1. Fixation stability: the patient has to stare at a static target on the screen (Fig.1).
2. Visual pursuit: the patient has to gaze-follow a target moving on the screen (Fig. 2).
3. Visual search and exploration: the patient have to visually search for a target that disappears and re-appears on the screen in different positions (Fig. 3).
4. Saccadic eye movements: the patient has to stare at a target on the screen and then he/she has to stare at another one (Fig. 4).

5. Visual attention: the patient has to verbally report details from a scene on the screen that changes (Fig. 5).
6. Visual-spatial-motor coordination: the patient has to describe the spatial orientation of a target (Fig. 6).
7. Eye-hand coordination: the patient has to indicate with the index finger the position of a static or mobile target on the screen (Fig.7).
8. Aid-training use: the patient is trained in the use of eyeglasses, speech synthesis instruments, visual magnifiers, etc. (Fig.8).

Moreover, reading exercises and eye-relaxation exercises could be implemented to complete and integrate the sessions.

Figure 1. Fixation stability.

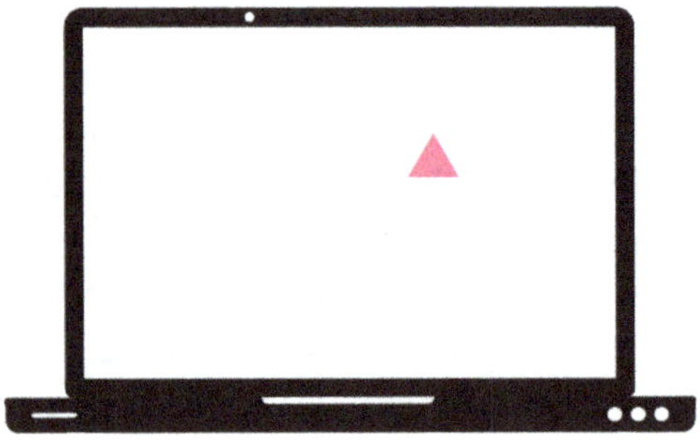

Figure 2. Visual pursuit.

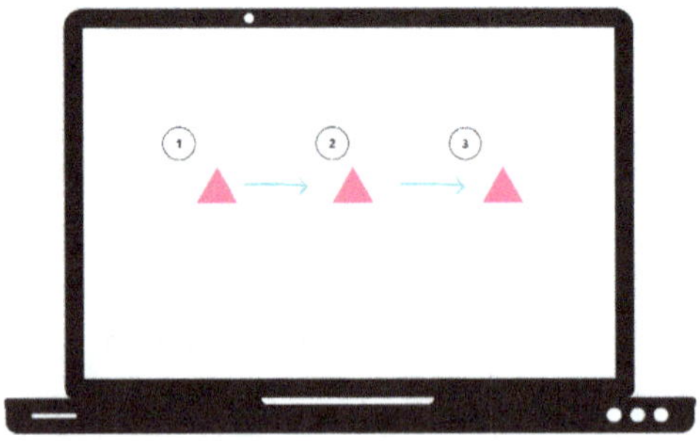

Figure 3. Visual search.

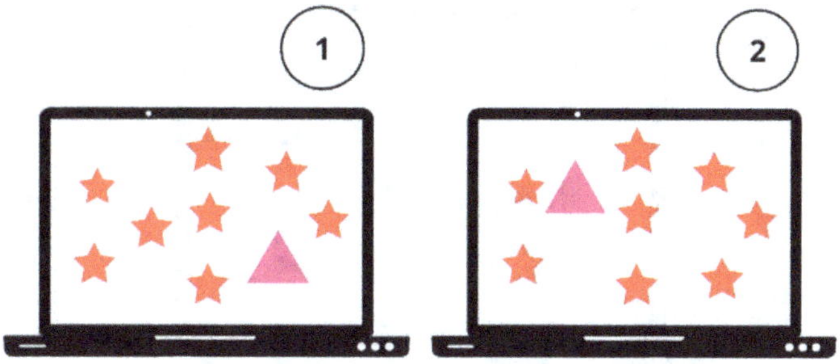

Figure 4. Saccadic eye movement.

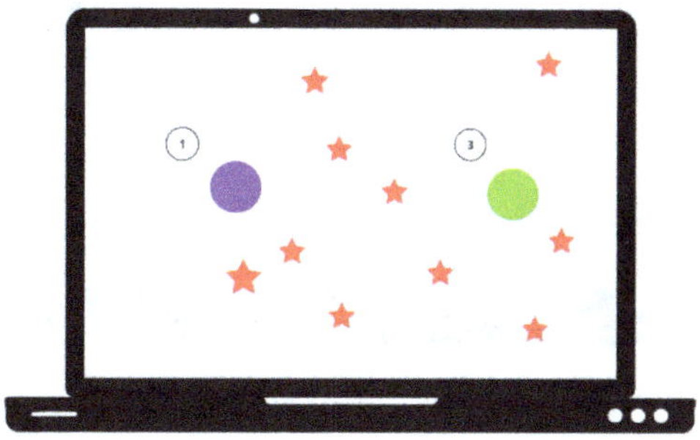

Figure 5. Visual attention.

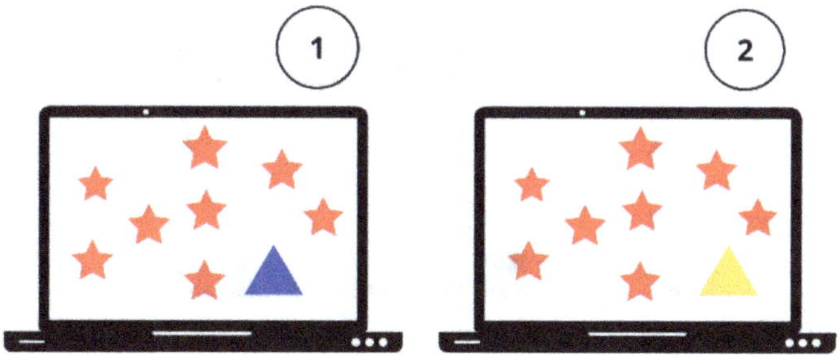

Figure 6. Visual-spatial-motor coordination.

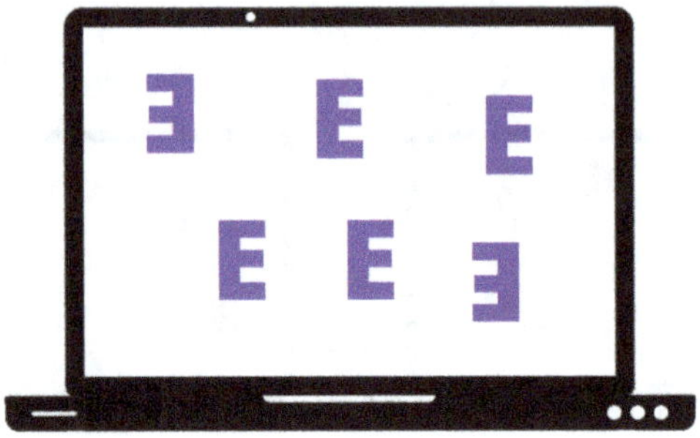

Figure 7. Eye-hand coordination.

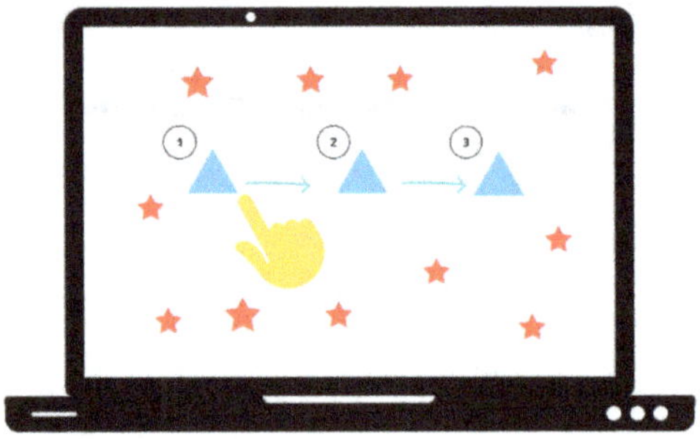

Figure 8. Aid-training use.

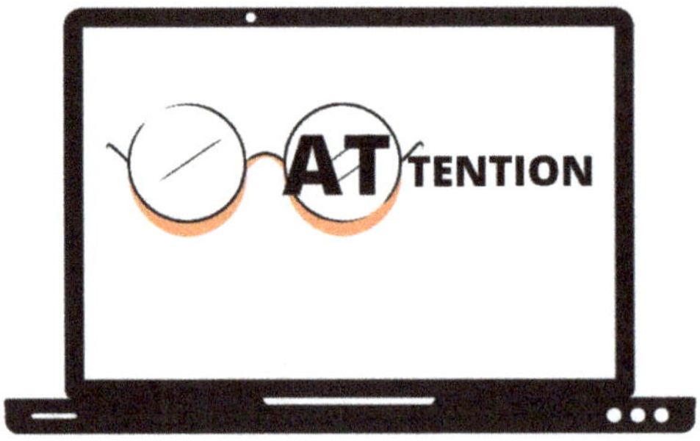

METHODOLOGY

This chapter presents evidence from a quantitative and qualitative methodological perspective. Respectively, the methodologies have been elected to respond to different objectives:

1. Explore the impact of the protocol on the patient in terms of reaction time.
2. Deepen the orthoptist's experience of telematic rehabilitation because this was the first time they implemented online rehabilitation.

Quantitative Study

The procedure was empirically tested to understand the true potential of the telematic rehabilitation intervention. Given the lack of previous studies in the field, no a-priori hypotheses were formulated. Thus, the study aimed at exploring and detecting which factors predicted telematic visual rehabilitation protocol's best outcomes (in terms of reaction time) among a constellation of factors including socio-demographical factors, residual vision, disability, rehabilitation time-length (i.e., duration of each session), collaboration, and support received by caregivers.

Sampling and Participants

The study included n=75 visually impaired participants who received the telematic visual rehabilitation protocol. Patients presented different diagnosis: Agenesis of the corpus callosum (n=1); Nistagmus retinal albinism (n=1), Leber optical atrophy (n=1); Cataract (n=3); Bilateral Colomboma (n=1); Age-related macular degeneration (n=16); Retinal detachment (n=1); Retinal distrophy (n=3); Encephalopathy (n=2); Glaucoma (n=3); Optic nerve glioma (n=1); Stroke (n=2); Derivative hydrocephalus (n=1); Stargardt maculopathy (n=1); Microphthalmic left eye and an ophthalmic right eye (n=1); Degenerative myopy (n=3); Degenerative myopy and Glaucoma (n=2); Occipital glioneural neoplasia (n=1); Nistagmus (n=10); Cerebral palsy (n=2); Spastic cerebral palsy (n=1); progressive supranuclear paralysis (n=1); Pigmental Retinitis (n=1); bilateral retinoblastoma (n=1); Retinopathy (n=6); Tracheostomy (n=1); Greig Syndrome (n=1); West Syndrome (n=2); Sickler Syndrome (n=1); Strabismus (n=3); Exudative vitreoretinopathy (n=1).

All the participants had already begun a traditional rehabilitation program with Chiossone institute's orthoptists before the Covid-19 pandemic outbreak. The total sample was composed of individuals between 2 and 89 years (mean age=32.68), including 45% females. Within the sample, two groups were included n=46 children (37% Females, mean age in years=7.48, SD=3.86, min=2, max=16) and n=29 adults (58% Females, mean age in years=72.66, SD=11.83, min=33, max=89). Totally, n=52 patients presented mono-disability, and n=23 presented pluri-disability. Within the children sample n=21 individuals had pluri-disability and n=25 individuals mono-disability. The adults' sample included n=2 individuals with pluri-disability and n=27 individuals with mono-disability.

Data Collection

Orthoptists completed an online self-report questionnaire (i.e., available on Google platform) by annotating participants' socio-demographical variables (i.e., gender, age), diagnosis, residual vision score (i.e., in tenth), level of disability, telematic session time-length (i.e., measured in minutes), evaluation of the reaction time, collaboration with the orthoptist, and the level of support received from the caregivers (see table 1). The mean between the level of support and the collaboration with the orthoptist was computed as a comprehensive index of the patient's compliance to the intervention.

Table 1. Measures and levels of patients' disability, reaction time, collaboration, caregivers' support.

Measure	Levels
Level of disability	1=mono-disability 2=pluri-disability
Reaction time	0=not sufficient 1=sufficient 2=good
Collaboration with the orthoptist	1=not collaborative 2=medium 3=highly collaborative
Support by caregivers	1=not helped 2=helped

Results

All the analyses were conducted considering the total sample (adults and children). The linear regression and moderation analyses were performed by using statistical software SPSS (IBM) with the macro-extension Process. Linear regression analysis is used to detect variables, named predictors, that associate with a specific outcome. Differently, moderation analysis is implemented to understand whether one or more variables, called moderators, impact the relationship between two variables. In this case, a linear regression analysis was implemented to analyze whether the reaction time after the intervention was predicted by two blocks of factors: (i) block 1: gender, age, disability level, residual vision; (ii) block 2: collaboration level, caregiver help, sessions' duration. In the sample ($n=75$), the linear regression model resulted to be statistically significant $F(7,73)=12.94$, $p<.001$, explaining 58% of the variance ($R2=.58$). The reaction time after the intervention resulted predicted by the duration of the sessions β =.230, p < .01 and the collaboration level β =.64, p < .001. The level of disability β =-.01, p >.05 and the residual vision β =.14, p >.05 do not predict the reaction time (see Table 1).

Table 2. Linear regression to predict reaction time of patients after the telerehabilitation intervention

	Unstandardized Coefficients		Standardized Coefficients		
	B	**SD Error**	**Beta**	**t**	**Sig.**
Constant	-.71	.44		-1.63	.11
Gender	.09	.11	.07	.86	.39
Age	.00	.00	-.18	-1.81	.07
Disability	.00	.12	.00	-.01	.99
Residual vision	.04	.02	.15	1.59	.12
Collaboration	.64	.11	.64	5.89	.00
Caregiver support	-.16	.11	-.13	-1.50	.14
Sessions duration	.02	.01	.23	2.32	.02

Note: Gender is coded Male=0, Female=1; Disability is coded 1=mono-disability, 2=pluri-disability; Collaboration with the orthoptist is coded 1=not collaborative, 2=medium collaborative, 3=highly collaborative; Support received from caregivers is coded 1= not-helped, 2=helped.

A moderation model (number 2 in Hayes template) was implemented to test the intervening factors in the association between the reaction time at the beginning of the procedure (t0) (X) and at the end of the intervention (t1) (Y). The moderating potential of compliance and sessions' time length were investigated, statistically controlling as covariates age, residual vision, and disability (see Table 2). The moderation model resulted statistically significant at F(8,65)=25.5, p<.001 (explaining 76% of the variance, R2=.76). The reaction time at t0 (X) significantly predicts reaction time at t1 (Y) (B=2.34, t=4.85, p<.001, LLCI=1.37, ULCI=3.31). Compliance also predicts the reaction time at t1 (B=.55, t=2.31, p<.05, LLCI=.07, ULCI=1.04). However, the interaction between reaction times at t0 and compliance (Int_1) is not statistically significant (B=-.31, t=-1.88, p>.05, LLCI= -.63, ULCI=.08). The compliance level does not moderate the relationship between reaction time a t0 and reaction time at t1. Sessions' time duration statistically predicted reaction time at t1 (B=.05, t=-1.88, p<.01, LLCI=.02; ULCI=.08). The interaction (Int_2) between reaction time at t0 and session's time duration resulted statistically significant (B=-.02, t=-.2.81, p<.01, LLCI=-.05, ULCI=-.01). Sessions' time duration resulted statistically moderating the relationship between reaction time at t0 and reaction time at t1 (see Table 3).

Table 3. Moderation model predicting patients' reaction time at t1

	B	se	t	p	LLCI	ULCI
constant	-2.3078	.6386	-3.6140	.0006	-3.5832	-1.0325
Time t0	2.3412	.4820	4.8576	.0000	1.3787	3.3038
Compliance	.5598	.2418	2.3150	.0238	.0769	1.0428
Int_1	-.3104	.1649	-1.8821	.0643	-.6398	.0190
Session time	.0526	.0155	3.3862	.0012	.0216	.0836
Int_2	-.0296	.0105	-2.8198	.0064	-.0505	-.0086
Age	-.0015	.0014	-1.0643	.2911	-.0042	.0013
Res. vision	.0226	.0183	1.2332	.2219	-.0140	.0592
Disability	.0356	.0931	.3825	.7033	-.1503	.2215

Note: Interaction 1 is reaction time (t0) X Compliance; Interaction 2 is reaction time (t0) x Sessions' duration.

Study Discussion

The present research points out the factors predicting good reaction times, after a visual telerehabilitation procedure, among visually impaired individuals who received the intervention during the Covid-19 first Italian lockdown (March 2020-May 2020). Findings highlight that higher collaboration and longer sessions of telematic rehabilitation are likely to predict good reaction time as an outcome. The association between the reaction time before and after the visual telerehabilitation intervention is impacted by the session's duration. The results highlight the importance of collaboration between the patient and the orthoptist. The alliance in this relationship emerges to be fundamental for successful outcomes (Fitzmaurice, 1996), and it also constitutes one of the main elements that guaranteed the visual rehabilitation protocol's resilience during the Covid-19 pandemic.

While space and distancing were the conditions of existence of the setting, time also emerged to be an influential factor. Longer sessions were associated with more fruitful outcomes in terms of reaction time. It is possible to speculate that giving the patient the right time to adapt to the virtual environment constitutes a key factor for successful outcomes in telematic visual rehabilitation. Moreover, as in-person visual rehabilitation sessions usually last between 40 and 60 minutes, keeping the same time length is an element of continuity between tradition and innovation. Noticeably, the age of the patients, the residual vision, the disability level (i.e., mono or pluri-disability) and the level of support provided by the caregivers did not predict the outcome. In this sense, the protocol effectiveness on reaction time is relevant besides patients' age since the orthoptists tailored different training activities and exercises on adults and children with visual disabilities. Residual vision and disability levels were not impacting the possibility to gain faster reaction time, proving that orthoptists could adapt to the individual's features going beyond his/her impairment. Noticeably, the illustrated research arises from an emergency context where conceptual framework and international standards were not available yet. Thus, the study could contribute to the development and dissemination of guidelines in the specific field of telehealth and telemedicine, following the recommended steps to create guidelines from practice and research (Berg et al., 1997).

RECOMMENDATION FOR FUTURE RESEARCH

Notwithstanding the strengths of this study, the research presents several methodological limitations that should be considered for future research in the field. Firstly, the visual telerehabilitation protocol was unexpectedly developed as a measure to respond to Covid-19 out-break. The urgency of keeping a continuous rehabilitation service for visually impaired individuals and the need to avoid patients' drop-out did not leave for David Chiossone Institute's orthoptists the time to test the procedure before its application. For these reasons, the research brings results from a group of patients recruited upon convenience sampling. Further studies should implement a-priori power analysis to establish sample size for recruitment. Random and cluster sampling are also vividly recommended for future studies about visual telerehabilitation. Another issue is related to the measures administered for data collection. The use of a self-report questionnaire completed by orthoptists as the main informants of patients' performance may generate social biases in the respondents. These issues could be controlled with the integration of pre and post telerehabilitation ergospirometry measures. The reaction time was considered the main parameter of improvement of patients in different areas (e.g., fixation, visual attention, visual pursuit, spatial coordination, eye-hand coordination, aid-training use) and it was measured as a qualitative score by orthoptists' evaluation (i.e., 0=not sufficient, 1=sufficient, 2=good). The study should be repeated enriching the methodology with the patients' reaction time clocked in milliseconds. Finally, the study has not been preceded by a review of literature on telematic rehabilitation of visually impaired individuals in time of pandemic: given the time-range of Covid-19 and the particular field of knowledge, literature sources were not yet compatible with such bibliographic study that it is recommendable to developed in post-pandemic time.

The present study detects an improvement in reaction time but does not compare the results between an intervention group and a control group. Further studies should test the spurious procedure's effect comparing a visual telerehabilitation group, with a group doing traditional visual rehabilitation, and a mixed group (i.e., alternatively doing traditional and telematic rehabilitation) and/or a waiting list group (i.e., not undergoing either traditional or telematic rehabilitation). Finally, a future direction in combining traditional and telematic rehabilitation for individuals with a visual disability is related to the importance of returning to the normal life precedent the pandemics. In fact, the two modalities should converge in re-establishing confidence in touch as a fundamental sense to explore the environment: Covid-19 may have hindered visually disabled children's and adults' use of tactile perception to avoid contagion (Rizzo et al., 2021). A mixed methodology rehabilitation could occur in restoring the complementary support of touch, after the pandemic.

Qualitative Investigation: The Orthoptists' Experience

Four orthoptists from David Chiossone Institute conducted the visual telerehabilitation intervention from March to May 2020. Overall, the group had a previous experience in the visual rehabilitation of an average of 10 years in a range from a minimum of 5 and a maximum of 16 years. Each professional had a mean of 20 patients during the four months of the Italian lockdown. Three professionals worked with children and one with adults. To detailly describe their professional experience during the pandemic, orthoptists were required to complete an online survey in which they had to answer the following questions with rates 1=not satisfying, 2=neutral, 3=satisfying:

1. How would you describe your work experience with the telematic approach?
2. How would you rate the relationship with the patients during telematic rehabilitation?
3. How would you describe the video-calling platforms you used for work?
4. How would you describe the protocol exercises and training activities you implemented online?
5. How would you describe the resources you have found on the web?

The majority (three orthoptists on a total of four) described the experience with the visual telerehabilitation protocol as satisfying as well as the relationship with their patients. Overall, the group (three orthoptists on a total of four) described as neutral the video-call platforms, the protocol exercises, and the web resources implied in the process.

After the lockdown, a focus group was held with the orthoptists to derive qualitative data regarding the visual rehabilitation protocol. Results were summarized in the following categories:

1. Satisfying elements of the online visual rehabilitation experience.
2. Challenging aspects of the online visual rehabilitation experience.
3. Potential improvements for future applications.
4. Anecdotes and observations.

Among the satisfying elements that emerged, all orthoptists highlighted the importance of not letting the patients down or drop-out during the sanitary emergency. Covid-19 lockdown months (i.e., from March to May 2020 in Italy) may have constituted a risk for visually impaired people due to the disruption of previous rehabilitation patterns and social isolation. Orthoptists also pointed out that the patients and the families were happy to continue the intervention from remote, welcoming the professionals in their everyday life and allowing them to know their home-life through the eye of the devices' camera.

Some of the professionals defined challenging to manage the Internet connection. For instance, weather conditions influencing connection stability disrupted the session and some patients found it difficult to restore it. Orthoptists working with children also found it difficult to engage the ones who were not actively supported by caregivers. Overall, all the orthoptists described as challenging the emergency itself:

"Suddenly, we have found ourselves in lockdown, without materials and tools to work with as they were in our office, at the institute… Which was closed! The possibility to exchange materials and experiences with colleagues was also hindered as we were all in the same situation! The only tools I had were my personal computer and my smartphone! Thus, the main challenge was to activate our technological knowledge, and most of all, our fantasy in creating a new work methodology that could be appreciated by the patients. However, in those months preparing ex-novo contents and materials was particularly demanding in terms of time."

The setting online was described as less controlled than the traditional one by the orthoptists. Although it guaranteed a more precise focus on the patients' eye movements through the camera, activities seemed less structured than in-person paper format exercises. Orthoptists working with children also referred that the triangulation among the child, the orthoptist, and the parent was an interfering factor: in some cases, parental intrusiveness could lead the child to listen to parents instead of following the orthoptist's prompts during the rehabilitation.

In regard to the suggestions for improving the protocol for future application, some professionals suggested using the same video-calling platform for all the patients and limiting the use of smartphones only in cases where a larger screen is not available. Shortening the session's length is suggested for younger children who were likely to easily be distracted. Screen dimensions standards should also be established. Moreover, all orthoptists agreed about the need to multidimensionally quantify patients' parameters before and after the session's cycle.
Finally, other significant observations emerged:

Orthoptist1: "In the first months, visual telerehabilitation was working. Children were enthusiastic because it was something new and the proposed activities were engaging. However, after two months, they began to show their tiredness. I think that in-person and remote therapy should be combined. At the stage we were, continuing with only telerehabilitation could not be sustainable for us and the patients."

Orthoptist2: "Patients referred that telematic rehabilitation exercises were stimulating they perceived themselves more reactive. On a relational level, I could feel that they were not perceiving themselves abandoned by us. Patients feeling lonely and isolated was our main concern for the four lockdown months. Fortunately, telematic rehabilitation guaranteed weekly meetings with patients, going beyond those months' confusion and uncertainty."

Orthoptist3: "I think that we will not forget this experience as we shared a particular historical period with the families, we have done the rehabilitation with during those months. We have learned a lot about our patients. We have learned things about their daily life that we do not get to see in the traditional setting. It was pleasing to see the parents enthusiastic about this new method. However, sometimes difficulties emerged. Once, one of the children I am rehabilitating was so frustrated by the connection problems that we had to interrupt the session!"

CONCLUSION

This chapter evaluated a visual telerehabilitation protocol that was implemented at the David Chiossone Institute's to respond to the challenges imposed by the Covid-19 outbreak in Italy. Its contribution constitutes an example of resilience and flexibility in the healthcare system, as this protocol promptly and adequately met the need for providing continuative assistance to the population through ICTs during the Covid-19 emergency. Resilience, indeed, is the capacity to bend without breaking, which is appliable to the illustrated contribution. Notwithstanding the limitations and issues brought to healthcare by Covid-19 pandemics, the combination of ICTs and orthoptic knowledge made it possible to offer assistance to visually impaired children and adults overcoming socio-behavioral restriction and isolation. Still, after the pandemic, the need to develop international guidelines and standards to implement telehealth is emerging future worldwide challenges, indeed, requires healthcare readiness in facing emergency through telemedicine and telehealth validated procedures.

REFERENCES

Ackland, P., Resnikoff, S., & Bourne, R. (2017). World blindness and visual impairment: Despite many successes, the problem is growing. *Community Eye Health*, *30*(100), 71. PMID:29483748

Banes, M. J., Culham, L. E., Crowston, J. G., Bunce, C., & Khaw, P. T. (2000). An optometrist's role of co-management in a hospital glaucoma clinic. *Ophthalmic & Physiological Optics*, *20*(5), 351–359. doi:10.1046/j.1475-1313.2000.00527.x PMID:11045243

Berg, A. O., Atkins, D., & Tierney, W. (1997). Clinical practice guidelines in practice and education. *Journal of General Internal Medicine*, *12*(S2, Suppl 2), S25–S33. doi:10.1046/j.1525-1497.12.s2.4.x PMID:9127241

Bieling, T. (2009). Design Research and Disability. In *ICERI2009 Proceedings* (pp. 5761-5763). IATED.

Bittner, A. K., Yoshinaga, P. D., Wykstra, S. L., & Li, T. (2020). Telerehabilitation for people with low vision. *Cochrane Database of Systematic Reviews*, 2. PMID:32102114

Bourne, R. R., Adelson, J., Flaxman, S., Briant, P., Bottone, M., Vos, T., ... Taylor, H. R. (2020). Global Prevalence of Blindness and Distance and Near Vision Impairment in 2020: Progress towards the Vision 2020 targets and what the future holds. *Investigative Ophthalmology & Visual Science*, *61*(7), 2317–2317.

Chiang, M. F., Cole, R. G., Gupta, S., Kaiser, G. E., & Starren, J. B. (2005). Computer and world wide web accessibility by visually disabled patients: Problems and solutions. *Survey of Ophthalmology*, *50*(4), 394–405. doi:10.1016/j.survophthal.2005.04.004 PMID:15967193

Das, A. V., & Christy, B. (2021). Commentary: Conquering insurmountable challenges: The importance of tele-rehabilitation. *Indian Journal of Ophthalmology*, *69*(3), 729. doi:10.4103/ijo.IJO_280_21 PMID:33595511

Edwards, R. S., Davis, A. R., & Shilling, J. L. (1999). The role of orthoptists in biometry. *The British Orthoptic Journal*, (56), 19–21.

Fitzmaurice, K. (1999). Low vision rehabilitation: An update. *Australian Orthoptic Journal, 34*, 9–14.

Fitzmaurice, K. (2000). A Method of Assessing Visual Performance Applicable to Multi-Handicapped Children: Response Mode. *Vision Rehabilitation*, 416.

Flaxman, S. R., Bourne, R. R., Resnikoff, S., Ackland, P., Braithwaite, T., Cicinelli, M. V., Das, A., Jonas, J. B., Keeffe, J., Kempen, J. H., Leasher, J., Limburg, H., Naidoo, K., Pesudovs, K., Silvester, A., Stevens, G. A., Tahhan, N., Wong, T. Y., Taylor, H. R., ... Zheng, Y. (2017). Global causes of blindness and distance vision impairment 1990–2020: A systematic review and meta-analysis. *The Lancet. Global Health, 5*(12), e1221–e1234. doi:10.1016/S2214-109X(17)30393-5 PMID:29032195

Fujita, J., Aoki, S., & Shimizu, K. (2000). Orthoptist in Low Vision Clinic. *Japanese Orthoptic Journal, 28*, 239–243. doi:10.4263/jorthoptic.28.239

Georgievski, Z., Koklanis, K., Fenton, A., & Koukouras, I. (2007). Victorian orthoptists' performance in the photo evaluation of diabetic retinopathy. *Clinical & Experimental Ophthalmology, 35*(8), 733–738. doi:10.1111/j.1442-9071.2007.01576.x PMID:17997777

Helveston, E. M. (2005). Visual training: Current status in ophthalmology. *American Journal of Ophthalmology, 140*(5), 903–910. doi:10.1016/j.ajo.2005.06.003 PMID:16310470

Horwood, A. M. (2018). What do we expect new graduate orthoptists to do? *The British and Irish Orthoptic Journal, 14*(1), 11–19. doi:10.22599/bioj.108 PMID:32999959

Iacobucci, I. L. (1991). The role and growth of orthoptics in the ophthalmologist's private practice: The orthoptist's view. *The American Orthoptic Journal, 41*(1), 15–18. doi:10.1080/0065955X.1991.11981846

Jarvis, S. N., Tamhne, R. C., Thompson, L., Francis, P. M., Anderson, J., & Colver, A. F. (1991). Preschool vision screening. *Archives of Disease in Childhood, 66*(3), 288–294. doi:10.1136/adc.66.3.288 PMID:2025002

Karmarkar, U. R., & Dan, Y. (2006). Experience-dependent plasticity in adult visual cortex. *Neuron, 52*(4), 577–585. doi:10.1016/j.neuron.2006.11.001 PMID:17114043

Martinez, M. S., Robinson, M. R., & Arora, V. M. (2020). Rethinking Hospital-Associated Disability for Patients With COVID-19. *Journal of Hospital Medicine, 15*(12), 757–759. doi:10.12788/jhm.3504 PMID:33231543

McCarry, B. (1999). Orthoptists' current shared care role in ophthalmology. *The British Orthoptic Journal*, (56), 11–18.

Muranaka, Y., Furuta, N., Aoki, S., & Gohke, K. (1985). Use of the simplified color video magnifier by young children with severely impaired vision. *Journal of Visual Impairment & Blindness*, *79*(9), 391–395. doi:10.1177/0145482X8507900902

Murphy, E., Kuber, R., McAllister, G., Strain, P., & Yu, W. (2008). An empirical investigation into the difficulties experienced by visually impaired Internet users. *Universal Access in the Information Society*, *7*(1), 79–91. doi:10.100710209-007-0098-4

Nilsson, U. L., Frennesson, C., & Nilsson, S. E. G. (2003). Patients with AMD and a large absolute central scotoma can be trained successfully to use eccentric viewing, as demonstrated in a scanning laser ophthalmoscope. *Vision Research*, *43*(16), 1777–1787. doi:10.1016/S0042-6989(03)00219-0 PMID:12818347

Novis, C. (2020). Orthoptists. *South African Ophthalmology Journal*, *15*(2), 44–46.

Panesi, S., Caruso, G., Earp, J., Ferlino, L., & Dini, S. (2020). Visually-impaired children and apps: sharing informal and formal information to guide choice. INNODOCT 2019.

Panesi, S. Caruso, G.P., Ferlino, L., & Dini, S. (2018). Choosing apps for rehabilitation, learning and leisure activities involving visually-impairedvisually impaired children. *Edulearn 2018.*

Parant, A., Schiano-Lomoriello, S., & Marchan, F. (2017). How would I live with a disability? Expectations of bio-psychosocial consequences and assistive technology use. *Disability and Rehabilitation. Assistive Technology*, *12*(7), 681–685. doi:10.1080/17483107.2016.1218555 PMID:27677931

Pattillo, S. T., Heller, K. W., & Smith, M. (2004). The impact of a modified repeated-reading strategy paired with optical character recognition on the reading rates of students with visual impairments. *Journal of Visual Impairment & Blindness*, *98*(1), 28–46. doi:10.1177/0145482X0409800104

Perasso, G., Bagino, C., Capris, E., Cocchi, E., Dini, S., Facchini, V., Panizzi, A., & Salvagno, S. (2021). Visual telerehabilitation in the Covid-19 era: tradition meets innovation. *INNODOCT*: Congress at University of Valencia, Spain, 27 October - 1 November 2021

Pilz, K. S., Braun, C., Altpeter, E., MacKeben, M., & Trauzettel-Klosinski, S. (2006). Modulation of visual stimulus discrimination by sustained focal attention: An MEG study. *Investigative Ophthalmology & Visual Science*, *47*(3), 1225–1229. doi:10.1167/iovs.04-1338 PMID:16505062

Rizzo, J. R., Beheshti, M., Fang, Y., Flanagan, S., & Giudice, N. A. (2021). COVID-19 and Visual Disability: Can't Look and Now Don't Touch. *PM & R*, *13*(4), 415–421. doi:10.1002/pmrj.12541 PMID:33354903

Salgueiro, C., Urrùtia, G., & Cabanas-Valdés, R. (2021). Available apps for stroke telerehabilitation during corona virus disease 2019 confinement in Spain. *Disability and Rehabilitation. Assistive Technology*, 1–11. doi:10.1080/17483107.2021.1883751 PMID:33576299

Saltes, N. (2018). Navigating disabling spaces: Challenging ontological norms and the spatialization of difference through 'Embodied Practices of Mobility'. *Mobilities*, *13*(1), 81–95. doi:10.1080/17450101.2017.1333279

Scheetz, J., Koklanis, K., McGuinness, M., Long, M., & Morris, M. E. (2019). A Randomized Trial to Increase the Assessment Accuracy of Glaucoma and Optic Disc Characteristics by Orthoptists. *The Journal of Continuing Education in the Health Professions*, *39*(3), 161–167. doi:10.1097/CEH.0000000000000258 PMID:31318721

Senjam, S. S., Manna, S., Vashist, P., Gupta, V., Varughese, S., & Tandon, R. (2021). Tele-rehabilitation for visually challenged students during COVID-19 pandemic: Lesson learned. *Indian Journal of Ophthalmology*, *69*(3), 722. doi:10.4103/ijo.IJO_2527_20 PMID:33595510

Shadrick, I. D. (2020). Social and Community Inclusion of People Withwith Blindness, Low Vision, and DeafBlindness. *Journal of Applied Rehabilitation Counseling*, *51*(4), 290–294. doi:10.1891/JARC-D-20-00026

Stanhope, J., Gregory, M., & Murphy, K. (2014). The current role of orthoptists: A systematic review. *The Internet Journal of Allied Health Sciences and Practice*, *12*(4), 6. doi:10.46743/1540-580X/2014.1501

Stent, A., Syrdal, A., & Mishra, T. (2011). On the intelligibility of fast synthesized speech for individuals with early-onset blindness. In *Proceedings of the 13th international ACM SIGACCESS conference on Computers and accessibility* (pp. 211-218). 10.1145/2049536.2049574

Supriya, S., & Senthilkumar, A. (2009). Electronic braille pad. In 2009 international conference on control, automation, communication, and energy conservation (pp. 1-5). IEEE.

Tamura, S., Yoshitake, S., Okano, M., Uchikawa, Y., Onitsuka, S., & Kawano, R. (2020). Benefits of consulting a certified orthoptist in a pediatric vision screening program. *Journal of American Association for Pediatric Ophthalmology and Strabismus*, *24*(6), 371–374. doi:10.1016/j.jaapos.2020.08.008 PMID:33246111

Training Cognitivo. (2020). *Game Center*. https://www.trainingcognitivo.it/

Trauzettel-Klosinski, S. (2011). Current methods of visual rehabilitation. *Deutsches Ärzteblatt International*, *108*(51-52), 871. PMID:22259642

Trzepacz, M., Łagodziński, P., & Grzegorzek, M. (2019). Electrooculography Application in Vision Therapy Using Smart Glasses. In *International Conference on Information Technologies in Biomedicine* (pp. 103-116). Springer. 10.1007/978-3-030-23762-2_10

Varela-Aldás, J., Buele, J., Ramos Lorente, P., García-Magariño, I., & Palacios-Navarro, G. (2021). A Virtual Reality-Based Cognitive TeleRehabilitation System for Use in the COVID-19 Pandemic. *Sustainability*, *13*(4), 2183. doi:10.3390u13042183

Vukicevic, M., Koklanis, K., & Giribaldi, M. (2013). Orthoptics: Evolving to meet increasing demand for eye service. Sydney: Insight News.

Wallace, M., & Shelkey, M. (2007). Katz index of independence in activities of daily living (ADL). *Urologic Nursing*, *27*(1), 93–94. PMID:17390935

White, J. M., & Bedell, H. E. (1990). The oculomotor reference in humans with bilateral macular disease. *Investigative Ophthalmology & Visual Science*, *31*(6), 1149–1161. PMID:2354915

Yang, S., Fichman, P., Zhu, X., Sanfilippo, M., Li, S., & Fleischmann, K. R. (2020). The use of ICT during COVID-19. *Proceedings of the Association for Information Science and Technology*, *57*(1), e297. doi:10.1002/pra2.297 PMID:33173819

KEY TERMS AND DEFINITIONS

Activities of Daily Living (ADLs): Activities of daily living are all the activities performed by individuals to take care of themselves and adapt to the environment. This label encompasses Basic ADLs and Instrumental ADLs. Basic ADLs include ambulating, dressing, feeding, personal hygiene, toileting, continence. Instrumental ADLs require more complex skills to interact with the environment: transportation and shopping, meal preparation, house cleaning, managing communication, managing finances, managing medications.

Assistive Technology (AT): Assistive or adaptive or rehabilitative technologies are devices and tools for elderly individuals or individuals with a disability, that help them to perform ADLs. Screen readers, braille pads, video magnifiers, tactile keyboards, wearable technologies, are examples of AT applications.

Optical Character Recognition (OCR): The terms optical character recognition or optical character reader (OCR) indicate electronic devices aimed at the mechanical conversion of images input (e.g., presenting printed or handwritten text) in the machined encoded text. The image inputs are scanned or photographed.

Orthoptist: Orthoptists are experts in the diagnosis and treatment of visual impairments. Orthoptists work with a various range of diagnoses and conditions as they are trained in procedures to correct visual deficits and help patients using their residual vision as best as possible.

Rehabilitation: Rehabilitation is a set of actions aimed at reducing psychophysical deficits, optimizing residual functioning, simplifying daily life, and the adaptation to the environment. It is tailored to individuals with congenital or acquired disability, or on individuals who underwent injury, surgery, illness, or on elderly people whose functioning declines with age.

Residual Vision: Residual vision is a subjective parameter measuring the remaining ability of the patient to see. It is quantified by perimetry testing.

Speech Synthesizers: Speech synthesizers are computerized tools that elaborate textual inputs and translate them in audible language outputs. These devices use a text-to-speech system (TTS) and symbolic-linguistic transcriptions to elaborate and convert inputs into outputs.

Telerehabilitation: Telerehabilitation or e-rehabilitation is the process of delivering rehabilitation through the use of telecommunications and the Internet. This method consents healthcare providers to remotely assist and train the patients. Telerehabilitation is commonly used in occupational therapy, psychology, audiology, speech-language rehabilitation, physical therapy. It includes sessions of exercises structured towards a goal. Video-calling applications, phone-calling, webcams, screen sharing make remote rehabilitation possible. However, the range of activities to practice in remote is more limited than the one professional in-person. Combined modalities (i.e., in-person and telematic therapy) are often used in the healthcare field.

Video Magnifier: Video magnifier is an electronic device provided with a camera and display screen (LCD or CRT). The camera captures the printed stimuli (e.g., a book page) and the display allows to enlarge them. It can include a lamp to lighten the material that has to be magnified.

Visual Impairment (VI): Visual impairment is the term used to describe total or partial vision loss. The entity of the deficit is not fixable by using glasses. A visual impairment becomes legal blindness when a person's better eye—under the use of corrective lens—has 20/200 or lower central visual acuity and 20 degrees or lower field of vision.

Chapter 2
Multimodal Representation of Hygiene Practices in Nigeria Under the COVID-19 Pandemic

Simon Shachia Oryila
https://orcid.org/0000-0003-3940-3328
Benue State University, Makurdi, Nigeria

Philip Chike Chukwunonso Aghadiuno
Isa Mustapha Agwai 1 Polytechnic, Nigeria

ABSTRACT

Disease outbreaks do not only create health challenges; they also potentially affect public health communication. To complement the efforts of medical and health workers, health communication professionals often try to design semiotic resources to advance the goal of health and medical practice. This chapter, therefore, explores the various semiotic resources created with the aid of digital technologies and deployed by the Nigeria Center for Disease Control across digital platforms to combat the COVID-19 pandemic. Applying Kress and van Leeuwen's social semiotic theory to 12 NCDC images sourced online, the chapter demonstrates that the semiotic resources shared by the NCDC on hygiene practices to fight COVID-19 have the potential of broadening the scope of interpretation, meaning, and understanding of COVID-19, health problems, and medical practices on account of the texts' representational, interactional, and compositional structures, thereby helping in building a vibrant healthcare system in Nigeria.

DOI: 10.4018/978-1-7998-8915-1.ch002

INTRODUCTION AND BACKGROUND

The need to maintain good health is not new to humankind. For centuries, people have practiced good health by keeping their environments clean, sometimes with the aid of disinfectants, regular cleaning of infected surfaces, hand washing, bathing and isolating infected persons. The recent outbreak of Coronavirus disease also called "Covid-19" raises the need to practice an improved hygiene culture as a way of dealing with the pandemic and associated diseases. In many societies, governments and other critical stakeholders have led massive campaigns and awareness programs to fight the disease. Nigeria is not left behind.

However, the outbreak of infectious diseases generally does not only create medical and health challenges in a city or country, it also creates new linguistic and communication problems for health and medical practitioners. This is because social and cultural differences, such as level of a society's educational attainment, religious beliefs, exposure, personal lifestyles, and psychological perceptions, among others, affect the way people understand health issues (World Health Organization, 1982; Hernandez & Blazer, 2006; Alves & Oliveira, 2018), as well as how they view and interpret health messages (Mateus, Santos, & Mari, 2005). Conservative adherence to sacred texts, culture or traditions may prevent some people from taking certain drugs, undergoing medical procedures, observing health guidelines, protocols or hygiene practices set out to deal with infectious diseases.

The resistance to new medical and health communication may be exacerbated by the modes and media of the messages. Messages which should be visually represented may only be linguistically represented; those that should be linguistically represented may only be visually represented; and, yet, those which should be co-deployed with multiple semiotic resources may utilize only a single modality of representation and, in all these cases, the affordances of the modes and media play a significant role in broadening or narrowing the scope of interpretation of the messages. To achieve a viable communicative result and improved public health objectives, health and medical communication practitioners often seek novel ways to design messages with "a distinctive 'look and feel'" (Walker, 2019, p.1) to convey the nature, prevention, and treatment of the diseases.

In times past, much information about Nigeria's public health, such as hygiene and sanitation, was circulated by the use of town criers, gongs, flutes and animal horns (Nwosu, 2013; Aghadiuno and Onyekweodiri, 2019. Nwosu (2013) notes that, in traditional African society, the primary indigenous modes and media of public communication used to share information and bring about development generally to the people include: idiophones, membranophones, aerophones, symbolography, signals, objectifics, color schemes, music, extra-mundane communication and symbolic displays. These indigenous modes of communication or cultural artefacts, such as the talking drums, proverbs, wooden gongs, live drama, puppet theatre, and folktales, are still very much in use alongside messages circulated via analogue devices, such as radios, television, gramophones, magazines, newspapers, as well as digital devices on diverse issues of public health and social life.

The traditional media, like their modern counterparts, play a role in disseminating ideas and information about government and community programs, instilling in the people various ethical or moral conducts, educating or raising the people's awareness about diseases and infections, as well as identifying the existing preventive, curative or treatment options available for the people. Information now travels faster with the presence of digital platforms, such as Facebook and Twitter, patronized by many organizations and government institutions. With the Covid-19 crisis, much effort, globally and locally, is geared towards raising public awareness and campaigns about the need to imbibe appropriate hygiene practices, through diverse media and multi-semiotic texts. In Nigeria, the national response to fight the Covid-19 pandemic through prevention, detection, and control of the spread of the disease is led by the Nigeria Center for Disease Control (NCDC) under the Federal Ministry of Health alongside various state ministries of health.

The Nigeria Center for Disease Control is a recent creation. According to Njidda et al. (2018), "the Nigeria Centre for Disease Control (NCDC) was conceived much earlier in 2007 as an attempt to establish an institution that can effectively mobilize its resources to respond to these outbreaks and other public health emergencies" (p.1). Its establishment came at a time many African countries, including Nigeria, were battling deadly diseases, such as Ebola, Lassa fever, bird flu, among others. With the outbreak of Covid-19, the centre has led aggressive mass media awareness and campaigns through the creation of semiotic resources to simplify Covid-19 messages for the benefit of the people. Health awareness and campaigns, as noted by Mustapha (2008), play significant roles in raising awareness on issues, enhancing knowledge and beliefs, as well as reinforcing existing attitudes. This underlines the importance of crafting public health messages carefully, especially about Covid-19 in Nigeria, where there is mass ignorance, myths, and pessimism about the disease.

At the linguistic level, the Covid-19 outbreak raises the challenge of creating new and appropriate words and concepts by medical and health communication practitioners to talk about Covid-19 in a language that the people can connect easily. Al-Salman and Haider (2021, p.28) note that the emergence of Covid-19 leads to a sudden upsurge in the use of neologisms, English words or expressions, such as "pandemic," "coronavirus outbreak," "spike in cases," "peaked," "face-masks," "test positive," "self-isolation," "super-spreader," "lockdown," "closures," "social-distancing," "self-isolating," among others, that emerged in the course of the Covid-19 crisis. These words, such as "pandemic," may not be new, but some of them are used in a way that they reflect or acquire meanings based on the social contexts that give rise to their being invented, deployed or simplified for the people to understand the nature, prevention and treatment of Covid-19. To deal with the Covid-19 crisis within the Nigerian healthcare system, the Nigeria Center for Disease Control and its partners in public health communication now try to devise various multi-semiotic resources in form of colourful flyers, posters, handbills, cartoons, graffiti, among others, enhanced by the appropriation of digital devices to amplify or lower the bar of the modalities for the interpretation of multimodal texts on Covid-19 and the required hygiene practices to deal with the disease, sometimes shared across digital platforms, hospital noticeboards, pharmaceutical stores, homes, and other public places. The semiotic resources are invariably hygiene practices requiring people to wear facemasks, observe physical distancing, avoid public gatherings, wash hands regularly with running water, use hand sanitizers, cough into a bent elbow, sneeze into a tissue or bent elbow, keep rooms ventilated, prevent contact with high-risk surfaces, and limit the risk of infection by being conscious of one's environment.

This chapter, therefore, seeks to explore these semiotic resources chiefly created with the aid of digital devices as a response to the Covid-19 crisis in Nigeria, as well as the varying messages they embody. The chapter seeks to identify the semiotic resources and analyze them in terms of the broad spectrum of communicative meanings they demonstrate in building vibrant health and medical practice in Nigeria. In conclusion, the chapter demonstrates the viability of deploying multimodal texts to enhance medical and healthcare delivery in Nigeria. However, because the analysis and interpretation of semiotic resources are often influenced by the social context in which they are created, this chapter employs Kress and van Leuween's (1996) social semiotic theory, its methodological and analytical frames to examine the aspects of the data's representational, interpersonal, and compositional structures which are multimodally orchestrated to deal with the pandemic.

THEORETICAL FRAMEWORK

Theoretical background influences the meaning and interpretation of multimodal texts. This is because, without recourse to any theoretical frame, it is impossible to account in a scientific and detailed manner, the network of choices authors of multimodal texts make in the representation of events and meaning.

Historically, there are many broad perspectives that have dominated the study of multimodal texts, namely, cognitive approach, social semiotic approach, systemic functional linguistic approach, among other emerging approaches. But, because of the interdependency of the field and given that every approach is concerned with the multimodal analysis of texts, Kress and van Leeuwen (2001) observe that analysis of multimodal communication shares "common principles" and that these "common semiotic principles operate in and across different modes" (p.2). It is in the light of this that this chapter adopts Kress and van Leeuwen's (1996) social semiotic theory, which is an expansion of Halliday's Systemic Functional Linguistic theory. The semiotic theory enables scholars interested in text analysis to bring together the different modes of making meaning, such as words, writing, image, colours, among others. Kress and van Leeuwen's social semiotic theory is fashioned after Halliday's Systemic Functional Linguistics model as follows:

Table 1. Visual-Verbal Analysis: Systemic Functional Linguistics and System Networks

Metafunction	Definition	SFL Tools
Ideational	What the image represents. The narrative, themes, logical relations. The view of the world the image conveys.	<u>Narrative Representations</u> Participant(s) Vector Actor/Goal Reactor/Phenomena <u>Conceptual Structures</u> Carrier/Possessive Attributes Taxonomies
Interpersonal	The interaction between the participant(s) in an image and the viewer. The mood an image conveys. The interactivity between software/hardware and user	Demand/Offer Modality Modality Scale (Cline of Instantiation) Color, light, depth, brightness, representation, contextualization Coding orientations (technological, sensory, abstract, naturalistic)
Textual	The arrangement or composition of an image.	Given/New Ideal/Real Star Tree Table Network Information value Salience

Source: Multimodal Analysis Toolkit (Kress & van Leeuwen, 1996)

Kress and van Leeuwen's social semiotic theory demonstrates that linguistic and visual texts fulfil Halliday's three metafunctions, namely, ideational, interpersonal and textual, which they call representational, interactional and compositional. According to Kress and van Leeuwen (2001), "Every semiotic fulfils both an 'ideational' function, a function of representing 'the world around and inside us' and an 'interpersonal' function, a function of enacting social interactions as social relations" (p. 13). In the case of the third metafunction in Halliday's theory, namely, the 'textual' function, Kress and van Leeuwen (2001, p. 14) note that semiotic resources fulfil "the way in which representations and communicative acts cohere into the kind of meaningful whole we call 'text.'"

The social semiotic theory demonstrates how each semiotic element in a text is selected and co-deployed with others as meaning-making devices. This means that each semiotic element contributes to the meaning of the multimodal text. The way human and non-human characters, objects, colours, layouts, illustrations, dress are co-deployed in medical posters, leaflets, or images, though independently, help in building the collective meaning of the multimodal text shared in representing hygiene practices to deal with Covid-19 pandemic and other related diseases. Kress and van Leeuwen (1996, pp.39 – 40) note thus:

The different modes of representation are not held discretely, separately, as autonomous domains on the brain, or as autonomous communicational resources in a culture, nor are they deployed discretely, either in representation or in communication; rather, they intermesh and interact at all times.

Kress and van Leeuwen (1996) state that semiotic resources, whether words or images, can *offer* or *demand* some form of interaction from the viewer, often *inviting* the readers or viewers into some transactional act. The presence of various human or non-human characters in the medical leaflets, flyers, or images are oriented as interactional acts or events to advance hygiene practices for the prevention and treatment of Covid-19 and other related health challenges. In addition, the interactional metafunction shows how authors of medical leaflets create a sense of connection or distance between the characters in the multimodal texts or viewers/readers of the multimodal texts. Kress and van Leeuwen (1996) specifically elucidate the import of the interactional metafunction by stating that, wherein the English language, the interactional meaning is realized linguistically, it is realized in image by the system of offer-and-demand gaze, making the participants, such as persons, objects, or animals represented in an image to look at the viewer to demand some action, or inviting the viewer to enter into some kind of imaginary relationships with the participants. Where such a gaze is not present, the image is an offer, represented by the participants, for example, the humans and non-human characters in the medical leaflets, looking away. Modality, in visual communication, refers to the degrees to which semiotic representation is real or not real. The authors of multimodal texts employ colour, light, and other interactional devices among other elements in an image to engage the viewers/readers of the texts.

Lastly, the compositional metafunction is realized through the position, colour, size, shape, and orientation of the semiotic devices used in the text and how these elements are combined. With advances in computer technology, the meaning of multimodal texts are varied and enhanced with novel principles of designs, which help health communication professionals to achieve their goal of creating awareness about effective hygiene practices for the prevention and treatment of diseases.

THE CONCEPT OF HEALTH AND EVOLUTION OF NIGERIAN HEALTHCARE

The concept of "health" is central to the understanding and evolution of Nigeria's healthcare and hygiene practices. Although it is not the aim of this chapter to go into the whole gamut of scholarly debates and discussions on the concept of health, it is important to note that "health" is perceived in different ways by different institutions and scholars, arising principally from the difficulty of defining or measuring health. This difficulty in defining or measuring health gives rise to various concepts of health, such as biomedical, ecological, psychological, and holistic.

The biomedical concept views health as "absence of disease" (Suls & Walston, 2003), the ecological concept views health as "the interrelationships between the environment and the individual's quality of life" (Boruchovitch & Mednick, 2002, p.176), the psychological concept views health as "a biological and social phenomenon" (Taylor, 1978), and the holistic concept views health as "the physical, emotional, social, economic, and spiritual needs of the person, his or her response to illness and the effect of the illness on the ability to meet self-care needs" (Ventegodt, Kandel, Ervin, & Merrick, 2016, p. 1935). All these scholars or schools of thought approach the concept of health from their own perspectives which, as may be noted, is not all-encompassing. The conceptualization of health as the absence of disease, the equilibrium between environment and individual's life, the product of biological and social make-up, or the interplay of individual's needs and responses to the needs holds promise, but it is defective in providing a comprehensive understanding about health.

In its attempt to provide a comprehensive definition of health, the World Health Organization defines "health" in 1948 as "a complete state of physical, mental and social wellbeing and not merely the absence of diseases or infirmity." Yet, this definition is also criticized. Smith (2008), for instance, argues that the conceptualization of health as a state of "complete" wellness is faulty because, apart from the fact that a state of perfect wellness can never be fully attained, people's state of wellness often fluctuates from time to time, and this does not mean that the individual does not enjoy a state of complete health. Even though the WHO's definition is criticized, the definition, nevertheless, shows the different levels of health, namely, physical health, social health, and mental health which reflect an individual's state of wellness. People who enjoy physical, social, mental or psychological wellbeing live healthy lives even though they occasionally fall sick and receive treatment. The sporadic periods where people fall sick should, therefore, be taken into consideration in determining what it means to be in a state of complete health.

Closely related to health is the concept of "healthcare." Healthcare is defined as "an avenue of improving the economy of a country" (Folorunso, Oyeyemi, Udoh, Ayodele, & Excellence-Oluye (2020, p.88). A healthy population translates to a vibrant economy as the people are healthy and strong to pursue their means of livelihood. It is as a result of this that Yamuah (2005, p.11) observes that, "Without good health, families, individuals, communities, and nations cannot hope to achieve their social and economic goals." An appropriate hygiene culture is, therefore, necessary to achieve such social and economic goals. Hygiene involves the formulation and implementation of practices and programs to ensure that facilities, homes, and public places meet the acceptable minimum standard of cleanliness by the removal of dirt, germs, infections, blood, urine, vomit, feces, and mucus to make the place suitable for use. Much of these programs and policies are coordinated by the Federal Ministry of Health in conjunction with the various states, local governments, and other critical stakeholders in Nigeria.

As it is officially known, the Federal Republic of Nigeria consists of thirty-six states, 774 Local Government Areas and the Federal Capital Territory called "Abuja." The country is structured into three tiers of government, namely, Federal, State and Local Government Areas. Nigeria is located in West Africa, bordering Niger in the north, the Republic of Benin in the west, and Chad and Cameroon in the east. Nigeria shares coastlines in the Gulf of Guinea and the Atlantic Ocean in the south. It is estimated to have 200 million people, requiring the authorities at different levels to enact laws, make regulations and policies to deal with the public health and safety of the population. Over the years, various forms of health reforms also have been undertaken in Nigeria to deal with emerging needs (Scott-Emuakpor, 2010). These include laws, regulations, policies and schemes, such as Public Health Laws (1917) currently known as Public Health Ordinance Cap 165 of 1958; the Standard Organization of Nigeria Degree No. 56 of 1971; the Food and Drug Act No.35 of 1974 (now Food and Drug Act Cap F32 Laws of the Federal Republic of Nigeria, 2004); the Animal Disease Control No. 10 of 1988; the Marketing of Breast Milk Substitute Decree No. 41 of 1990 (now Marketing Milk Act Cap M5 LFN, 2004); the National Agency for Food and Drugs Administration and Control Decree No.15 of 1993 (Now NAFDAC Act Cap No.1 Laws of the Federal Republic of Nigeria, 2004); National Health Insurance Scheme (NHSIS); National Immunization Coverage Scheme (NICS), among others, which are advancing the goal of quality healthcare.

The Nigerian healthcare system, as may be observed from the preceding discussion, evolves over the century from its traditional background to its current mixed modern and traditional state. During its purely traditional state, which covers the pre-colonial era, that is, before the arrival of the British colonialists, healthcare services in the different communities of the geographical entity which came to be known today as "Nigeria" were primarily in the hands of the traditional institutions, such as community leaders or village chiefs, who officially appointed medicine men, native doctors, fortunetellers, soothsayers or traditional birth attendants to superintend over the people's wellbeing and also deal with health and medical emergencies, such as influenza, fever, diarrhoea, chickenpox, smallpox, ill-luck, spiritual attacks, and all emerging health threats. In some cases, native doctors who distinguished themselves assumed symbolic status as the community's native doctors. During epidemics, the native doctors made rules of hygiene for treatment or prevention of the infections, such as abstinence, isolation of infected persons, wearing ash all over the body, and so on. But, as with most cases of traditional medicine or complementary alternative medicine, the lack of precision in diagnosis and prescription of treatment often created health and medical challenges for the patients.

The coming of the British and Christian missionaries as far back as the 18th century to communities, as well as the subsequent merging of the Northern and Southern Protectorates and the Crown Colony of Lagos in 1914, heralded the building of medical centres, the introduction of immunization and vaccination, and other periodic healthcare services to deal with communicable and non-communicable diseases. The period brought about massive improvements in healthcare and medical services as orthodox medicine found its way into the hinterlands and city centers. While traditional medicine was still patronized, the introduction of western and orthodox medicine for the diagnosis and treatment of diseases brought about precision and quick diagnosis and treatment.

With the attainment of independence in 1960, the provision of healthcare and medical services became the responsibility of the federal government and the states and local governments (Akhtar, 1991). The Federal Government of Nigeria, through the Federal Ministry of Health, establishes tertiary hospitals across the federation to offer advanced medical and healthcare services and formulate policies and programs to deal with health and medical crises, such as infant mortality, poliomyelitis, river blindness, guinea worm disease, Ebola Virus Disease, HID/AIDS, tuberculosis, Lassa fever, and Covid-19, among others. Through the various state hospital boards and primary healthcare boards, general hospitals, specialist hospitals, and primary healthcare centers are built to attend to the people's health and medical needs.

Although hygiene and sanitation are considered effective ways of dealing with health and medical emergencies, the practices have regressed over the years in Nigeria. In its grim report about the poor state of sanitation and hygiene in Nigeria, the World Bank notes thus:

A large body of evidence suggests that limited or no access to water supply, sanitation, and hygiene (WASH) services adversely affects individuals' health, hinders their access to educational and economic opportunities, and affects their work efficiency and labor productivity (p. xvii).

It is, perhaps, as a result of this that the Nigeria Center for Disease Control (NCDC) engages in aggressive health awareness and campaigns on viable hygienic behaviors to fight the dreaded Covid-19 using various mass media and digital platforms. The mass media channels, as noted by Abone (2003, p.190), are a key component of global strategy for sustainable health issues. Through these health campaigns, people come to know how best to prevent and treat Covid-19.

A viable healthcare delivery goes hand in hand with effective and successful health information and communication tradition. This is because the way health and medical information and communication is handled could significantly impact the functioning of a country's healthcare system, patients' health needs and the population's response to health matters. It is on this note that the National Cancer Institute and the Centers of Disease Control and Prevention (2010, p.2), for example, defines "health communication" as "the study and the use of communication strategies to inform and influence individual and community decisions that enhance health." In other words, health communication involves the adoption of effective principles, methods, and practices of communication that produce positive outcomes in the country's healthcare delivery.

According to the National Cancer Institute and the Centers of Disease Control and Prevention (2010, p.3), such communication strategies increase the intended audience's knowledge and awareness of health issues, problems, or solutions; influence perceptions, beliefs, and attitudes that may change social norms; stimulate prompt action; demonstrate or illustrate healthy skills; reinforce knowledge, attitude or behavior; show the benefits of behavioral change; advocate positions on health issues or policies; increase demand or support for health services; refute myths and misconceptions; and strengthen organizational relationships. It is in line with this that the NCDC employs various semiotic resources to advance the course of health in Nigeria.

ORIGIN AND DEVELOPMENT OF MULTIMODAL COMMUNICATION

Before going into the origin of multimodal communication, it is important to understand what the concept is all about. The concept of "multimodal communication" or "multimodality" calls into question a number of associated terms and concepts, such as mode, modality or multi-semiotic resources. In brief, "mode is a socially shaped and culturally given semiotic resource for making meaning" (Kress (2010), p.79). This means that a mode is any semiotic artefact, such as speech, writing, signs, symbols, illustrations, images, colors, layouts, sounds, or anything created or shaped by someone to convey meaning.

Page (2009, p.6) categorizes mode as "a system of choices used to communicate meaning. What might count as a mode is an open-ended set," meaning that a mode is any semiotic resource which is designed manually or with the aid of technology for the purpose of representation in a given context. Thus, with advances in science and technology, there can be no limit to the multiple semiotic systems or modes that can be created for the purpose of representing meaning. Therefore, modes have contexts and, as Gibbons (2011, p.10) observes, "modes are fluid, and determining what counts as a mode must be based on their context of use." It then means that what functions as a mode has relevance to the context in which particular semiotic devices are deployed. For example, modes created to aid health communication, such as hygiene and public safety, would be different from those created to depict dangers of conflicts, classroom learning, or new farming methods. It is in the light of this that Lyons (2016) characterizes "mode" thus:

A set of socially and culturally shaped resources for making meaning. Modes, rather than fixed, are created through social processes, and thus fluid and context-dependent. In order for a particular resource to be a mode, the community in which it is used needs to recognize it as a mode and share a cultural sense of how this resource can be organized to construct and convey meaning. The choice of mode is a central aspect of interaction and meaning-making. Mode is often contrasted with medium, i.e., the substance through which texts are disseminated, e.g., a printed book or an audio file.

Within the literature, multimodality or multimodal communication is treated as a field, discipline or concept which came to the limelight in the twentieth century, principally by advances in science and technology, such as smartphones and computer applications. It is, however, important to note that the tradition of multimodal communication was in existence long before the emergence of Information and Communication Technology. As early as the eighteenth century, people had used multi-semiotic resources for the purpose of making meaning in various socio-cultural contexts, such as marriages, burials, wars, ritual practices, among others. For instance, clothes were made embroidered with symbolic patterns, signs or symbols for the purpose of conveying meaning. Among Africans, especially Nigerians, indigo patterns were made on wrappers to depict the richness of the fabric and the social status of those who wear them. Marks were made on faces or objects to convey meaning. The so-called talking drums, songs, music, dance and all the other art forms had a multimodal character.

This was a period of time scholars, such as Ferdinand de Saussure, Charles Sanders Peirce, and Roland Barthes devoted their scholarship to the classical study of the signs and symbols and process of signification. This chapter does not intend to go into a full account of their individual contributions on signs or classical semiotics. However, it should be understood that the classical notion of sign which they pursued is grossly inadequate to elucidate the meaning of semiotic resources, and this is why scholars, such as Kress and van Leeuwen (1996, 2001) came up with their social semiotic theories to account for the social aspects of meaning made by semiotic systems in diverse socio-cultural contexts. Following advances in computer technology, the field of social semiotics has become highly revolutionized. O'Halloran et al. (2010, p.3) capture this development more succinctly thus:

The twentieth century was a time of rapid change and growth in the study and understanding of human meaning systems. Whereas scholars prior to the mid-twentieth century were on the whole in the relatively safe position of being able to restrict themselves to the study of (for the most part written) language, the ongoing revolution in multimedia design and digital technology within contemporary society at large has led to a proliferation of multimodal documents (using media such as graphics, digitized photographs, audio and video texts, contemporary digital media, in particular web-based media, and three-dimensional virtual objects). Meanwhile, the twentieth century has seen a profusion of disciplinary and theoretical perspectives upon human communication in general and multimodal communication in particular.

This makes it possible to study texts across genres while appropriating the interdisciplinary techniques, theoretical, and methodological practices from language and other fields of human endeavour.

In Nigeria, the increased use of multimodal communication through the appropriation of digital technology is also linked to twentieth-century development. Olateju and Oyebode state that:

One of the main reasons for the study of multimodal discourse in the 20th century was the increasing power of computers to handle multimodal data. This generated a lot of online images, music, videos, animation etc all in dazzling colors (Olateju & Oyebode, 2014, p.92).

With more and more texts now incorporating various semiotic systems as means of representation in Nigeria, Oryila and Aghadiuno (2021, p.33) note that:

The Digital Revolution, which has seen the expansion of the Nigerian digital environment since the 1990s, has significantly moved the modes and media of communication away from the indigenous art forms and the overly alphabetic system of the earliest centuries to other semiotic systems incorporating traditional modes, as well as computer-generated multimodal texts."

This is why health and medical communication professionals now use modern technology to design semiotic resources, not only for the benefit of patients but also as a way to build a strong health system in the country. According to Jewitt (2005, p.321), "the new technologies emphasize the visual potential of writing in ways that bring forth new configurations of images and writing on the screen: font, bold, italic, colour, layout, and beyond" in order to reinforce the meaning of the message being conveyed. In fact, as may soon be noted in the figures of images in this chapter, the "visual and verbal modes co-occurring in page-based multimodal text complement each other semantically to produce a single textual phenomenon in a relationship which can be referred to as intersemiotic complementarity" (Royce, 2007, p.103). That is, each mode in an image complements one another—for example, writing complements pictures, typography contributes to framing elements and salience in multimodal texts.

MULTISEMIOTIC REPRESENTATION OF COVID-19 AND HYGIENE PRACTICES

The upsurge of Covid-19 in Nigeria has given rise to the use of various multimodal texts to represent hygiene practices to fight the pandemic. These multimodal texts include:

Figure 1. The Power to Stop Covid-19
Source: https://www.facebook.com/104295201243448 8/photos/pb.100064649291568.-2207520000../4614898731906447/?type=3

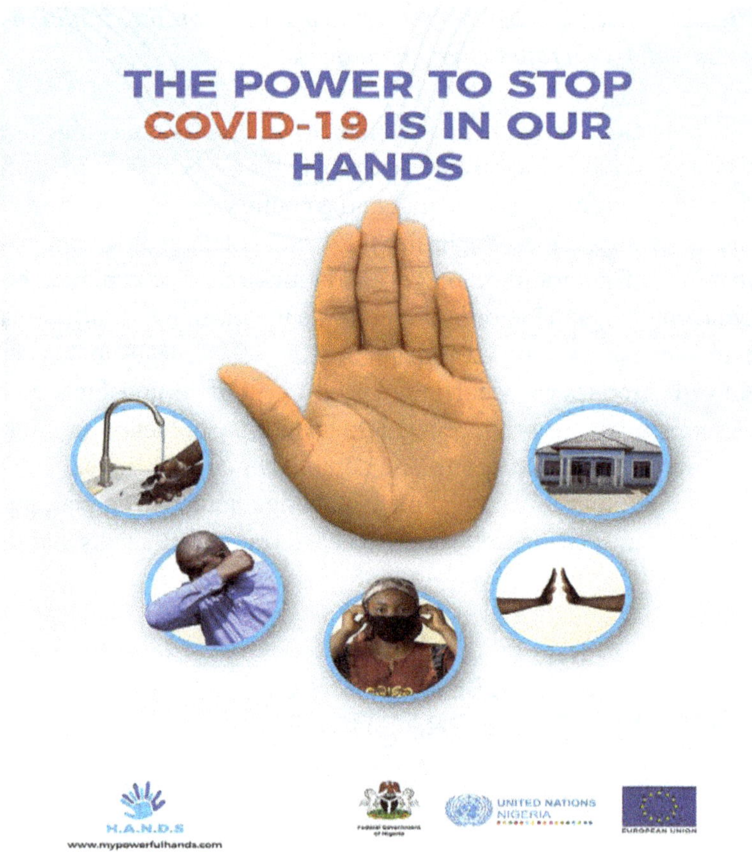

Figure 1 is an image consisting of participants, such as hands washing at a tap, a man coughing into a bent elbow, a woman wearing a facemask, a symbolic handshake, a home, and an open palm at the center. From the representational metafunction, the image shows that the prevention of Covid-19 lies in our "hands" and our personal hygiene practices at "home." At the interactional level, the hand at the middle and the picture of the woman are oriented as demand acts for the reader/viewer to take action by preventing the spread of Covid-19.

There is nothing in the image to suggest that there is some kind of interaction going on between the represented participants in the image. However, the system of expression for the interpersonal meaning is the mood consisting of nominal type elements (the power, Covid-19, our hands), and verbal type element, that is finite (process, e.g., is) to convey a declarative mood. The image reveals various compositional structures: Covid-19 is cast in red, and red highlights the infectious and dangerous nature of the disease. "Hand" acquires salience by being projected in the middle, and it is connected to every activity we do at home. So, washing hands is crucial; coughing into the elbow prevents the "hands" from being infected; using a mask is required and not having a handshake are at the core of preventive practices to fight Covid-19.

Figure 2. The Power to Stop Covid-19 is in our Hands
Source: https://www.facebook.com/104295201243448/photos/pb.100064649291568.-2207520000../4633547313374922/?type=3

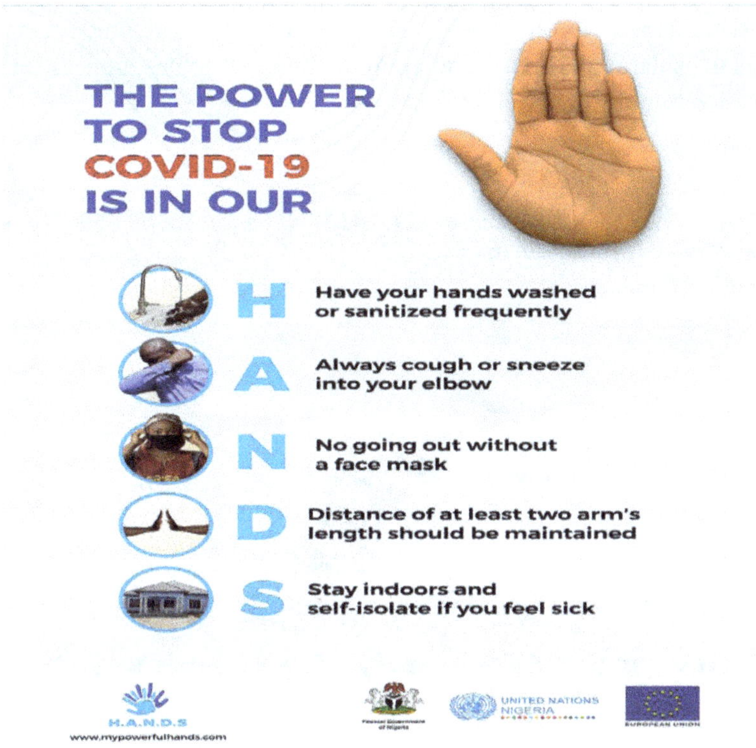

Just like Figure 1, Figure 2 retains the same semiotic elements but, in addition, carries an abbreviation of HANDS, with each alphabet representing an action expected from the reader/viewer. The points that have been made about the representational and interactional metafunctions in Figure 1 can also be made about Figure 2. The use of the modality of writing through abbreviation is done to enhance the reader's understanding of the message. The creation of the image is thus in line with the observation of Wysocki (2004) that designing a visual text "involves choosing strategies for shaping what is on a page or screen to direct a reader/viewer/browsers' attention, within the context of the other texts." (p.126) Although the symbol of hand stands out, it is the writing that further consummates the text's interactional meaning, imploring the reader/viewer to "Have" their hands washed, "Always" cough or sneeze into the bent elbow, "Not" to go out without a facemask, keep "Distance" of at least two arm's length, and "Stay" indoors.

The framing of the abbreviation fortifies the interactional demand of the writing by ascribing a definitive action to each of the letters in HANDS. The expression of meaning in the image is further achieved by an imperative mood system that requires action from the reader or viewer (have, cough or sneeze, not to go, distance, stay). The process involves the use of finite constructions (is) and non-finite constructions (have, washed, sanitized; cough, sneezed; going out; distance, should be, maintained; and stay, self-isolate, and feel). The compositional structure amplifies the visual elements already built by the linguistic meaning of the text.

Figure 3. Parents and Families
Source: https://www.facebook.com/1042952012434488/photos/pb.100064649291568.-2207520000../4467564643306524/?type=3

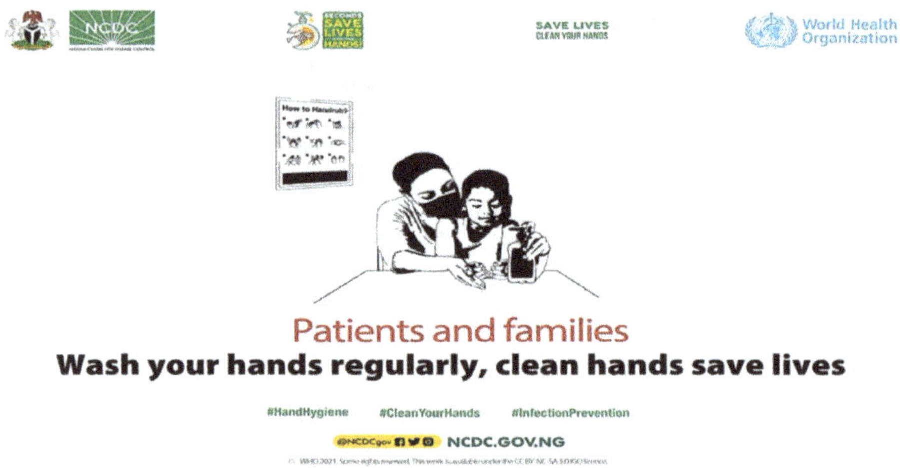

Figure 3 reflects parental and family hygiene. From the representational level, the image shows a mother teaching her child how to use hand sanitizer. Beneath the mother-and-child picture, the words, "Wash your hands regularly, clean hands and save lives" come in dark lettering against the largely white background. Both the woman and her child are not looking directly at the reader or viewer, indicating there is no demand in the picture. Yet, the interactional metafunction is encoded by a system of imperative, “wash your hands regularly,” “clean hands,” and “save lives.” This shows that, in spite of the fact that the visual is used to achieve meaning as seen in this image, it does not mean that the linguistic components of the image no longer serve any useful purpose. Clarifying this misconception about writing and image generally, Jewitt et al. (2001) note that “we are not suggesting that the linguistic realization of meanings is no longer important, we are, however, suggesting that the visual realization of meaning is important.” (p.17)

At the compositional level, the closeness of the masked woman with her daughter depicts filial attachment, the rendering of the words “parent and families” in red highlights those to whom the message is directed, and the imperatives are ordered to show hierarchical relationship—parent, family and their role in improving hygiene behaviour.

Figure 4. Low Risk Isn’t No Risk
Source: https://www.facebook.com/1042952012434488/photos/pb.100064649291568.-2207520000../4535286876534300/?type=3

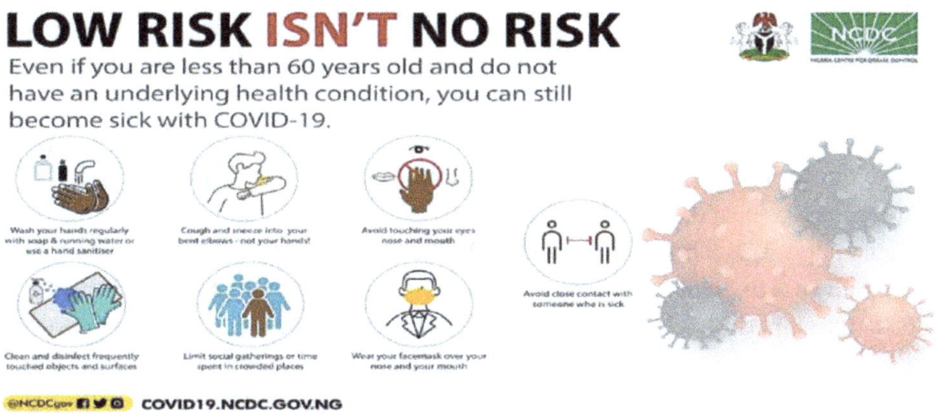

In Figure 4, the image carries the caption: “LOW-RISK ISN’T NO RISK.” At the bottom, the words, “Even if you are less than 60 years old and do not have an underlying health condition, you can still become sick with COVID-19.” There are seven circles with words written under each circle thus: a circle with hands washing at a flowing tap—Wash your hands regularly with soap and running water; circle with a cartoon character coughing or sneezing into the elbow—cough and sneeze into bent elbow; a circle with eyes, nose, and mouth—avoid touching your eyes, nose, and mouth; a circle with hands touching surfaces—clean and disinfect frequently touched objects and surfaces; a circle with many cartoon characters—limit social gathering or time spent in a crowded place; a circle with masked face—wear your facemask over your nose and your mouth, and a circle with two-meter distance spaces—avoid close contact with someone who is sick. There is also the magnified structure of the coronavirus.

From the representational angle, the image together with the words helps in further illuminating the possible ways one could be infected with Covid-19 and the possible preventive measures. It also makes the case that, contrary to the popular belief that Covid-19 affects older people mostly with existing medical conditions, the image shows that there is no exception. All the characters in the image are non-human, but they exemplified human activities, inviting the reader/viewer to take preventive measures outlined to avoid infection. The distance and spatial distribution of the circles demonstrate the role of proximity to infection, spread, and control of Covid-19. In highlighting the role of space in designing comics generally, Khordoc (2001, p.171) observes that:

Reading text and looking at pictures are two important ways of appropriating comics, but these two activities are not independent of each other, and furthermore, readers must draw links between words and images, as well as perceive and understand other coded components of comics, such as pictorial symbols, zip ribbons … and the space between panels.

The circles initiate interaction, not only with the represented participants (the cartoon characters and others objects) in the image, but the outside world on how to fight the pandemic. Through the imperative mood in the image (Wash your hands; cough and sneeze; avoid touching your eyes, nose and mouth; clean and disinfect; limit social gathering; wear your facemask; avoid close contact), as well as the verbal processes (are, have, do, can, become), the obligation to take preventive measures to deal with the circumstances are activated and solidified. Thus, both the writing and images are framed as playing a complementary role in understanding Covid-19 and its preventive measures.

Figure 5. Ways to Clean Contact Surface
Source: https://m.facebook.com/NCDCgov/posts/4408347769228212

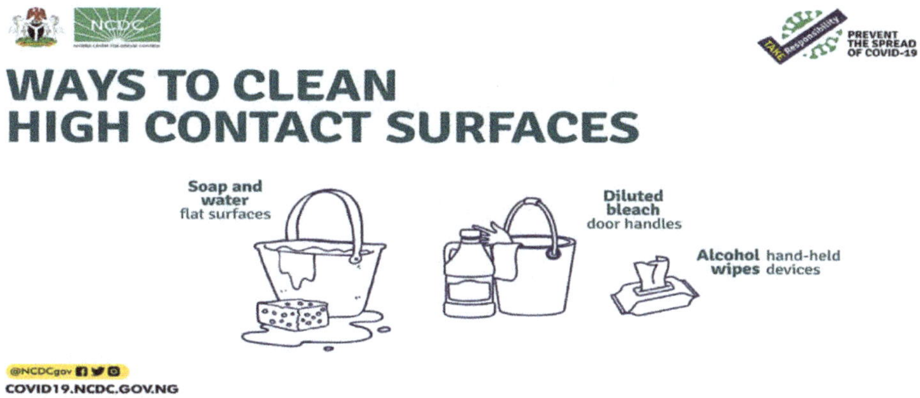
NCDC
PREVENT THE SPREAD OF COVID-19
TAKE Responsibility
WAYS TO CLEAN HIGH CONTACT SURFACES
Soap and water flat surfaces
Diluted bleach door handles
Alcohol wipes hand-held devices
@NCDCgov
COVID19.NCDC.GOV.NG

The way high surfaces should be cleaned is the subject of Figure 5. As may be noted, contact is one of the easiest transmission channels of Covid-19. The representational metafunction, therefore, depicts participants, such as buckets, detergents and reagents used in cleaning vulnerable contact surfaces (flat surfaces, door handles, hand-held devices). The words, "WAYS TO CLEAN HIGH CONTACT SURFACES," acquire salience and initiate interaction with other represented participants in the image as well as the reader/viewer on the things needed for effective cleaning of high contact surfaces. The presence of the buckets, water, reagents, are all hygienic means to help the reader/viewer prevent Covid-19 infection. As products of a compositional structure, the intermodal relations—between the writing and pictorial representation—ease the interpretation and meaning of the image.

Figure 6. Hand Washing Moments
Source: https://www.facebook.com/photo.php?fbid=228295876002054&set=pb.100064649291568.-2207520000..&type=3

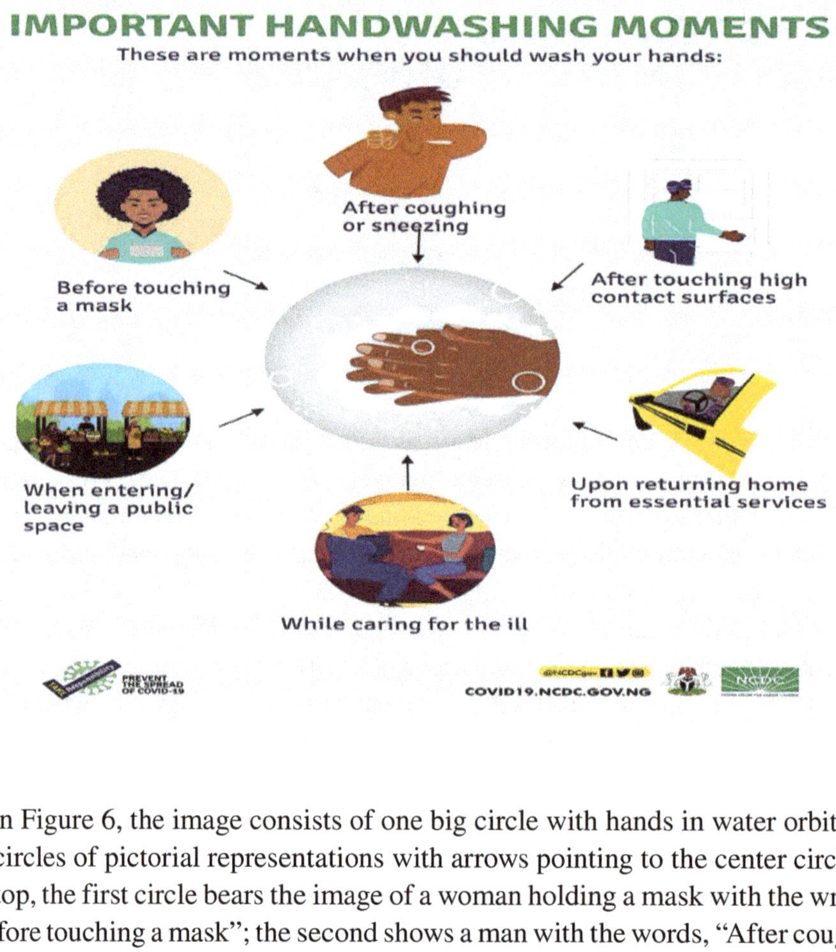

In Figure 6, the image consists of one big circle with hands in water orbited by six circles of pictorial representations with arrows pointing to the center circle. At the top, the first circle bears the image of a woman holding a mask with the writing, "Before touching a mask"; the second shows a man with the words, "After coughing or sneezing"; the third depicts a man touching a door's handle followed by the words, "After touching high contact surfaces"; the fourth reflects cartoon characters in a public place with the words, "When entering or leaving a public place"; the fifth demonstrates two characters with the words, "While caring for the ill"; and the last illustrates a man returning home in his car with the words, "Upon returning home from essential services."

From the semiotic devices used in the image, the representational metafunction seeks to enlighten the people on how to keep a handwashing hygiene culture during the pandemic among the commonest possible human activities. "IMPORTANT HANDWASHING MOMENTS" with its rider, "These are moments when you should wash your hands," invite the reader to adopt appropriate hygiene behaviors to fight Covid-19. The pictorial representations are relevant as they initiate appropriate behavioral and cognitive reactions from the reader/viewer. The image is framed around hands as it is a key semiotic device in attaining an overall hygiene practice during the pandemic

Figure 7. Covid-19 Prevention
Source: https://www.facebook.com/photo.php?fbid=218663956965246&set=pb.100064649291568.-2207520000..&type=3

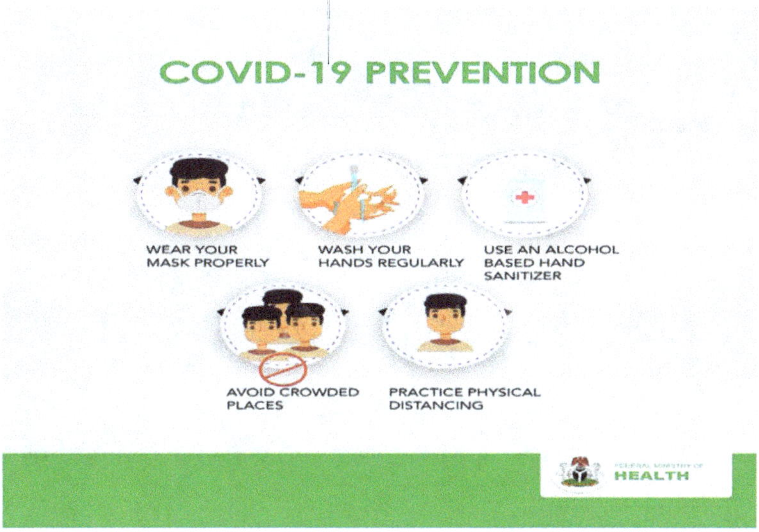

Figure 7 reproduces some of the protective hygiene practices NCDC and its partners, such as the World Health Organization, use to fight Covid-19. The primary semiotic devices in the image are hands, cartoon characters, facemasks, among others. Five circles carry different representational information; first circle: masked face with writing—wear your facemask; second circle: hands being washed at a flowing water tap—wash your hands regularly; third circle: a reagent—use an alcohol-based hand sanitiser; fifth circle: prototype crowd—avoid crowded places; last circle: a character in a single space—practice physical distancing. The image is cast in-demand position, with the cartoon characters looking directly at the reader/viewer through imaginary vectors. The imperative mood--achieved through "wear," "wash," "use," "avoid," and "practice"— helps in concretizing the necessary action expected from the reader or viewer of the image. Through the various signs, such as a sign of danger or hospital sign, the reader or viewer is not in doubt about the expected response from the image. The compositional structure of the image ties the hygiene message to acts that could cause the spread of Covid-19.

Figure 8. Protect Your Customers and Business
Source: https://www.facebook.com/104295201243448/photos/pb.100064649291568.-2207520000../4636584436404543/?type=3

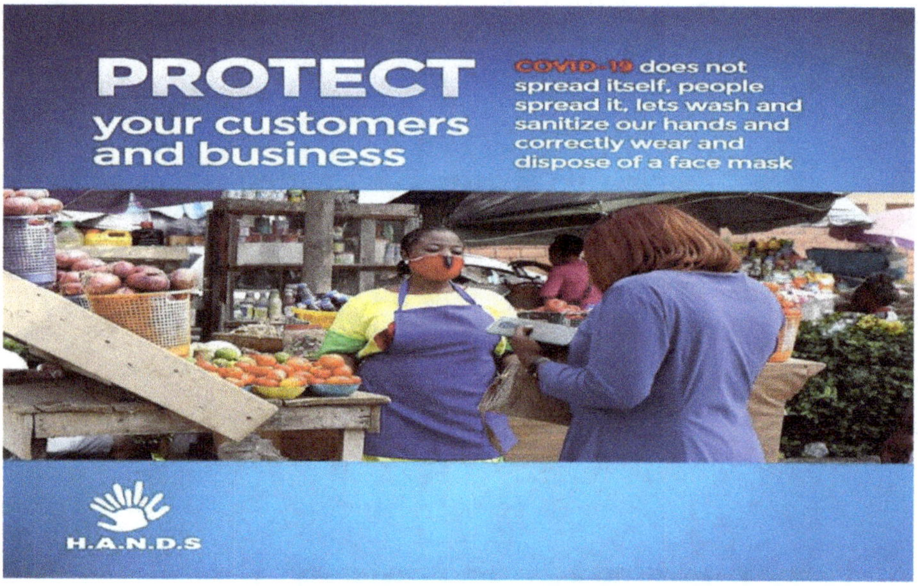

One of the places people could be easily infected with Covid-19 is market, where customers come in contact. The semiotic resources used in Figure 8 are human characters, articles for sale, colors, writing, font size, among other typographical elements. From the representational angle, two customers are depicted at the market buying and selling. At the top, there is extended font-sized writing, saying "PROTECT your customers and business." Close to the writing is another sentence in reduced font-size: "COVID-19 does not spread itself, people spread it, let's wash and sanitize our hands and correctly wear and dispose of a facemask." "PROTECT" and the pictorial representation of the unidentified customers acquire salience in advancing the meaning of the image, which primarily is to invite business owners and their customers, from the interactional metafunction, to embrace hygiene practices, such as hand washing, using hand sanitizer, wearing a facemask, and disposing them after use to stop the spread of Covid-19 among customers. Shot in its naturalistic setting and rich in the modality of colors, the image and the various semiotic elements they embody heighten the bar of the message as a realistic representation of human activities which pose a challenge in the fight against Covid-19. The recourse to the use of the imperative mood “Protect yourself…” is associated with the change of behavior. Also, through the finite processes (does, wash, sanitize, dispose) the image shows how words and image complement each other in meaning making.

Figure 9. Covid-19 and Age
Source: https://www.facebook.com/photo.php?fbid=230890085742633&set=pb.100064649291568.-2207520000..&type=3

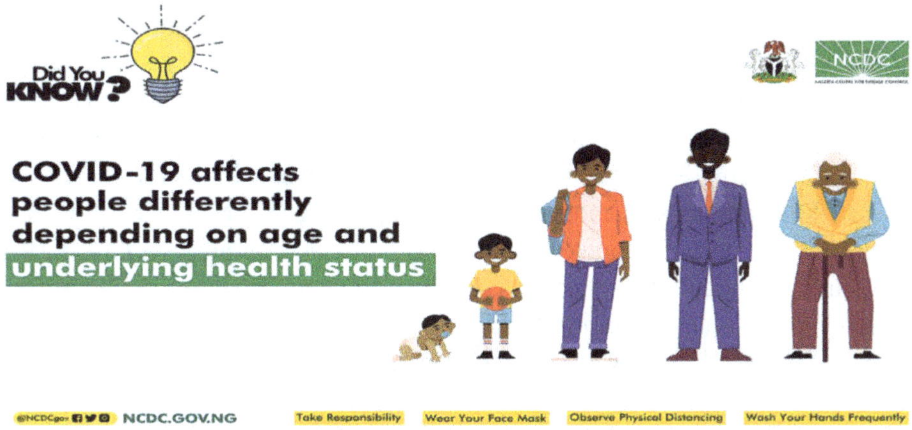
Did You KNOW?
NCDC
COVID-19 affects people differently depending on age and underlying health status
@NCDCgov
NCDC.GOV.NG
Take Responsibility
Wear Your Face Mask
Observe Physical Distancing
Wash Your Hands Frequently

Figure 9 consists of words rendered in black and white against a green and white background. At the topmost part of the image, the words “Did you know?” followed by “COVID-19 affects people differently depending on the age and underlying health status.” At the opposite end of the words, five cartoon characters at various stages of human life is represented by a crawling child, a child of school age, a young person, a mature adult, and an old man with a walking stick.

The representational metafunction narrates how Covid-19 infection affects all, irrespective of age. From the interactional angle, all the characters are looking directly at the reader or viewer in a demand function, inviting the reader or viewer into some kind of action against Covid-19. The presence of the writing supports the visual expression about the nature of Covid-19 infection. Through the interrogative (Do you know?), the finite process (affects) and circumstance of the image, both the linguistic and pictorial structure of the message are amplified.

FEATURES OF NCDC MULTIMODAL TEXTS ON HYGIENE PRACTICES UNDER COVID-19

Multimodal texts shared by the Nigeria Center for Disease Control to fight Covid-19 embody different semiotic devices. These semiotic devices follow a consistent design trajectory that needs to be isolated and discussed. These semiotic devices include:

- **Use of Human Characters**: The use of human characters as the represented participants is a prominent feature of NCDC multimodal texts on hygiene practices on the Covid-19 pandemic. A look at the figures of images (1, 2, and 8) shows human characters are integrated with other semiotic elements to convey the meaning embedded in the images. These human characters, though positioned differently, are oriented to serve the function of achieving a realistic representation of the semiotic acts or events in the images.
- **Use of Cartoon Characters**: NCDC exploits cartoon characters to their great advantage in representing information and messages on Covid-19 in their multimodal texts. In fact, cartoon characters, representing humans or non-humans, as seen in the figures of images (3, 4, 5, 6, 7, and 9) help to create a neutral identity around represented participants, yet give the readers/viewers an idea of the action humans need to take to practice an acceptable hygiene culture, fight disease, or stay healthy.
- **Use of Health and Medical Supplies**: Since the use of health and medical facilities is central to the prevention of Covid-19, much of NCDC's multimodal texts on hygiene practices embody health and medical consumables, such as reagents, detergents, facemasks, wipes, among others, as seen in the figures of images (3, 4, 5). The pictorial representations help those who do not know the use of those consumable to understand how to use them.
- **Use of Colors**: Colors play a key role in conveying messages, and the NCDC utilizes the use of primary colors like red (figure, 1, 2, 3), black (figure 4), blue (1, 2, 9) in order to sediment the meaning of their multimodal texts. Red, as in western and most global cultures, symbolizes danger, death. It is, therefore, not a coincidence to have the name "Covid-19" written in red in figures 1, 2, and "parents and family" in figure 3 also cast in red because they are the primary units of human society where the message on Covid-19 should be received and acted upon before the larger society. Black, like red, possesses attributes of danger, death, and sadness. This is why the magnified image of the Covid-19 virus is represented in both red and black colors in NCDC multimodal texts.
- **Use of Home and Public Setting**: The need to develop a suitable hygiene culture in the home and public places is key to securing an efficient measure

against the Covid-19 pandemic. That is why the figures of images dwell so much on home and public hygiene practices that will help to prevent the spread of Covid-19 among the people—from the home to the larger part of the society. As seen in figures 1, 2, 3, 6, 7, and 8, the multimodal texts specifically use hygiene practices in the home and public setting to show Covid-19 can be prevented by the people.

- **Use of Writing, Signs or Symbols**: Writing, signs, and symbols are carefully exploited to enrich visual communication. In its multimodal texts on hygiene practices, NCDC uses words, phrases, clauses, and sentences to provide linguistic and visual supports to messages in the figures of images. The use of hand/palm (figure 1, 2), danger sign (7), among others, help to crystalize the meaning of the text.
- **Use of Typography:** Typography is an essential feature of NCDC's multimodal text. Typography plays a crucial role in highlighting the main information and backgrounding less important ones. In asserting typography as a semiotic mode in multimodal texts, Bringhurst (2004, p.19) states that "typography exists to honor the content." This means that typographical elements, such as large font size, boldface, and capitalization contribute to the meaning of the content of multimodal texts. Thus, the writing on the multimodal texts shared by NCDC on their platforms often varies in font size according to the relevance of the information. Information with high modality acquires salience and dominance in the image. As noted in figures 1 (THE POWER TO STOP COVID-19 IS IN OUR HANDS), 2 (THE POWER TO STOP COVID-19 IS IN OUR HANDS), 4(LOW RISK IS ISN'T NO RISK), 5 (WAYS TO CLEAN HIGH CONTACT SURFACES), 6(IMPORTANT HANDWASHING MOMENTS), 7(COVID-19 PREVENTION), and 8 (PROTECT your customers and business), the characters of the writing is not only cast in large font size but also coloured in boldface to reinforce the meaning of the message.

SIGNIFICANCE OF NCDC'S MULTIMODAL TEXTS ON COVID-19 PANDEMIC

The multimodal texts shared by NCDC on their digital channels play very significant roles in diverse ways. These include:

- **Summarize Hygiene Practices**: NCDC multimodal texts summarize basic information on Covid-19 in just a small space. If all the information on hygiene practices were to be written in words, it would be very difficult or impossible to achieve that brevity. A picture, they say, is worth more than a thousand words. Therefore, images and other semiotic devices help health communication professionals to condense the information for the benefit of the reader/viewer.

- **Simplify Information on Covid-19**: Understanding technical information is often difficult for most people. By using multimodal texts embodying diverse semiotic systems, NCDC seeks to simplify information about hygiene and Covid-19 for the benefit of the reader/viewer. These images will help medical and health workers to explain the nature of Covid-19 and various hygiene behaviors to their patients with ease.
- **Use Local Semiotic Resources**: NCDC deploys local multisemiotic resources in constructing texts that the local Nigerian digital population can easily identify with. The use of bodily parts, such as hands, mouth, nose, and eyes to depict the contact channels of Covid-19 work well with the local population where myths about the disease are rife. Using local settings, such as markets, to create multimodal texts can make the reader/viewer easily connect with the message.
- **Convey Ideological Stance on Health Issues**: The various semiotic resources circulated by NCDC help them to create and reinforce ideological positions on Covid-19 and hygiene practices. According toStockl (2004, p. 10), the use of a semiotic resource in a multimodal text is "guided by socially determined intentions and realizes group interests, subjective points of view or ideological stances." (Cited in Serafini & Clausen, 2012). The goal of NCDC in sharing these multimodal resources on Covid-19 and the expected hygiene practice is to fight the pandemic, create awareness on the danger of the disease, educate the people on improved hygiene culture, prevent the spread of Covid-19, as well as achieve a better public healthcare.

CHALLENGES

In spite of the rich potential of multimodal communication, there are many challenges associated with it within the Nigerian local context.

- **Finance**: Designing multimodal texts involves money. The cost of printing is prohibitive, just like the cost of data. Since the NCDC needs to constantly keep the people informed about Covid-19 and hygiene practices to curtail Covid-19, they must ensure that the agency is adequately funded to perform its role.

- **Absence of Multimodal Literacy Skills**: The lack of multimodal literacy skills among a greater majority of the Nigerian populace constitutes a serious setback to creating or understanding multimodal texts. Most people lack the basic skills to understand semiotic resources, such as signs, colors, illustrations, and what they represent. The problem is compounded by the fact that multimodal literacy is not taught in schools as a basic reading skill compared to writing, leaving learners with the feeling that t*o read* is to only understand linguistic texts.
- **Obscurity**: Many semiotic resources circulated by NCDC are obscure. Yet, as Kress and van Leeuwen (1996) observe, "the visual, like all semiotic modes, has to serve several communicational (and representational) requirements, in order to function as a full system of communication" (p.40). In addition, it is necessary to fix the context of the text. However, the wall poster in Figure 4, for instance, is obscure and leaves the reader/viewer guessing what it represents. The obscurity of semiotic resources will hamper many people from making sufficient meaning from the multimodal texts.
- **Misapplication of Colors**: Colors are not to be used indiscriminately. Looking at the colors in many of the multimodal texts, it appears that they are not meant to serve the purpose of advancing the meaning of the texts. They are just there and nothing more.
- **Poor Conceptualization of Multimodal Texts**: Designing multimodal texts is governed by certain principles. Often, knowledge of this skill is lacking, ending in creating texts which do not sufficiently address the problem.
- **Draught of Competent Graphic Designers**: In many parts of the world, graphic designers are in short supply. The cost of paying available ones is also high. As a result, people patronize those who are still learning the art. A close look at some of the multimodal texts shared by NCDC appears to lack the fine-grained touches of an experienced graphic designer.

SOLUTIONS

In spite of the challenges highlighted in this chapter, there are possible solutions to the challenges. These include:

- **Need for Adequate Funding**: As an agency of the government, the Nigerian Government must ensure adequate funding of the agency to perform its duties.
- **Promotion of Multimodal Literacy Skills**: Schools must redefine the concept of reading to include the ability to reader multimodal texts—and not just linguistic texts.

- **Creating Appropriate Context for Multimodal Texts**: In the creation of multimodal texts, appropriate steps must be taken to ensure that the context is not hazy, vague or ambiguous.
- **Training and Retraining of Graphic Artists**: More and more training should be organized for graphic artists to sharpen their skills and knowledge.

DIRECTION FOR FURTHER RESEARCH

The field of multimodal communication is relatively new, but it is rich in theory and practice to investigate diverse semiotic resources used in depicting social problems. In recent times, the use of multimodal texts, such as colored placards, flags, signs, illustrations, dress, music, dance, hashtags, among others, appear to be pervasive in many parts of the world during protests, strikes, and rallies. Research on flags *per se* is not new. But, integrating flags and other meaning-making devices as articles of mobilization and mass action are recent trends. The study of the meaning these semiotic resources make have largely remained neglected or understudied. Research is required to uncover the salient messages and meaning they embody and their effective roles as tools of social change.

Closely related to the use of multimodal communication as a tool for social action, it will serve a useful purpose to examine how cartoons and other semiotic resources are used to depict repressive regimes and as means to bypass censorship and promote freedom of expression.

CONCLUSION

From the preceding discussion, the outbreak of the deadly coronavirus has, not only severely brought about health and medical challenges and altered the way people live and work, it has also tasked health communication professionals on how to create novel multisemiotic resources embodying a vast array of meaning to deal with the pandemic. Much of the problems created by Covid-19 raises the need to bring messages on Covid-19 and hygiene practices popularized by the Nigeria Center for Disease Control and accessible to every segment of the society, such as the need to wash hands regularly, use a facemask and dispose of correctly, cough or sneeze into bent elbow, avoid crowds, observe physical distancing, keep two-meter distance between two persons, use hand sanitizers to wash hands or clean high contact surfaces. Many figures of images embodying semiotic resources, such as signs, illustrations, colors, human and cartoon characters, detergents and reagents alongside writing are co-deployed and, from the systemic functional analysis, the semiotic resources, created by digital devices, fulfill the representational, interactional, and compositional metafunctions. The images serve the useful purpose of conveying messages about the improved culture of hygiene and general health and medical practice in Nigeria.

REFERENCES

Abone, C. (2003). Mass media: Effective instrument for promoting health programs in Africa. In I. E. Nwosu (Ed.), *Sustainable development in Nigeria*. Rhyce Kerex Publishers.

Aghadiuno, P. C., & Onyekweodiri, N. E. (2019). Social media for information dissemination in the digital era. In K.I. Igwe, S.A. Sadiku, & I.B. Edam-Agbor (Eds.), Themes and trends in information science (pp. 241-250). Ikorodu, Nigeria: Zeh.

Akhtar, R. (1991). *Healthcare patterns and planning in developing countries*. Greenwood Press.

Al-Salman, S., & Ahmad, S. H. (2021). COVID-19 trending neologisms and word formation processes in English. *Russian Journal of Linguistics*, *25*(1), 24–42. doi:10.22363/2687-0088-2021-25-1-24-42

Alves, S. A. A., & Oliveira, M. L. B. (2018). Sociocultural aspects of health and disease and their pragmatic impact. *Journal of Human Growth and Development*, *28*(2), 183–188. doi:10.7322/jhgd.147236

Boruchovitch, E., & Mednick, B. R. (2002, July/December). The meaning of health and illness: Some considerations for health psychology. *Psico-USF*, *7*(2), 175–183. doi:10.1590/S1413-82712002000200006

Bringhurst, R. (2004). Elements of typographical style. Roberts Point, WA: Hartley and Marks.

Folorunso, G. I., Oyeyemi, A. I., Udoh, O. D., Ayodele, O. T., & Excellence-Oluye, N. O. (2020). Rethinking the role of traditional media on migration issues in Nigeria. In N. Okorie, B. R. Ojebuyi, & J. W. Macharia (Eds.), *Handbook of Research on the Global Impact of Media on Migration Issues* (pp. 85–95). IGI Global.

Hernandez, L. M., & Blazer, D. G. (2006). *Genes, behavior, and the social environment: Moving beyond the nature/nurture debate*. National Academies Press.

Jewitt, C. (2005). Multimodality, "reading," and "writing" for the 21st Century. *Discourse (Abingdon)*, *26*(3), 315–331. doi:10.1080/01596300500200011

Jewitt, C., Kress, G., Ogborn, J., & Tsatsarelis, C. (2001). Exploring learning through visual, actional and linguistic communication: The multimodal environment of a science classroom. *Educational Review, 53*(1), 5–18. doi:10.1080/00131910123753

Khordoc, C. (2001). The comic book's soundtrack: Visual sound effects in Asterix. In R. Varnum & C. T. Gibbons (Eds.), *The language of comics: Word and image* (pp. 156–173). University Press of Mississippi.

Kress, G. (2010). *Multimodality: A social semiotic approach to contemporary communication*. Routledge.

Kress, G. R., & van Leeuwen, T. (1996). *Reading images: The grammar of visual design*. Routledge.

Kress, G. R., & van Leeuwen, T. (2001). *Multimodal discourse: The modes and media of contemporary communication*. Arnold.

Mateus, M. D., Santos, J. Q., & Mari, J. J. (2005). Popular conceptions of schizophrenia in Cape Verde, Africa. *Revista Brasileira de Psiquiatria (Sao Paulo, Brazil), 27*(2), 101–107. doi:10.1590/S1516-44462005000200006 PMID:15962133

Mustapha, L. (2008). Mass media and optimization of health policy, the participating option. In R. A. Akinfeleye (Ed.), *Mass media and society: A multiperspective approach*. Department of Mass Communication University of Lagos.

National Cancer Institute and the Centers for Disease Control and Prevention. (2010). *Making health communication programs work*. National Cancer Institute and the Centers for Disease Control and Prevention.

Njidda, A. M., Oyebanji, O., Obasanya, J., Ojo, O., Adedeji, A., Mba, N., Oladejo, J., & Ihekweazu, C. (2018). The Nigeria Centre for Disease Control. *BMJ Global Health, 3*(2), e000712. doi:10.1136/bmjgh-2018-000712 PMID:29707246

Nwosu, I. A. (2013). Indigenous communication as an enabling factor for rural development in Nigeria. *International Journal of Development and Management Review, 8*(1).

O'Halloran, K. L., Tan, S., Smith, B. A., & Podlasov, A. (2010). Challenges in designing digital interfaces for the study of multimodal phenomena. *Information Design Journal, 18*(1), 2–21. doi:10.1075/idj.18.1.02hal

Oryila, S. S., & Aghadiuno, P. C. (2021). Multimodal communication practice in Nigeria's digital space. In P. Ndayizigamiye, G. Barlow-Jones, R. Brink, S. Bvuma, R. Minty, & S. Mhlongo (Eds.), *Perspectives on ICT4D and socio-economic growth opportunities in developing countries* (pp. 31–61). IGI Publications. doi:10.4018/978-1-7998-2983-6.ch002

Royce, T. D. (2007). *Intersemiotic complementarity: A framework for multimodal discourse analysis. In New directions in the analysis of multimodal discourse.* Routledge.

Scott-Emuakpor, A. (2010). The evolution of healthcare systems in Nigeria: Which way forward in the twenty-first century. *Nigerian Medical Journal*, *51*, 53–65.

Serafini, F., & Clausen, J. (2012). Typography as semiotic resource. *Journal of Visual Literacy*, *31*(2), 1–16. doi:10.1080/23796529.2012.11674697

Smith, R. (2008). The end of disease and the beginning of health. *BMJ Group Blogs 2008*. Retrieved September 10, 2021 from https://blogs.bmj.com/bmj/2008/07/08/richard-smith-the-end-of-disease-and-the-beginning-of-health/

Suls, J., & Wallston, K. A. (2003). Introduction. In J. Suls & K. A. Wallston (Eds.), *Social psychological foundations of health and illness*. Blackwell Publishing. doi:10.1002/9780470753552

Taylor, S. (1978). A developing role of social psychology in medicine and medical practice. *Personality and Social Psychology Bulletin*, *4*(4), 515–524. doi:10.1177/014616727800400404

The World Bank. (2017). *A wake up call: Nigeria water supply, sanitation, and hygiene poverty diagnostic*. World Bank Publications.

Ventegodt, S., Kandel, I., Ervin, D. A., & Merrick, J. (2016). Concepts of holistic care (1935-1941). In *Healthcare for people with Intellectual and developmental disabilities across the Lifespan*. doi:10.1007/978-3-319-18096-0_148

Walker, S. (2019). Effective antimicrobial resistance communication: The role of information design. *Palgrave Communications*, *5*(24), 24. doi:10.105741599-019-0231-z

World Health Organization. (1982). *Medium term program*. World Health Organization.

Wyscocki, A. (2004). The multiple media of texts: How onscreen and paper texts incorporate words, images, and other media. In C. Bazerman & P. Prior (Eds.), *What writing does and how it does it: An introduction to analyzing texts and textual practices* (pp. 123–163). Lawrence Erlbaum.

Yamuah, L. (2005). *Towards healthy nations with ICT wealth.* Information for Development. Retrieved October 10, 2021, from www.i4d.csdms

Chapter 3
A Systematic Review of eHealth Studies on the COVID-19 Pandemic

Macire Kante
https://orcid.org/0000-0001-5425-4549
University of Johannesburg, South Africa

Patrick Ndayizigamiye
https://orcid.org/0000-0001-5721-6070
University of Johannesburg, South Africa

ABSTRACT

In the current context of the COVID-19 pandemic, many healthcare institutions have resorted to eHealth to manage the disruption in healthcare brought by the pandemic. However, the extent to which eHealth has been used in the context of the COVID-19 pandemic has not been widely investigated. It is in this context that this study sought to systematically review research trends on the use of eHealth in the context of the COVID-19 pandemic era, the theoretical underpinnings of the studies on the use of eHealth in the context of the COVID-19 pandemic, and the contributions made by these studies. Findings revealed that most studies focused on the 'health in our hands' and 'interacting for health' components of eHealth while none of the studies focused on the 'data enabling health' component. In addition, none of the reviewed studies used a theoretical framework. Albeit with limitations, these studies shed light on the use of eHealth applications for patients' data management and the provision of telemedicine in the fight against COVID-19.

DOI: 10.4018/978-1-7998-8915-1.ch003

INTRODUCTION AND BACKGROUND

Electronic Health (eHealth) can be defined as "the use of technologies such as mobile phones or the Internet to provide or enhance health services (Kante & Ndayizigamiye, 2021, p.1). Rothman and Malster (2021, p.24) further elaborated on the eHealth definition and stated that eHealth can be defined as "the use of information and communication technologies for health and can include the use of email, text messaging, push notifications, websites, and mobile-based applications". Many studies have been conducted on the adoption or use of eHealth to provide public healthcare services (Ndayizigamiye & Maharaj, 2016a; Ndayizigamiye & Maharaj, 2016b; Ndayizigamiye, 2016; Ndayizigamiye & Maharaj, 2017; Ndayizigamiye, Hangulu & Akintola, 2017; Imaja, Ndayizigamiye & Maharaj, 2017; Ndayizigamiye & Maharaj, 2018; Matiyabu & Ndayizigamiye, 2019; Kante & Ndayizigamiye, 2021); promote healthy lifestyles (Ndayizigamiye, Kante & Shingwenyana, 2020); for self-healthcare monitoring (Ndayizigamiye, Soni, & Jere, 2018; Soni, Ndayizigamiye, & Kante, 2019), to name a few.

In the context of the current Coronavirus pandemic (Covid-19), many studies have been conducted on the use of eHealth in the fight against the pandemic (Scott et al., 2020). Scott et al. (2020) further highlighted that many of these studies have synthesized the literature to highlight the current trend on eHealth research and how eHealth could be used to address future emergencies. Similarly, Vokinger et al. (2020) reviewed the literature and argued that despite a high number of health applications being developed and implemented, there was a need to assess them as their usefulness remains somehow questionable. They then proposed a framework for assessing such applications in the fight against Covid-19. Another synthesis of the literature has been provided by Neubeck et al. (2020) on the remote provision of healthcare to cardiovascular patients during the Covid-19 pandemic era.

Despite these syntheses of the literature on the use of eHealth, the literature that portrays the nexus between eHealth and Covid-19 is still accumulating and hence there is a need to be acquainted with new developments in the fight against Covid-19. Furthermore, most of the literature reviews focused only on some areas of application of eHealth. For instance, the review of Neubeck et al. (2020) focused on cardiovascular patients whilst Scott et al. (2020) investigated the evaluation of eHealth applications. Therefore, there is need for a synthesis of eHealth research that provides a comprehensive understanding of eHealth research in the context of the Covid-19 pandemic. It is in this context that the following objectives of this study were formulated:

1. To highlight the current research trend on eHealth components and Covid-19.

2. To synthesize the theoretical underpinning studies on the use of eHealth in the context of the Covid-19 pandemic.
3. To synthesize the contributions made by studies on the use of eHealth in the context of the Covid-19 pandemic.

METHODOLOGY

This study was conducted using a systematic literature review approach. Systematic literature review has been recognised as the most appropriate method in establishing a generalisable and informative evidence-based conclusion (Boland et al., 2017; Hanson & Heeks, 2020). In this study, the systematic literature review was conducted using Google Scholar, which, according to Khabsa & Giles (2014, 15), covers a wide variety of multidisciplinary literature. This study adopted the Preferred Reporting Items for Systematic Reviews and Meta-Analysis (PRISMA) as the underpinning methodology. The PRISMA model is one of the most popular guidelines for conducting systematic reviews (Shamseer et al., 2015). The PRISMA model comprises 4 phases namely: identification, screening, eligibility, and inclusion as depicted in Figure 1.

Figure 1. PRISMA Guidelines Flow.
Adopted from Buthelezi, Ndayizigamiye, Twinomurinzi & Dube (2022)

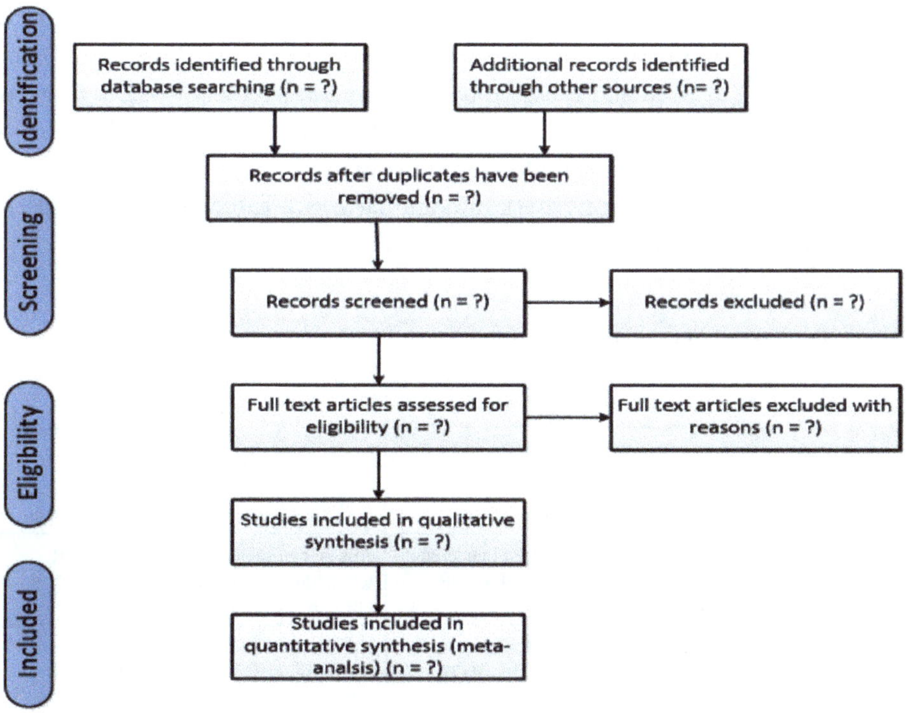

Indeed, a systematic literature review holds an important place in healthcare. In healthcare, a systematic literature review forms the basis for developing practice guidelines and can highlight gaps in knowledge, thus informing future research efforts (Shamseer et al., 2015). Thus, findings from a systematic review could benefit many stakeholders across healthcare systems. The rigour and trustworthiness of systematic reviews is, in large part, based on the a priori planning and documentation of a methodical approach (also known as protocol) to conduct the review. The process that was followed to conduct this systematic review using the PRISMA guidelines is described below:

IDENTIFICATION, SCREENING AND ELIGIBILITY

The search was performed using the key terms "(eHealth OR mHealth) AND (Covid-19 OR COVID)". The first key term search resulted in the collection of 1590 papers. Another criterion was applied to the data set, namely the time range. In this case only papers published in 2019 and 2020 were considered. This resulted in the exclusion of 1276 papers. Furthermore, 33 papers were not available for downloading, thus we excluded them for further analysis. Only 314 papers were carried on to the eligibility stage. Then, we removed posters, short papers, pre-prints, and reports. The remaining full papers were analysed based on the research objectives. Additionally, there were some review papers (full papers) that were part of the search results. These reviews were further assessed following the Overview Quality Assessment Questionnaire (OQAQ) of Greaves et al. (2011) and Oxman & Guyatt (1991) as used and reported by Lwoga & Sangeda (Lwoga & Sangeda, 2019) (see Appendix A). A review paper was included for further analysis only if its OQAQ score was 10 or above (from a range of 0–18).

The inclusion and exclusion criteria are summarized in Table 1 while the selection process and the results thereof are depicted in Figure 2.

Table 1. Inclusion and Exclusion Criteria

Description	Inclusion	Exclusion
Research paper sources	Google Scholar	Not from the Google scholar
Publication year	Published in 2019 or 2020	Published before 2019 and after 2020
Words in the text	(eHealth OR mHealth OR telemedicine OR telehealth) AND (Covid-19 OR Covid)	Absence of (eHealth OR mHealth OR telemedicine OR telehealth) AND (Covid-19 OR Covid)
Words in the title or Abstract	(eHealth OR mHealth OR telemedicine OR telehealth) AND (Covid-19 OR Covid)	Absence of (eHealth OR mHealth OR telemedicine OR telehealth) AND (Covid-19 OR Covid)

Figure 2. Selection Process

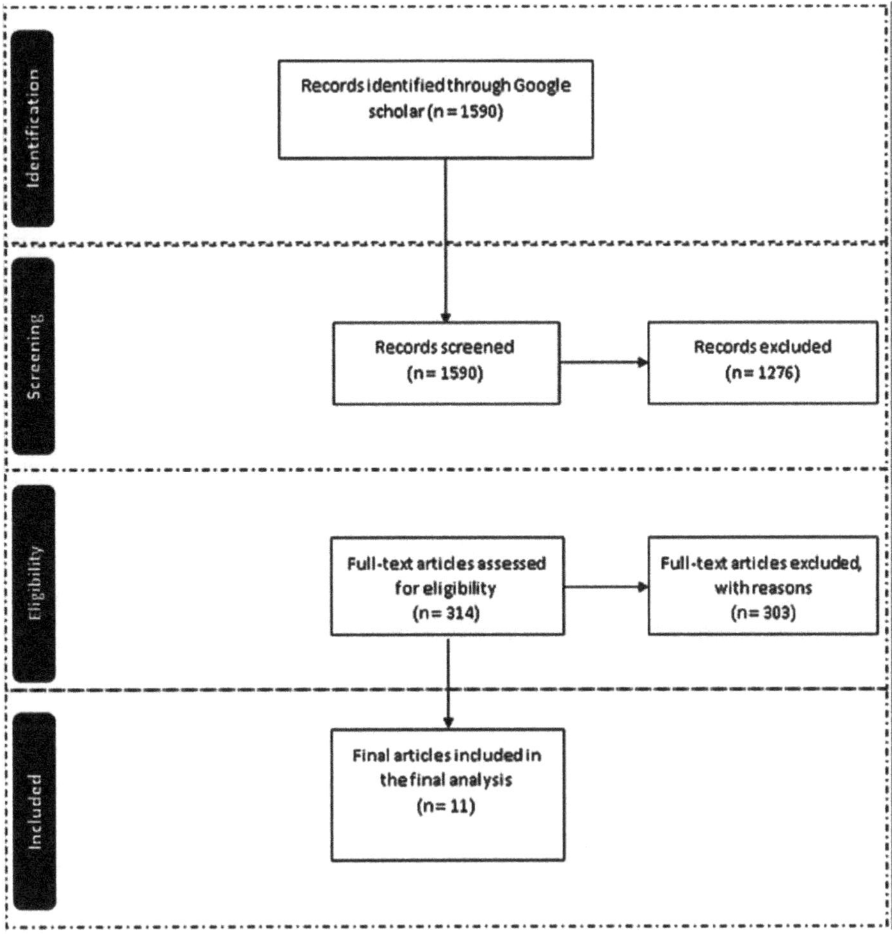

DATA EXTRACTION AND ANALYSIS PROCESS

A template was developed for the data extraction from the selected studies. The template is displayed below in Table 2. A variable, named as extraction variable in this study, consisted of a data item and a value as suggested by the literature (Petersen et al., 2015). The extraction variables were purposefully defined to answer the research objectives.

Table 2. Data Extraction Form

Data Item	Value	Research Objectives
Article Title	Name of the article	
Author Name	Set of Names of the authors	
Country	In which country has the study been done	
Field of study	What was the field of study	Research Objective 1
Theories/models used	What other theories/models have been used	Research Objective 2
Findings	What contributions were made	Research Objective 3

TOOLS USED IN THE ANALYSIS PROCESS

The selection process was managed using the open-source desktop-based application Mendeley, as used and suggested by Kante & Ndayizigamiye (2020a) and Zewge & Dittrich (2017). The Mendeley tool was used to classify, tag, and reference each paper using the data extraction form (Table 2) as a guide. After the selection and pre-processing phases, articles that were selected for further analysis were exported to a Microsoft Excel 2019 file.

RESULTS AND DISCUSSIONS

This section presents and discusses the results of this study. It starts by characterizing the collected data and then goes on with answering the first specific objective to identify the current research trend on the use of eHealth in the context of the Covid-19 pandemic. Lastly, the second and third research specific objectives' results are presented and discussed.

Data Characterization

Eleven (11) research papers were selected for final analysis. These consisted of five review papers and six full research papers. Six papers were published from the United States of America (Barney et al., 2020; Contreras et al., 2020; Jethwa et al., 2020; Marra et al., 2020; Punia et al., 2020; Scott et al., 2020); one from the United Kingdom (Neubeck et al., 2020); one from Spain (Rabuñal et al., 2020); one from Italy (Giudice et al., 2020); one from the People's Republic of China (Ren et al., 2020) and one from Switzerland (Vokinger et al., 2020). This means that 90.9% of the selected papers were from developed countries, with the United States of America accounting for 60% of the papers. This shows the trend of eHealth's research related to the Covid-19 pandemic. This trend could be explained by the fact that these countries have been more affected by the Covid-19 than the developing world. For instance, as of 22nd July 2020, 144,000 (Wikipedia, 2020) deaths related to Covid-19 were reported in the United States of America whilst 4,653 (Wikipedia, 2020) deaths related to Covid-19 were reported in China (mainland).

Health Component

Oh et al. (2005) defined health as "a state of complete physical, mental, and social wellbeing and not just the absence of disease or infirmity". The use of technology (Information Technology) to enhance healthcare is known as electronic health (eHealth) (Oh et al., 2005). This definition has evolved from health-based technology to the communicative functions of eHealth, specifically the use of networked digital technologies, primarily the Internet, thus differentiating eHealth from the field of medical informatics (Pagliari et al., 2005). The definition of eHealth encompasses mobile health (mHealth), Internet of Things (IoT) for healthcare, mobile based Internet of Things for Healthcare (m-IoT) and Internet of Medical Things (IoMT) (Kante & Ndayizigamiye, 2020b); blockchain in healthcare (Girardi et al., 2020); telemedicine or telehealth (Oh et al., 2005). eHealth comprises three main components (Shaw et al., 2017) namely, (a) 'health in our hands' (the use of technology for monitoring, tracking, and informing), (b) 'interacting for health' (using technology to enable health communication among practitioners and between health professionals and clients or patients), and (c) 'data enabling health' (collecting, managing, and using health data with the help of technology). Thus, we divided the selected papers into these three components as reported below:

Health in Our Hands

These represent studies that focused on the use of eHealth to monitor, track and provide information on Covid-19. About 26% of the selected papers were classified in this category. Rabuñal et al. (2020) examined the usefulness of a telemedicine tool (TELEA) in the management of Covid-19. Vokinger et al. (2020) on the other hand, reviewed eHealth applications for monitoring Covid-19. Giudice et al. (2020) conducted a pilot study to assess the monitoring of patients using telemedicine. What can be drawn here is that there is little research regarding this health component in the context of Covid-19. However, the World Health Organization recommends that the control of the spread of Covid-19 requires the breaking of the chains of human-to-human transmission (WHO, 2020). Hence, more research should be done regarding the component 'health in our hands' to shed more light on how to break the chains of transmission using e-health.

Interacting for Health

This component represents the most researched area in the selected papers. Almost 63.6% of the papers investigated this component. Neubeck et al. (2020) synthesized the literature on delivering healthcare remotely to cardiovascular patients in the context of Covid-19 pandemic. Punia et al. (2020) reviewed the literature on delivering healthcare using telemedicine during the Covid-19 pandemic era. Ren et al. (2020) investigated the application of mobile telehealth system to facilitate patient information management. Marra et al. (2020) explored the delivery of neuropsychology using telehealth. Contreras et al. (2020) studied the provision of healthcare using telemedicine during Covid-19 pandemic era. Contreras et al. (2020) mostly focused on the environment that is conducive for an effective utilization of telemedicine. Barney et al. (2020) researched the implementation of telemedicine to deliver healthcare to adolescent and young adults in the context of Covid-19 pandemic era. Jethwa et al. (2020) implemented a virtual clinic for Covid-19 screening and treatment and report the preliminary results of the implementation.

The fact that most of the research focused on this component, could mean that most of the research focused on treatment rather than prevention, as prevention is normally the focus of the first component, i.e., health in our hands.

Data Enabling Health

There was not even a single paper that researched this area. The implication of this is that research on Covid-19 health data is still scanty. This is understandable as at the time this study was conducted data pertaining to Covid-19 was still scarce to allow meaningful data-enabled decision making.

THEORETICAL UNDERPINNING OF THE STUDIES

All the research papers were not anchored on a theoretical framework or model. This is a gap that needs to be addressed by future studies. According to Mueller & Urbach (2013, p.2), a study without a theoretical underpinning lacks the synthesis and integration needed for knowledge-based claims and can be compared to a "heap of leaves without a tree". Furthermore, without a theoretical lens, the description, prediction and explanation of a phenomenon may not be comprehensive (Kante et al., 2018).

RESEARCH CONTRIBUTION

In terms of research contribution, the reviewed papers did bring some new insights into healthcare delivery using digital technologies in the context of Covid-19. The reviewed papers provided an understanding on how to deliver cardiovascular operations remotely during Covid-19 (Neubeck et al., 2020); develop a framework for the evaluation of mHealth applications for epidemic control or mitigating its effects, proposed new applications to support the fight against Covid-19 (Vokinger et al., 2020); suggested technologies that could be used in fighting Covid-19 (Scott et al., 2020); the use of Teleneuropsychology during Covid-19 (Marra et al., 2020), and the environmental factors of the utilization of telemedicine during Covid-19 (Contreras et al., 2020).

Some studies developed and implemented eHealth (including mHealth and telemedicine) applications. These applications help in the fight against Covid-19. Rabuñal et al. (2020) implemented an application (TELEA) and reported its usefulness in the management of Covid-19 patients. Similarly, Punia et al. (2020), after implementing an online clinic, reported that the virtual clinic could be useful in maintaining a seamless transition of outpatient care during the pandemic (Covid-19). Ren et al. (2020) also developed a mobile telehealth system (MTS) to present patient information and case discussion. They reported that the MTS was beneficial for the healthcare professionals as it considerably reduced face-to-face contacts. Jethwa et al. (2020, p.1) reported that results of their implementation of a drive through Covid-19 testing and virtual clinic enabled them to deliver "high-quality care in an anxious time without consuming excessive personal protective equipment or unnecessarily exposing health care workers". They further argued that their paper could serve as a guide to future similar research. These contributions remain empirical as they were not grounded into theory.

CONCLUSION

This paper sought to summarize the literature on eHealth and Covid-19. The study had three specific research objectives: a) to highlight the current research trend on eHealth components and Covid-19, b) to synthesize the theoretical underpinning of studies on the use of eHealth in the context of the Covid-19 pandemic and c) to synthesize the contributions made by studies on the use of eHealth in the context of the Covid-19 pandemic. On the first research objective, the results showed that most of the research (63%) investigated the use of e-health to communicate among health practitioners and between health professionals and patients. On the second research objective, the study revealed that there was a lack of theoretical grounding of the identified studies on the use of eHealth in the context of the Covid-19 pandemic. Lastly, on the research objective 3, the studies made contributions on the use of eHealth applications for patients' data management; provision of telemedicine in the fight against Covid-19; and related policy recommendations. This study suggests that more studies should be conducted on some components of eHealth such as the 'health in our hands' (technology enabling monitoring, tracking Covid-19, and informing healthcare professionals). This study may have left out some published papers and more research may have been published since the completion of this study. Hence, we recommend further investigation into the covered research objectives of this study.

REFERENCES

Barney, A., Buckelew, S., Mesheriakova, V., & Raymond-Flesch, M. (2020). The Covid-19 Pandemic and Rapid Implementation of Adolescent and Young Adult Telemedicine: Challenges and Opportunities for Innovation. *The Journal of Adolescent Health*, (2), 1–8. doi:10.1016/j.jadohealth.2020.05.006 PMID:32410810

Boland, A., Cherry, G., & Dickson, R. (2017). Doing a systematic review: A student's guide. *Sage (Atlanta, Ga.)*.

Buthelezi, B.E., Ndayizigamiye, P., & Twinomurinzi, H., & Dube. (2022). A Systematic Review of the Adoption of Blockchain for Supply Chain Processes. *Journal of Global Information Management.*

Contreras, C. M., Metzger, G. A., Beane, J. D., Dedhia, P. H., Ejaz, A., & Pawlik, T. M. (2020). Telemedicine: Patient-Provider Clinical Engagement During the Covid-19 Pandemic and Beyond. *Journal of Gastrointestinal Surgery*, *1*(7), 1692–1697. Advance online publication. doi:10.100711605-020-04623-5 PMID:32385614

Girardi, F., De Gennaro, G., Colizzi, L., & Convertini, N. (2020). Improving the Healthcare Effectiveness: The Possible Role of EHR, IoMT and Blockchain. *Electronics (Basel)*, *9*(6), 884. doi:10.3390/electronics9060884

Giudice, A., Barone, S., Muraca, D., Averta, F., Diodati, F., Antonelli, A., & Fortunato, L. (2020). Can teledentistry improve the monitoring of patients during the Covid-19 dissemination? A descriptive pilot study. *International Journal of Environmental Research and Public Health*, *17*(10), 1–9. doi:10.3390/ijerph17103399 PMID:32414126

Greaves, C. J., Sheppard, K. E., Abraham, C., Hardeman, W., Roden, M., Evans, P. H., & Schwarz, P. (2011). Systematic review of reviews of intervention components associated with increased effectiveness in dietary and physical activity interventions. *BMC Public Health, 11*(1), 1–12. doi:10.1186/1471-2458-11-119 PMID:21333011

Hanson, W., & Heeks, R. (2020). Impact of ICTs-in-Agriculture on Rural Resilience in Developing Countries. In *Development Informatics* (No. 84; Working Paper Series, Issue July). doi:10.13140/RG.2.2.31885.90084

Imaja, I. M., Ndayizigamiye, P., & Maharaj, M. (2017). A design of a mobile health intervention for the prevention and treatment of Cholera in South Kivu in the Democratic Republic of Congo. In *2017 IEEE Global Humanitarian Technology Conference (GHTC)* (pp. 1-5). IEEE. 10.1109/GHTC.2017.8239251

Jethwa, T., Ton, A., Paredes Molina, C. S., Speicher, L., Walsh, K., Knight, D., Davlantes, T., & Francis, D. (2020). Establishing Mayo Clinic's Coronavirus Disease 2019 Virtual Clinic: A Preliminary Communication. *Telemedicine Journal and E-Health : The Official Journal of the American Telemedicine Association.* . doi:10.1089/tmj.2020.0145

Kante, M., Chepken, C., & Oboko, R. (2018). Partial Least Square Structural Equation Modelling' use in Information Systems: An Updated Guideline of Practices in Exploratory Settings. *Kabarak Journal of Research & Innovation, 6*(1), 49–67. http://eserver.kabarak.ac.ke/ojs/

Kante, M., & Ndayizigamiye, P. (2020a). A systematic mapping of the adoption of Internet of Things to provide healthcare services in developing countries. In P. Ndayizigamiye, G. Barlow-Jones, R. Brink, S. Bvuma, R. Minty, & S. Mhlongo (Eds.), *Perspectives on ICT4D and Socio-Economic Growth Opportunities in Developing Countries* (pp. 99–126). IGI Global. doi:10.4018/978-1-7998-2983-6.ch004

Kante, M., & Ndayizigamiye, P. (2020b). An analysis of the current status of Internet of Medical Things policies in developing countries. *NPG. Neurologie, Psychiatrie, Gériatrie, 20*(119), 259–265. doi:10.1016/j.npg.2020.03.002

Kante, M., & Ndayizigamiye, P. (2021). Internet of Medical Things, Policies and Geriatrics: An Analysis of the National Digital Health Strategy for South Africa 2019-2024 from the Policy Triangle Framework Perspective. *Scientific African*, e00759.

Khabsa, M., & Giles, C. L. (2014). The number of scholarly documents on the public web. *PLoS One, 9*(5), e93949. doi:10.1371/journal.pone.0093949 PMID:24817403

Lwoga, E. T., & Sangeda, R. Z. (2019). ICTs and development in developing countries: A systematic review of reviews. *The Electronic Journal on Information Systems in Developing Countries*, *85*(1), e12060. doi:10.1002/isd2.12060

Marra, D. E., Hamlet, K. M., Bauer, R. M., & Bowers, D. (2020). Validity of teleneuropsychology for older adults in response to Covid-19: A systematic and critical review. *The Clinical Neuropsychologist*, *0*(0), 1–42. doi:10.1080/13854046.2020.1769192 PMID:32519594

Matiyabu, I. I., & Ndayizigamiye, P. (2019). The potential use of Social Media for Healthcare Advocacy in the Democratic Republic of Congo. In *Proceedings of 4th International Conference on the* (*Vol. 12*, pp. 105-111). Academic Press.

Mueller, B., & Urbach, N. (2013). The why, what, and how of theories in is research. In *Thirty Fourth International Conference on Information Systems* (*Vol. 192*, Issue 111, pp. 181–192). AISel.

Ndayizigamiye, P. (2016). *Potential adoption of mobile health technologies for public healthcare in Burundi* (Doctoral dissertation).

Ndayizigamiye, P., Hangulu, L., & Akintola, O. (2017). A design of a mobile health intervention to enhance home-carers' disposal of medical waste in South Africa. In *2017 IEEE Global Humanitarian Technology Conference (GHTC)* (pp. 1-6). IEEE. 10.1109/GHTC.2017.8239241

Ndayizigamiye, P., Kante, M., & Shingwenyana, S. (2020). An adoption model of mHealth applications that promote physical activity. *Cogent Psychology*, *7*(1), 1764703. doi:10.1080/23311908.2020.1764703

Ndayizigamiye, P., & Maharaj, M. (2016a). Mobile health adoption in Burundi: A UTAUT perspective. In *2016 IEEE Global Humanitarian Technology Conference (GHTC)* (pp. 613-623). IEEE. 10.1109/GHTC.2016.7857342

Ndayizigamiye, P., & Maharaj, M. (2016b). *Applying bridges framework to investigate challenges to the adoption of mHealth in Burundi. In 2016 IST-Africa Week Conference*. IEEE.

Ndayizigamiye, P., & Maharaj, M. (2017). Determinants of mobile health adoption in Burundi. *The African Journal of Information Systems*, *9*(3), 1–23.

Ndayizigamiye, P., & Maharaj, M. (2018). *A Systematic review of mHealth interventions for public healthcare in East Africa in AMCIS 2018 proceedings*. AIS.

Ndayizigamiye, P., Soni, T. C., & Jere, N. (2018). *Factors Motivating the Adoption of Self-Healthcare Monitoring Mobile Applications by the South African Youth. In 2018 IST-Africa Week Conference (IST-Africa).* IEEE.

Neubeck, L., Hansen, T., Jaarsma, T., Klompstra, L., & Gallagher, R. (2020). Delivering healthcare remotely to cardiovascular patients during Covid-19: A rapid review of the evidence. *European Journal of Cardiovascular Nursing*, *0*(0), 1–9. doi:10.1177/1474515120924530 PMID:32380858

Oh, H., Rizo, C., Enkin, M., & Jadad, A. (2005). What Is eHealth (3): A Systematic Review of Published Definitions. J Med Internet Res, 7(1). doi:10.2196/jmir.7.1.e1

Oxman, A. D., & Guyatt, G. H. (1991). Validation of an index of the quality of review articles. *Journal of Clinical Epidemiology*, *44*(11), 1271–1278. doi:10.1016/0895-4356(91)90160-B PMID:1834807

Pagliari, C., Sloan, D., Gregor, P., Sullivan, F., Detmer, D., Kahan, J. P., Oortwijn, W., & MacGillivray, S. (2005). What Is eHealth (4): A Scoping Exercise to Map the Field. J Med Internet Res, 7(1). doi:10.2196/jmir.7.1.e9

Petersen, K., Vakkalanka, S., & Kuzniarz, L. (2015). Guidelines for conducting systematic mapping studies in software engineering: An update. *Information and Software Technology*, *64*, 1–18. doi:10.1016/j.infsof.2015.03.007

Punia, V., Nasr, G., Zagorski, V., Lawrence, G., Fesler, J., Nair, D., & Najm, I. (2020). Evidence of a Rapid Shift in Outpatient Practice During the Covid-19 Pandemic Using Telemedicine. *Telemedicine Journal and e-Health*, *00*(00), 1–3. doi:10.1089/tmj.2020.0150 PMID:32429769

Rabuñal, R., Suarez-Gil, R., Golpe, R., Martínez-García, M., Gómez-Méndez, R., Romay-Lema, E., Pérez-López, A., Rodríguez-Álvarez, A., & Bal-Alvaredo, M. (2020). Usefulness of a Telemedicine Tool TELEA in the Management of the Covid-19 Pandemic. *Telemedicine Journal and e-Health*, *00*(00), 1–4. doi:10.1089/tmj.2020.0144 PMID:32501747

Ren, X., Zhai, Y., Song, X., Wang, Z., Dou, D., & Li, Y. (2020). The Application of Mobile Telehealth System to Facilitate Patient Information Presentation and Case Discussion. *Telemedicine Journal and e-Health*, *26*(6), 725–733. doi:10.1089/tmj.2020.0084 PMID:32298208

Rothman, C., & Maltser, S. (2021). Exercise while living with breast and gynecological cancers. In A. Cristian (Ed.), Breast cancer and gynecologic cancer rehabilitation (pp. 19-38). Elsevier.

Scott, B. K., Miller, G. T., Fonda, S. J., Yeaw, R. E., Gaudaen, J. C., Pavliscsak, H. H., Quinn, M. T., & Pamplin, J. C. (2020). Advanced Digital Health Technologies for Covid-19 and Future Emergencies. *Telemedicine Journal and e-Health, 00*(00), 1–8. doi:10.1089/tmj.2020.0140 PMID:32456560

Shamseer, L., Moher, D., Clarke, M., Ghersi, D., Liberati, A., Petticrew, M., Shekelle, P., Stewart, L. A., Altman, D. G., Booth, A., Chan, A. W., Chang, S., Clifford, T., Dickersin, K., Egger, M., Gøtzsche, P. C., Grimshaw, J. M., Groves, T., Helfand, M., … Whitlock, E. (2015). Preferred reporting items for systematic review and meta-analysis protocols (prisma-p) 2015: Elaboration and explanation. *BMJ, 349*(February), 1–25. . doi:10.1136/bmj.g7647

Shaw, T., McGregor, D., Brunner, M., Keep, M., Janssen, A., & Barnet, S. (2017). What is eHealth (6)? Development of a Conceptual Model for eHealth: Qualitative Study with Key Informants. *Journal of Medical Internet Research, 19*(10), e324. doi:10.2196/jmir.8106 PMID:29066429

Soni, T. C., Ndayizigamiye, P., & Kante, M. (2019). *Determinants of the Adoption of Self-healthcare Monitoring Mobile Applications. Fortieth International Conference on Information Systems (ICIS)*, Munich, Germany.

Vokinger, K. N., Nittas, V., Witt, C. M., Fabrikant, S. I., & von Wyl, V. (2020). Digital health and the Covid-19 epidemic: An assessment framework for apps from an epidemiological and legal perspective. *Swiss Medical Weekly, 150*(May), w20282. doi:10.4414mw.2020.20282 PMID:32418194

WHO. (2020). Contact tracing in the context of Covid-19. In *WHO Guidelines* (Vol. 2019, Issue May 10). https://www.who.int/publications-detail/contact-tracing-in-the-context-of-Covid-19

Wikipedia. (2020). *Covid 19 stats mali - Google Search*. https://www.google.com/search?client=firefox-b-d&q=covid+19+stats+mali

Zewge, A., & Dittrich, Y. (2017). Systematic mapping study of information technology for development in agriculture (the case of developing countries). *The Electronic Journal on Information Systems in Developing Countries, 82*(2), 1–25. doi:10.1002/j.1681-4835.2017.tb00602.x

KEY TERMS AND DEFINITIONS

COVID-19: Coronavirus disease (COVID-19) is an infectious disease caused by the SARS-CoV-2 virus.

eHealth: The use of information and communication technologies for health and can include the use of email, text messaging, push notifications, websites, and mobile-based applications.

Health Systems: Also known as health care system or healthcare system, is the organization of people, institutions, and resources that deliver health care services to meet the health needs of target populations.

Model: A system of statements targeted at describing, explaining, and predicting real-world phenomena. A scientific model is a system composed of two core constituents that have been tested and validated: (1) factors and (2) hypotheses.

Systematic Review: It is a form of evidence synthesis. It is the method used to collect, collate, and present research evidence.

Theory: A system of statements targeted at describing, explaining, and predicting real-world phenomena. A scientific theory is a system composed of two core constituents: (1) factors and (2) hypotheses.

APPENDIX A: OVERVIEW QUALITY ASSESSMENT QUESTIONNAIRE (OQAQ)

1. Were the search methods used to find evidence on the primary question(s) stated?
    a. **Yes**, description of databases searched, search strategy, and years reviewed. **2 pts**.
    b. **Partially**, descriptions of methods not complete. **1 pt**.
    c. **No**, no description of search methods. **0 pts**.
2. Was the search for evidence reasonably comprehensive?
    a. **Yes**, at least one computerized database searched and also a search of unpublished or non-indexed literature. **2 pts**.
    b. **Can't tell**, search strategy partially comprehensive, at least one of the strategies performed. **1 pt**.
    c. **No**, search not comprehensive or not described well. **0 pts**.
3. Were the criteria used for deciding which studies to include in the review reported?
    a. **Yes**, inclusion and exclusion criteria clearly defined. **2 pts**.
    b. **Partially**, reference to inclusion/exclusion criteria can be found but are not defined clearly enough. **1 pt**.
    c. **No**, no criteria defined. **0 pts**
4. Was bias in the selection of articles avoided?
    a. **Yes**, issues influencing selection bias were covered. Both of the following bias-avoiding strategies were used: (1) two or more assessors independently judged study relevance, (2) assessors selected studies using predetermined criteria. **2 pts**.
    b. **Can't tell**, only one of the strategies used. **1 pt**.
    c. **No**, selection bias was not avoided or was not discussed. **0 pts**.
5. Were the criteria used for assessing the methodological quality of studies reviewed reported?
    a. **Yes**, criteria defined and used addressed the major factors influencing bias. **2 pts**.
    b. **Partially**, some discussion or reference to criteria. **1 pt**.
    c. **No**, validity or methodological quality criteria not used or not described. **0 pts**.
6. Were study quality assessment criteria used to inform the review analysis?
    a. **Yes**, criteria were used to inform the analysis, either by exclusion from the analysis if low quality or through sensitivity analysis. **2 pts**.

   b. **Partially**, some discussion but not clearly described application of criteria. **1 pt**.
   c. **No**, criteria not used or not described. **0 pts**.
7. Were the methods used to combine the findings of the relevant studies (to reach a conclusion) reported?
   a. **Yes**, qualitative and quantitative methods are acceptable. **2 pts.**
   b. **Partially**, partial description of methods to combine and tabulate; not sufficient to duplicate. **1 pt**.
   c. **No**, methods not stated or described. **0 pts**.
8. Were findings of the relevant studies combined appropriately relative to the primary question of the overview?
   a. **Yes**, combining of studies appears acceptable. **2 pts**.
   b. **Can't tell**, should be marked if in doubt. **1 pt**.
   c. **No**, no attempt was made to combine findings, and no statement was made regarding the inappropriateness of combining findings. **0 pts**.
9. Were the conclusions made by the author(s) supported by the data and/or analysis reported in the overview?
   a. **Yes**, data were reported that support the main conclusions regarding the primary question(s) that the overview addresses. **2 pts**.
   b. **Partially**. **1 pt**.
   c. **No**, conclusions not supported or unclear. **0 pts**.

Chapter 4
COVID-19 Digital Technology Response in Sub-Saharan African Countries

Abiodun Alao
https://orcid.org/0000-0001-6288-2991
University of Johannesburg, South Africa

Roelien Brink
University of Johannesburg, South Africa

ABSTRACT

This chapter investigated the use of digital technologies as a response to the COVID-19 pandemic in Sub-Saharan African countries. The study explored possible ways towards building an open, inclusive, and secure digital ecosystem using digital technologies to create awareness of the coronavirus pandemic. The qualitative approach and critical discourse analysis were adopted to critically analyze the effects of digital technologies in the healthcare sector of the Sub-Saharan African region, while the technology determinism theory was used as the theoretical lens of the study. This study advocated the use of digital technologies as an effective tool to disseminate information about infectious diseases to the citizens of the Sub-Saharan African region.

INTRODUCTION

The Coronavirus infection primarily transmitted via contact and respiratory droplets (Gates, 2020; Kuca, 2020) was declared a global pandemic by the World Health

DOI: 10.4018/978-1-7998-8915-1.ch004

Organization (International Labour Organization, 2020) on the 11th of March 2020 (Haman, 2020). Eight months into the COVID-19 pandemic, there was an average of 54, 014, 420 confirmed infection cases and 1, 313, 563 deaths globally (International Labour Organization, 2020). The African continent recorded its first case of COVID-19 in Egypt on February 14, 2020, and thereafter, there have been reported COVID-19 infection cases in a total of 52 African countries (World Health Organization, 2020; Kalantaryan and McMahon, 2020). The realization is that the efforts made towards eradicating poverty are being forfeited as the pandemic has increased global poverty, given that many Sub-Saharan African countries just like many other nations in the world are experiencing a drastic economic recession (Sumner et al., 2020). Due to this many people were rendered jobless without a meaningful livelihood (International Labour Organization, 2020), while small to medium-sized enterprises (SMEs) were unable to operate causing some to eventually fold up, while big organizations were forced to change their business operations to use digital means to guide and adapt to new company measures (Dwivedi et al., 2020).

This study reflects on one of the targets of sustainable development goal (SDG) 9, which is to significantly increase the access to information and communications technology (ICT) to different sectors such as the healthcare sector, educational, government, and private organizations, and strive to provide universal and affordable internet access in the least developed countries by 2030. The several levels of strict lockdown strategies implemented by governments globally to limit the COVID-19 pandemic compelled organizations to encourage their staff to work from home (Dwivedi, et al., 2020). While essential sectors like the health systems in the Sub-Saharan Africa region faced many challenges such as equipment, data and service inadequacy, staffing, lack of medical infrastructure, poor deployment to meet medical outcome demands, lack of maintenance of medical equipment and instruments, management of clinical data, lack of new medical innovation and designs, lack of access to treatment and communication before the COVID-19 pandemic occurrence (Walsham, 2020; Ben, 2020). Hence, the lack of health information systems increased during the COVID-19 pandemic and the existing degeneration of the health sector became overwhelming due to the demand for medical treatment caused by the pandemic hazard (Walsham, 2020).

In adherence to this directive, the citizens of many Sub-Saharan African countries and the staff of many organizations have adopted the use of Wi-Fi connections in their homes, which in turn have promoted the use of digital technologies in both organization and human lives (Katz et al., 2020). In addition, the education sector across the world is compelled to replace in-person classrooms with online lesson delivery (Said et al., 2020; Mpungose and Khoza, 2020). While Sub-Saharan African countries such as South Africa, Kenya, Nigeria, Zimbabwe, etc. declared national health emergencies, broad travel restrictions, and border closure to reduce the spread and death rate caused by the coronavirus (World Economic Outlook, 2018). Many organizations ordered the closure of offices and the global stock market were declined which affected the economies of their countries (World Economic Outlook, 2018).

The efforts made to curtail the spread of the pandemic across nations included testing, strict quarantine, evaluation of interventions with mobility data and communication with the public, contact tracing, early population surveillance, and the creation of vaccination sites (Whitelaw et al., 2020). Amidst the pandemic, many of these Sub-Saharan African countries were able to seek for solutions to navigate their economies, while adhering to the lockdown directive of their government (Ozili, 2020). Also, many of the Sub-Sharan African countries relapsed into a recession that had not occurred in more than 50 years in the year 2020 due to the COVID–19 pandemic, as many of these countries GDP declined by 2.1% and might increase by 3.4% or more in the future if the issue is not adequately addressed (Ozili, 2020).

International donors such as the United Nations Educational, Scientific and Cultural Organization (UNESCO), the World Bank, the Department for International Development (DFID), and the Gates Foundation, have all made financial donations to the World Health Organization (WHO) and low- and middle-income countries to tackle the COVID-19 pandemic (see **Table 1** adapted from Ozili, 2020).

Table 1. Showing the list of COVID-19 foreign aid for African countries (adapted from Ozili, 2020).

S/N	African Countries	International Aid	Amount
1	Egypt	World Bank	US$7.9 Million
2	Sao Tome and Principle	The World Bank's IDA	$2.5 million grant
3	Gambia	The World Bank's IDA	$10 million grant
4	Congo	World Bank ($47m) and the US Government ($6m)	US$53 million
5	Libya	US government	$6 million
6	Rwanda	World Bank	$14.25 million
7	Malawi	UK's DFID	$2.24 million
8	Kenya	World Bank	US$60 million
9	Senegal	World Bank	$20 million
10	Djibouti	World Bank	US$5 million
11	South Sudan	World Bank	$7.6 million
12	Somalia	U.S. government	$7million
13	Sierra Leone	World Bank	$7.5 million

These funds were earmarked for the capacity development of health systems, relief for SMEs in terms of job and workers protection; the development of programs on social welfare legislation; and support for the agricultural sector in many Sub-Saharan African countries (see **Table 2**).

Table 2. COVID-19 relief packages for African countries (adapted from Ozili, 2020).

S/L	Country	Opportunities
1	Tanzania	Use legislation to pass an economic relief bill into law
2	South Africa	• Make private health care affordable to poor citizens. • Create a digital learning platform.
3	Ghana	• Use of legislation to pass on economic relief bill into law.
4	Mauritius	• Preserve the existing social welfare system. • Use of legislation to pass an economic relief bill into law. • Expand the capacity of the country's health system.
5	Guinea	• Use legislation to pass an economic relief bill into law. • Preserve the social welfare system.
6	Sierra Leone	• Create a well-functioning distance learning education system. • Use legislation to an economic relief bill into law.
7	Kenya	• Improve self-sufficient food production. • Improve the health care system. • Use of legislation to pass an economic relief bill into law.
8	Nigeria	• Repair the public health system. • Use legislation to create a national welfare system. • Create a well-functioning digital economy. • Establish a digital learning platform.

THE OBJECTIVE OF THE STUDY

This study aims at using COVID-19 digital technologies response for the resilience of health systems in selected Sub-Saharan African countries. The essence is to utilize digital technologies response to create awareness of the coronavirus pandemic in the Sub-Saharan African region. The present health systems in this region have pending societal issues caused by the COVID-19 pandemic which digital technologies are utilized as suitable measures to create awareness of the hazards caused. This study objective utilized digital technologies such as social media, mobile phones, e-commerce, internet, fiber optic technology, and different digital tools for the resilience of health systems to tackle the COVID-19 pandemic in the Sub-Saharan African region.

PROBLEM STATEMENT

The COVID-19 pandemic is a global health issue that caused the economic meltdown of many countries (Ben, 2020). However, the World Health Organization (2020) report has shown that the African continent was least affected by the COVID-19 pandemic compared to other continents in the world. This is because of the commendable efforts of the healthcare sector in the continent which was mostly attributed to the rapid transition to online platforms and the adoption of digital technologies by the government and health systems to create awareness of the coronavirus (Budd et al., 2020). However, some Sub-Saharan African countries struggled to take adequate efforts and measures to limit the widespread of the COVID-19 pandemic (Walsham, 2020). This limited effort has slowly proven productive in slowing down the spread of the coronavirus in this region (Ben, 2020). Therefore, the need to transition into using digital technologies such as e-commerce, e-health, and e-education has increased with the urgency to slow down the coronavirus pandemic (Ben, 2020). This study focuses on utilizing digital technologies response for the resilience of the health systems against the COVID-19 pandemic in selected Sub-Saharan African countries.

Research has shown that some Sub-Saharan African countries went into economic recession during the pandemic lockdown, while some were resilient (Victor Oluwole, 2021; Sumner et al., 2020; Ozili, 2020). While the Eastern African region was most resilient during the pandemic due to minimal reliance on primary commodities and greater diversification. As many countries in this region accumulated 5.3% growth in 2019 and an estimated 0.7% growth in the year 2020 (Oluwole, 2021). While in 2021, the growth of real GDP was viewed at 3.0% and 5.6% in 2022. However, the GDP of the Southern African region mostly struggled during the ongoing pandemic having an economic contraction of 7.0% in the year 2020 which is assumed to grow by 3.2% in 2021 and 2.4% in 2022. While the GDP of the Western African region was estimated to have contracted by 1.5% in the year 2020, and improved than the initial estimation of a 4.3% decline in June 2021 (Oluwole, 2021). Nevertheless, many Western African countries had an increase in GDP growth in 2020 with minimal restrictive lockdowns (Oluwole, 2021). But, the Central African, GDP was estimated to have contracted 2.7% in the year 2020, and the GDP of the Northern African region contracted by an estimated 1.1% in 2020 because of Egypt, which maintained its country's GDP 3.6% growth despite the decline of the health impact of the virus in the country.

The Sub-Saharan African economies can utilize digital technologies such as multimedia, social media, mobile phones, online mediums like large online datasets, advanced machine learning, and language processing digital health technology, and low-cost computing resources for public-health response to improve the aspects of the COVID-19 pandemic that has affected their economies (Research Africa, 2020).

Digital technologies are electronic tools, devices, and systems that generate store, or process data (Research Africa, 2020). Hence, the government of Sub-Saharan African countries needs to make considerable efforts to use digital technologies to ensure that the health systems in their countries respond rapidly to addressing the widespread COVID-19 pandemic and other hazardous health issues (Walsham, 2020). Citizens of these countries need to be aware of the importance of getting vaccinated against the deadly COVID-19 virus and the creation of vaccination sites in different designated location need to be propagated through the utilization of digital technologies (Research Africa, 2020).

Research Africa report (2020) has shown that the COVID-19 pandemic caused the economic crisis in the Southern African region i.e. South Africa to increase. This caused the digitization of the health systems in this region to have a slow response in tackling the pandemic. The country required an innovative digital solution that can develop online healthcare delivery models such as making use of smart health gadgets, increasing online pharma-retail and the doctor to patient telehealth services that can boost the public telehealth systems ensuring that quarantine measures are strategically placed for the long term to prepare the country for future pandemics. While in the Western African region, countries like Nigeria were affected by the COVID-19 pandemic and the economic sector had problems, while the public health sector consisted of poor ICT infrastructure and insufficient primary healthcare systems, ineffective national health insurance systems facilities that have often been linked to high mortality rates in the country (Ozili, 2020; Muhammad et al., 2017).

MAIN FOCUS OF THE CHAPTER

Scope of the Study

This study focuses on the Covid-19 digital technologies response for the resilience of health systems in selected Sub-Saharan African countries. The chapter focuses on the adoption of COVID-19 digital technologies as an essential awareness tool to disseminate information on how to address issues of the coronavirus pandemic to regulate the proper operations of many Sub-Saharan African economies. However, despite growing anticipation for accelerated change in the healthcare systems and economic sectors, the government, private businesses, and organizations are realizing a slow change in their operations and actual transformation has been confoundingly slow (McGowan, 2020).

In recent times, the role out of vaccination centers has been created, but people have responded slowly to receiving the approved COVID-19 vaccination due to the lack of trust by citizens of many countries. Therefore, digital technologies should be used to propagate the awareness and benefits of the administered COVID-19 vaccination to save lives. Therefore, the issue of digitization is a significant challenge in the Sub-Saharan African countries that need to be addressed to overcome the hazards caused by the COVID-19 pandemic and other future pandemics.

The Sub-Saharan African economies need to ensure sustainable adoption and use of broad bandwidth internet for essential services to improve health services, conduct businesses for e-commerce, e-health, and e-education to recover their economies after the COVID-19 crisis has ended. Therefore, this study posed the research question: How can Covid-19 digital technologies response be used for the resilience of health systems in selected African countries? The chapter explores the importance of digital technologies for the awareness of the COVID-19 pandemic in Sub-Saharan African countries, further in-depth explanation was highlighted in the literature review section.

LITERATURE REVIEW

Appraisal of ICT Response to the COVID-19 Pandemic

The 2020 COVID-19 originated from the coronavirus 2 (SARS - CoV-2) and was reported to have spread from Wuhan in the Hubei Province of China, to become a global pandemic that fatally impaired the human respiratory system (Baumgart, 2020). This fatal ailment has greatly overworked the healthcare system and impaired the normal operations of other economic sectors worldwide (*ibid*; Zu et al., 2020). The global effect of the pandemic has been challenging and resulted in uncertainties in economic operations, and growing numbers of infections and fatalities with threats of impending second waves.

The situation caused a global order imploring social distancing, a total ban of super-spreader gatherings and events, washing of hands, the use of alcohol-based hand sanitizers, and the mandatory wearing of facial masks as preventive measures to curb the spread of the virus. To evaluate the main source of information and news of the pandemic for individuals across the world, Haman (2020) used least square regression models to analyze 50,872 tweets about COVID-19 by 143 country leaders who used their Twitter accounts frequently. This study found that the state leaders received a significant increase in Twitter followers between January – May 2020 when there was a widespread rise in the COVID-19 pandemic globally in comparison with the pre-pandemic months. This study implies that citizen's interest in the pandemic was stimulated by the frequent update from their leading politicians about remedial measures towards curbing the spread of the coronavirus i.e. The establishment of testing and vaccination sites.

Impact of Digitization on Health Care Systems

International bodies such as Save the Children, Global Medix change for combating COVID-19, a partnership between the Alibaba Foundation and the First Afflicted Hospital of Zhejiang University, that brings together relevant research on virus prevention and treatment on resource portal, World Health Organization (WHO) and numerous humanitarian organization used digital technologies to propagate and create awareness about the deadly virus globally through health-specific online training courses and simulation exercises that relate to the COVID-19 pandemic to the general public (CDAC Network, 2018).

The use of the Strategic Preparedness and Response Plan (SPRP) along with UNHCR Risk Communication and Community Engagement guidance was used to outline the public health-specific measures needed to be undertaken to prepare for the COVID-19 pandemic through online platforms (World Health Organization, 2020). Social media tools such as WhatsApp, Facebook, Instagram, and many others were used to spread information about the pandemic to the public to prevent the spread of the coronavirus (CSEA, 2020). The government of developing countries used mobile phones as a medium to text COVID-19 related messages on how people can stay safe from the pandemic (CSEA, 2020). Additionally, traditional media like the radio and television were adequately used to spread the severity of the coronavirus to the public (CSEA, 2020).

GLOBAL HUMANITARIAN RELIEF USING DIGITAL TECHNOLOGIES PLATFORM FOR PREVENTIONS OF COVID-19 INFECTION

The dissemination of information on the effects of the coronavirus is crucial and decision-makers have embraced digital technology to distribute timely information about the coronavirus to health workers and the global community on how to protect themselves and their families. The World Health Organization (WHO) has been the main hub of the coronavirus response that has created the awareness of the virus globally and developed health-specific online training courses and a stimulation exercise relating to the COVID-19 pandemic. The WHO also implemented a Strategic Preparedness and Response Plan (SPRP) coupled with the Risk Communication and Community Engagement guidance for response and readiness to outline the public health-specific measures that need to be undertaken during the ongoing COVID-19 pandemic. These initiatives have been delivered using media and digital technology tools such as online information.

According to 2018 Communicating with Disaster Affected Communities (CDAC) Network, various digital platforms were used in response to the COVID-19 pandemic. For instance, the US Centre for Disease Control and Prevention website, information about the dangers of the virus; the "Save the children" a free online training platform focused on equipping humanitarians and local responders on ways to respond to the COVID-19 pandemic; the "Global Medix change" was established for combating COVID-19, and a partnership between the Alibaba Foundation and the First Afflicted Hospital of Zhejiang University collated the latest research on virus prevention and treatment on the resource portal.

Digital platforms are consistently being used for global humanitarian relief, for instance, the United Nations (UN) Office for Coordination of Human Affairs (OCHA) developed and curated key UN guidance for those working in the cluster system through their pre-existing platform. A typical example is 'Disaster Ready', which is a 2013 program of the Cornerstone On Demand Foundation non- governmental organization aimed at preparing and providing humanitarian and development professionals with free high-quality relevant online learning resources. This platform utilized a series of learning resources relating to COVID-19 for general use in the English and French language with a portal of resources specific to health workers that can be accessed and downloaded.

Also, the United Nations International Children's Emergency Fund (UNICEF) has online platforms to create some key messaging for the prevention of the spread of COVID-19 in schools (CDAC Network, 2018). The Humanitarian to Humanitarian (H2H) Network has funded the British Broadcasting Corporation (BBC) Media Action, and the interviews, Evidence Aid, and Translators Without Borders to lead projects to fight misinformation around the coronavirus using messaging and communications such as email. These humanitarian organizations have used their resources to create awareness and information on how to prevent the spread of COVID-19 through online platforms.

According to the 2020 Centre for Study of the Economies of Africa (CSEA) report, social protection programs have been rolled out in many African regions to provide relief to the less privileged through the provision of makeshift shelters, food banks, free medical care, and welfare packages. Many African countries such as South Africa, Zimbabwe, Togo, and Malawi have issued government relief such as tax breaks, business sustenance, and extended loans repayment periods with zero interest rates to their citizens who have lost their source of incomes and livelihoods due to the COVID-19 pandemic.

These relief packages are strictly delivered using digital technologies such as online and mobile banking platforms *(ibid).*

DEVELOPING POLICIES FOR COVID-19 HEALTH AWARENESS IN SUB-SAHARAN COUNTRIES

Table 3. Policy measures of African countries (Ozili, 2020)

S/N	Policy Measures	African Nations
1	State loans or credit guarantees for companies.	Nigeria, South Africa.
2	Tax suspensions.	South Africa.
3	Income Subventions for the affected worker.	South Africa.
4	Regulatory self-control to banks and corporate debtors.	South Africa, Nigeria.
5	Social security rearrangements of aids.	South Africa.
6	Bank grants debts repayment holidays e.g. loan suspensions.	Egypt, Nigeria.
7	Salary pay-cut by public officials and organizations towards coronavirus fund relief.	Rwanda, Kenya, Malawi, Nigeria, South Africa.
8	Pay cut from the nation's president and salary donation.	South Africa, Algeria, Mali, Rwanda, Malawi.
9	Provision of free water supply, donations of food parcels by government and private-owned organizations e.g. Media.	South Africa, Ghana, Rwanda.
10	Tax holiday.	Ghana.
11	Support from local philanthropists and wealthy citizens.	Nigeria, South Africa, Zimbabwe, Ethiopia, Rwanda, Cameroon.
12	Support from foreign philanthropists.	Nigeria, South Africa.
13	Cash relief pay-out to citizens to aid financial difficulty caused by the pandemic lockdown.	Malawi. Nigeria, South Africa.
14	Corporate and small business cash injection bailout	South Africa, Nigeria.
15	Assistance with debt relief to ease the economic effects of the pandemic.	Sub-Saharan African countries.
16	Implementing monetary policies by the country's central banks to reduce interest rates.	Congo, Nigeria, Egypt, Kenya.
17	Good Samaritans and philanthropists aid.	South Africa, Nigeria.
18	Countries with the United Nations and UNESCO aid.	Angola.
19	Release of prisoners to avoid prison congestion due to COVID-19.	Nigeria, South Africa, Cameroon.

Many African countries are familiar with managing infectious diseases due to their past experiences with pandemics such as Ebola, HIV, and Bird flu. Despite being classified as developing, countries in this region have adopted measures to address the problem and create awareness on the COVID-19 pandemic using mobile phones, large online datasets, advanced machine learning, and language processing digital health technology, low-cost computing resources, digital technologies and public-health response by the government and health systems in developing countries (Budd et al., 2020). In the globe, measures were made to assist SMEs, airlines service providers, hotels, and citizens to sustain the economic loss due to the pandemic and mandatory lockdowns of economic activities (Ozili, 2020). The Central Bank of Nigeria released a credit relief of $137 million to businesses affected by the COVID-19 pandemic (Anadolu Agency, 2020), and several other African countries have executed policies and pay-outs to assist citizens of their country (see **Table 3**) during the pandemic (Ozili, 2020).

Impact of Covid-19 Digital Technologies Response in Sub-Saharan African Countries

The pandemic affected the socio-economic activities of many Sub-Saharan African countries as many citizens lost their jobs and several small businesses and large organizations were affected by the strict lockdown ordered by their government (Papadopoulos et al., 2020). Furthermore, the COVID-19 lockdown action had negative effects on many African economies, as the pandemic limited the government from generating sufficient tax income from citizens. Also, many Africans encountered economic hardship and increased poverty due to strict lockdown measures (Ozili, 2020). The lockdown resulted in the loss of many jobs and the workers who were lucky to retain their jobs, have adopted the work from home and resulted to using the internet. Hence, unemployed citizens that depended on remittances tackled monetary problems (Ozili, 2020).

The 2020 International Labour Organization (ILO) report states that despite the alarming coronavirus infection rate and job loss in countries globally, the government, international donors, private organizations, health, and social care workers in developing countries have used digital technologies to tackle issues of the pandemic that has caused a high rate of unemployment, and suspension of socio-economic activities in private-owned and government organizations, as well as face-to-face educational agendas.

The CSEA (2020) report, access to digital technologies could be used to overcome ICT exclusion and increase social and economic development. The CSEA further highlights digital communication tools such as social network platforms; mass media communication tools e.g., radio and television jingles; and text messages via mobile phones as tools for disseminating the importance of keeping safe and ways to prevent the spread of the Coronavirus in the societies. The report also iterates that monitoring of cross-border activities within the African Union has played a huge role in controlling the spread of the coronavirus, and the healthcare sectors in the region have endeavored to provide effective support with the assistance of the African Centres for Disease Control and Prevention.

Lastly, the CSEA (2020) report commended some Sub-Saharan African countries (i.e., Nigeria, Ghana, Burkina Faso, Ivory Coast, Togo, Kenya, Tanzania, and the Gambia) on deploying the Surveillance, Outbreak Response Management and Analysis System (SORMAS), which is a digital solution for eHealth and mHealth involving contact tracing of an infected person. The CSEA reports further state that the COVID-19 digital technologies response solution such as mobile tracing application via WhatsApp chat service in many local dialects deployed by South Africa and Ugandan has been significantly effective in digital responses in tackling the coronavirus pandemic. The digital response of most African countries includes the rolling out of a toll-free mobile online tool that assists their citizens in accessing relevant COVID-19 information. Nigeria has put in place an online self-assessing health risk-based option for people to checklist any symptoms they have and travel history; this helps to reduce the number of calls to the disease control office hotlines.

OVERVIEW OF DIGITAL TECHNOLOGIES ON COVID-19 GLOBALLY

The immediate lockdown due to the COVID-19 pandemic encouraged citizens of many Sub-Saharan African countries to adopt the use of Wi-Fi in their homes, and all institutions have converted to using online tools to disseminate and tackle the pandemic (Katz et al., 2020). Thus, considering the effected change due to the strict lockdown, the coronavirus pandemic, therefore, serves as a great catalyst that significantly motivates digital transformation across all economic sectors in Africa (See Figure 1).

Ozili (2020) iterates how the COVID-19 pandemic has negatively impacted the lives of people in many Sub-Saharan African countries. The study states that despite strict lockdowns involving restrictions on movement, and social gatherings, a record increase in economic hardship, unemployment, increase in crime rates, domestic violence, mental health complications, and death is observed. Concerning how the pandemic affects the financial system of some Sub-Saharan African nations, research by ICTworks (2020) shows that the spread of the coronavirus has resulted in a declining stock market. A Geopoll (2020a) survey on the impact of COVID-19 on the economy, employment, and income was conducted between June 11th - July 6th, 2020 on five Sub-Saharan Africa countries like Kenya, South Africa, Nigeria, Côte D'Ivoire, and Mozambique. Geopoll (2020a) survey shows the results for the data obtained via interactive SMS sessions from a total of 2500 respondents that despite the swift implementation of strict lockdowns and other restrictions to stop the spread and save the lives of their citizens, the COVID-19 pandemic undoubtedly negatively impacted economic and employment growth in these Sub-Saharan African countries (Geopoll, 2020a).

Figure 1. Coronavirus serves as an accelerant for digital (human) transformation (Adapted from McGowan, 2020).

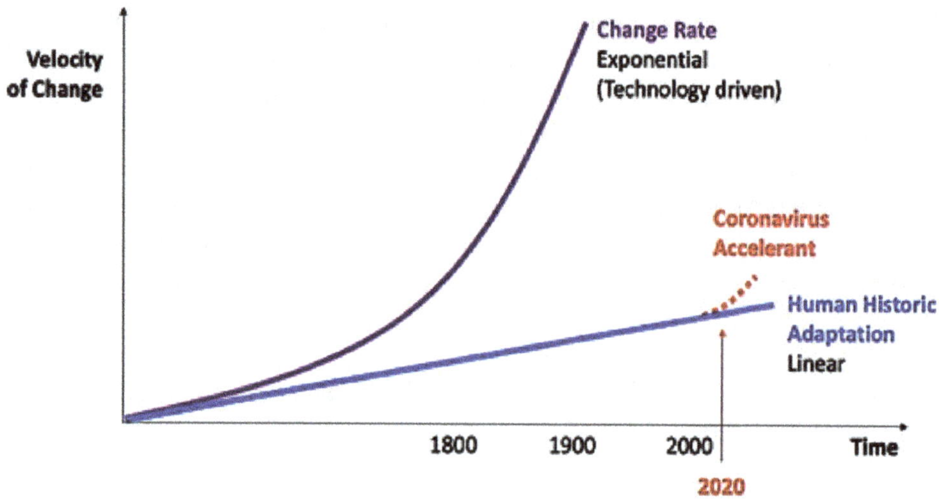

Also, the survey revealed that these Sub-Saharan countries have been successful in preventing a wide spread of the virus and low infection cases and deaths were recorded in the region compared to the high number of infection cases recorded in the developed countries like the United States, United Kingdom, Germany, Italy, and Brazil (Geopoll, 2020a). A Subsequent Geopoll (2020b) survey was conducted to show how the citizens of 12 nations in the Sub-Saharan African region respond to the COVID-19 outbreak. The findings of the study show that 94% of the respondents were aware of the coronavirus pandemic indicating that 72% South Africans, 71% Kenyans, and 69% Nigerians rated their concerns of the coronavirus pandemic as very high due to the risk of exposure and physical contact in public places and transportation (Geopoll, 2020b).

The Geopoll (2020b) survey further revealed that 25% of respondents from Nigeria and South Africa were not confident in their government health awareness, while 35% were confident of the government health awareness of their country's response to COVID-19, and Kenya recorded that 40% were not confident in their government health awareness, while 30% were confident of the government health awareness of the coronavirus. Further findings of the Geopoll (2020b) survey from developing countries show that 79% of Kenyans were concerned about the financial impact of the coronavirus, whereas 57% of Nigerian and South African respondents claim their countries were affected financially due to the spread of the coronavirus. Furthermore, results from the survey show that 25% of the retail store of most countries ran out of groceries as many people engaged in panic buying before the commencement of the lockdown, and 40% of respondents claims that some goods were out of stock due to the pandemic, buying of food and other necessities in anticipation of self-quarantines (Geopoll, 2002b).

Most of the concerns of many Sub-Saharan African citizens were based on the level of awareness and response of their government to the coronavirus pandemic. Thus, countries like South Africa, Nigeria, and Kenya used the results of the Geopoll (2020b) survey to examine their country's awareness levels, primary information sources, and knowledge of how to prevent the coronavirus. Thereafter, most of the respondents (53-56%) from most countries claim that their government was giving clear communication on how to limit the spread of the COVID-19 pandemic, especially through social distancing, and closure of public and economic activities (Geopoll, 2020b).

EFFECTS OF DIGITAL TECHNOLOGIES MITIGATION IN SUB-SAHARAN AFRICAN ECONOMIES

Many Sub-Saharan African countries experienced delay and mitigation phases of the COVID-19 pandemic control and needed urgent measures to address socioeconomic activities and critical health matters caused by the spread of the pandemic (Bakibinga-Gaswaga et al., 2020). The adoption of digital technologies was used as a strategy to support COVID-19 responses to contribute towards attaining universal health coverage. The aim is to facilitate communication, disseminate information to citizens and manage the continuous operations of many African countries (Bakibinga-Gaswaga et al., 2020). However, access to digital technologies was unequal due to inequality, exclusion, poor health systems, poor ICT infrastructure, limited or lack of electricity, high cost of ICT installation infrastructure, and poverty (Bakibinga-Gaswaga et al., 2020).

ICTs have mitigated the effects of covid-19 in many African countries due to the rise in inequalities among disadvantaged communities. Especially in the aspect of access to networks or connectivity, access to technology devices, and ICT skills (Beaunoyer et al., 2020). The issue of inequality and the digital divide has been a problem in many African countries, however, the COVID-19 pandemic is a significant contributor to the widening digital divide in poor areas where there is a lack of ICT access and affordability (Beaunoyer et al., 2020).

Gabbiadini et al. (2020) study has shown that the use of digital technologies minimized the feelings of isolation and loneliness, irritability, and anger among people during the COVID-19 pandemic lockdown. The pandemic restricted the social relations of the global populations, however, digital technology was used as a medium of communication to facilitate the maintenance of meaningful social relationships and promote social support (Gabbiadini et al., 2020). Despite the insistence of social distance to prevent the spread of COVID-19, technologies were used to bridge the gap of the lack of social interaction and communication with people. The use of digital technologies was a resourceful medium used by many company staff to work from home and have conferences and virtual meetings which mitigated negative psychological states during the pandemic (Gabbiadini et al., 2020).

Many schools were able to use digital technologies to have remote online learning and continue with students during the pandemic lockdown (Mhlanga and Moloi, 2020; Armitage and Nellums, 2020). In countries like South Africa, the COVID-19 instigated digital transformation through the use of digital tools at primary, secondary, and higher educational institutions (Mhlanga and Moloi, 2020). Although access to education has been a challenge in many Sub-Saharan African countries because of the limited educational resources, inequality, poverty, and availability of classroom spaces (Mhlanga and Moloi, 2020). However, the pandemic has presented the government of many African countries an opportunity to experience success and failures in providing technology access to schools despite the high costs of technology deployment to the educational systems to improve access (Mhlanga and Moloi, 2020).

Tin et al. (2020) says digital technologies are reliable tools that can be used to reduce the clinical load of physicians, reduce the physical crowding of patients in hospitals and clinics. This would allow patients to continue to receive standard clinical care through virtual clinics' using telemedicine consultations with imaging data, for example, chest X-ray and CT of the thorax) uploaded from peripheral sites and interpreted remotely (Ting et al., 2020). Other perks that digital technology can provide to healthcare systems include virtual e-learning platforms to eliminate physical meetings, and the possibilities for clinical research (Ting et al., 2020).

Conceptual Framework: Technology Determinism

The theory of technological determinism explains that human beings are active agents capable of identifying, achieving, modifying, and creating technology usability in pursuit of meaningful objectives (Smith et al., 1994). This study explores how digital technologies are used for the awareness of the COVID-19 pandemic. The use of digital technologies is essential to the operations of any society and helps to solve social problems (Smith et al., 1994). The **process** of using digital technologies to create awareness about the spread of COVID-19 pandemic health hazards has assisted citizens of many Sub-Saharan African countries to know how to manage the crisis like the rest of the globe. Technology is known as the basis of human activity and it is assumed to change how people think and act in situations (Smith et al., 1994). The internet, social media, digital media, and mobile phones are powerful tools that have been used by the health care sector to disseminate vital information about the seriousness of the pandemic.

Technological determinism theory proposes an observation of the world that assumes that technology can 'fix' social problems (Van Dijk, 2020). Nevertheless, technologies are 'owned' and how technology can be used to solve societal issues is not predictable (Silverstone, 2005). Technologies can not emerge without the functional interest of users, that accept the use of technology as being a relevant and useful component in their lives (Silverstone, 2005). It is assumed that people shape technology to fit appropriately into their lives before they can adapt to the change that it reaps socially and economically.

The framework reveals that the impacts of technology on society as a 'social shaping' that establish technology as a product of social interaction. Knopke (2013) explains that technology needs to be viewed as part of the social fabric that holds society together. In essence, society's technology use determines the development, **social structure,** and cultural values of that society. According to Haynes et al. (2009:484), technology is a socio-material product, 'a seamless web or network combining artifacts, people, organizations, cultural meanings, and knowledge'. Therefore, this chapter proposes the use of digital technologies as a suitable medium that can be used to disseminate information about the negative effects of the COVID-19 virus on humanity.

The technology determinist theory views technology as the determinist for societal change (Smith et al., 1994). Technology is viewed as an independent, driving component that determines the social and economic relationship (Smith et al., 1994). In other words, digital technologies are viewed as determining the development of social structures (Smith et al., 1994). Digital technologies can be adopted within the healthcare sector to inform society and organizations of the adverse health issues about the COVID-19 pandemic. This is because technology is a determining factor that directs, transforms, and changes societal ways of thinking (Smith et al.,1994). Hence, there is the possibility that the use of digital technologies can allow the healthcare sector to be resilient in managing the pandemic and other health issues.

CONCEPTUAL MODEL

The adaption of digital technologies in the health system is vital for the dissemination of information that can prevent the spread of the COVID-19 pandemic, and transform the socio-economic activities of the global community through the execution of normal activities that were disrupted by the coronavirus pandemic. The governmental and private organizations have transitioned to the adaption of digital technologies to create awareness of the severity of the pandemic and the preventive measures of the spread of the virus while trying to reach some form of balance and normalcy of their operations during the pandemic. The emergence of the COVID-19 pandemic has accelerated human and organizational technology use (see **Figure 1**), for example, citizens of nations, healthcare sectors, small and medium-sized organizations, international bodies, global humanitarian relief, government, and private organizations are forced to work from their respective homes using the internet. A conceptual model (see **Figure 2**) was developed from the reviews and appraisals of studies focused on the impact of digital technologies' response on combating the COVID-19 pandemic in Africa. The model shows how the COVID-19 pandemic has affected different sectors and how digital technologies can be used as a tool to create awareness of the pandemic.

Figure 2. Conceptual model for this study.

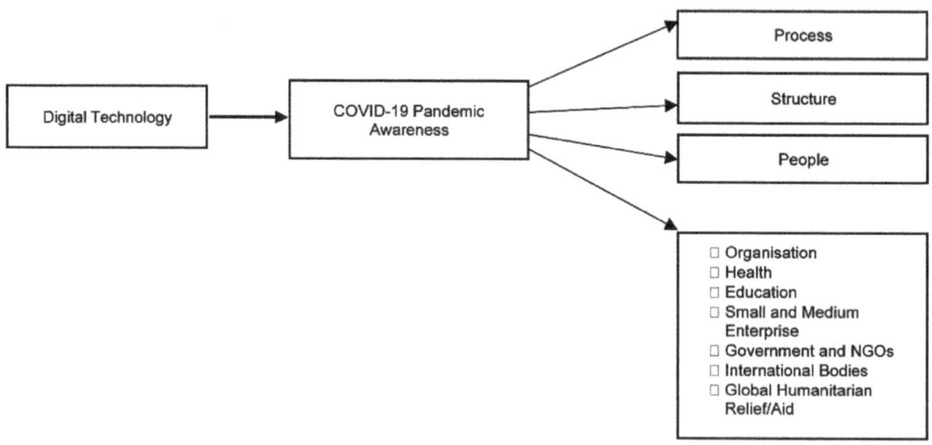

METHODOLOGY

The qualitative approach was used to understand the empirical situation of the study (Walsham, 2017). For example, how digital technologies can be used for the resilience of health systems in the Sub-Saharan Africa region. This study utilized critical discourse analysis to understand the societal problems caused by the COVID-19 pandemic. The research methodology used for the study was conceptual analysis using a qualitative research technique (Mullet, 2018; Cronin et al., 2008). A conceptual analysis was conducted to compare studies that used ICTs for the resilience of the health system during unexpected global pandemics. Hence, the study is a critical discourse study which is a written approach that relates to the functions of the social context that is used to investigate the meanings of societal situations (Mullet, 2018). The study used qualitative content analysis to understand the correlations and patterns of how digital technology are utilized as a communication tool in the different contexts used to tackle the COVID-19 pandemic.

The study used scholarly studies as backings to justify the research question posed: How can Covid-19 digital technologies response be used for the resilience of health systems in selected African countries? This study conducted a critical analysis to identify the themes from scholarly studies on how digital technology is utilized for the resilience of the healthcare systems and economic sustainability in the Sub-Saharan Africa region. Studies that focused on the suitability of digital technologies for the resilience of the health systems and economic development of the Sub-Saharan African region were presented in the study (see **Table 4**).

Table 4. Studies using ICTs for the health systems resilience of COVID-19.

Concepts	Themes Description	References
ICT impact on health systems.	The impact of ICTs on health systems performance.	Bloom et al. (2017). Making mHealth Work for All.
Digital technologies for health sustainability	How digital health technologies can contribute to the sustainable attainment of universal health coverage in Africa?	Olu et al. (2019). How can digital health technologies contribute to the sustainable attainment of universal health coverage in Africa?
Telemedicine adoption for COVID-19 pandemic health system resilience program.	The adoption of telemedicine as a health system resilience and an integral part of the public health response to the COVID-19 pandemic globally.	Bhaskar et al. (2020). Telemedicine across the globe-position paper from the COVID-19 pandemic health system resilience.
ICTs to improve the capacity of health care systems.	The use of ICTs in digitization, digital economy databases, and other ICT applications as a driver of sustainable and inclusive growth in the African health system.	Masłoń-Oracz et al. (2020). Digital Economy as a Driver of Sustainable and Inclusive Growth in Africa—Case Study.
ICTs for eHealth solutions.	The use of ICTs for eHealth solutions in global health	Muneene. (2020). eHealth Solutions in Global Health.
ICT is used to improve health systems.	The role of ICTs to improve healthcare systems in developing countries. Using Information systems to reduce healthcare costs and improve outcomes	Akinyemi et al. (2021). A qualitative exploration of the health system response to COVID-19 pandemic applying the WHO health systems frame. A case: A case study of a Nigerian state.
Digital health response to COVID-19.	The deployment of digital health for the management of crucial health crises such as the COVID-19 pandemic in Africa	Dehbi et al. (2021). Moroccan digital health response to the COVID-19 crisis.
ICTs to build health system resilient in response to COVID-19 pandemic.	The use of ICTs to build resilient health system in Africa to tackle COVID-19 pandemic response.	Gebremeskel. (2021). Building resilient health systems in Africa beyond the COVID-19 pandemic response.

This study appraises previous studies and reports from international bodies such as the World Health Organizations (WHO), websites, business and government documents. This study presents a descriptive report of the adoption of digital technologies and their impact on a real-life societal event. Furthermore, this research focused on the effects of the ongoing global pandemic, and the effects of digital technologies response in tackling the COVID-19 pandemic in the Sub-Saharan African region. The researchers identified the significant effects of digital technologies on the policy response, and digital information provided to tackle the COVID-19 cases in the Sub-Saharan African region where strict lockdown rules were implemented to limit the spread of the pandemic. This study shows how digital technologies were utilized for the health systems resilience of the COVID-19 pandemic to create awareness and cultivate preventive measures in the selected Sub-Saharan African countries (see **Table** 5).

Table 5. List of Sub-Saharan countries using ICTs for COVID-19 preventive measures

S/L	Country	Digital Technologies	References
1	Tunisia	Artificial Intelligence, Robotics.	Mogessie, Ntacyabukura, Mengesha, Musa, Wangari, Claude, and Lucero-Prisno, (2021). Digital health and COVID-19: challenges of use and implementation in Sub-Saharan Africa.
2	Nigeria.	Social Media e.g. Twitter; Mobile phones, Bluetooth, and device GPS location technology.	Adepoju. (2020). Africa's COVID-19-health technologies' watershed moment.
3	South Africa.	Mobile Applications; Social Media, GPS for contact tracing; Drones, Internet.	Chitungo et al. (2021). Digital technologies and COVID-19: reconsidering lockdown exit strategies for Africa.
4	Ethiopia.	Internet, e-Learning, Mobile Applications.	Marks. (2020). Ethiopian diaspora champions digital apps in the fight against COVID-19.
5	Sierra Leone, Morocco.	Drones, Mobile phones, Internet (E-Pass), 3D Printing.	Maharana et al. (2020). Use of technology and innovations in the COVID-19 pandemic response in Africa.
6	Ghana.	Internet, Mobile phone.	Sarfo and Karuppannan (2020). Application of geospatial technologies in the COVID-19 fight of Ghana.
7	Rwanda.	Drones, Mobile phones, Robotics.	World Health Organization Regional Office for Africa. (2020). COVID-19 in Rwanda: a country's response.
8	Kenya.	3D Printing, Mobile phone.	Quartz Africa. (2020). Kenya's 3D printing community making Covid-19 equipment.

INSIGHTS ON THE FACTORS OBSTRUCTING DIGITAL TECHNOLOGIES USED IN THE SUB-SAHARAN AFRICAN REGION

Despite the importance of digital technology's response to disseminate information to citizens of the Sub-Saharan African countries, this region unlike the developed countries is yet to fully enjoy the benefits of the fourth industrial revolution, especially in areas of infrastructure, technology access, and utilization. Some existing situations have hampered the use of technologies and affected the efforts of the government, non-governmental organizations (NGOs), and health sectors towards tackling the pandemic in the Sub-Saharan African region. According to CSEA (2020), the following issues are the main hindrances:

- **Online fake news:** This has been disseminated on social media platforms and mass texting of harmful disinformation that misled the citizens of many Sub-Saharan African countries to consume damaging products thereby sabotaging the efforts made by the government to manage the coronavirus using technologies.
- **Lack of ICT access:** A lack of ICT access is experienced in some Sub-Saharan African countries. For example, many citizens of these countries are unable to afford digital tools such as smartphones and computers or purchase a mobile bundle to use the internet to access online information or websites on COVID-19 prevention. This poverty has resulted in many African countries causing digital divide (Marinoni et al., 2020). In addition, about 66% of Sub-Saharan African schools lack communication facilities that can be used to disseminate information on the COVID-19 pandemic preventive measures, unlike in other continents such as Asia and Pacific where there is 99%, the Americas with 97%, and Europe where 97% of schools have adequate communication infrastructure to disseminate information on the pandemic to higher education institutions (HEIs) (Marinoni et al., 2020).
- **Lack of digital skills:** The lack of digital skills is among the contributing factors affecting many Sub-Saharan African citizens who are unemployed or who work in the informal sector. These include small business owners, farmers, and petty traders who rely on day-to-day incomes as their main source of livelihood. The population of these informal workers is about 85.5% of the labor force in many Sub-Saharan African countries, and they mostly depend on their daily income to sustain themselves and their families (CSEA, 2020).
- **Lack of digital biometric identity:** Many Sub-Saharan African countries have not adopted the use of online digital biometric identity to verify the personal information of their citizens. This legal form of identification is

expected to link to the government and health sectors of many countries but has not been adopted by many Sub-Saharan African countries due to poor governance, mismanagement of funds, and widespread corruption. Unfortunately, this has prevented the citizens of many Sub-Saharan African countries from fully accessing the necessary welfare packages during the ongoing COVID-19 pandemic era.

- **Restrictions of online educational resources:** Many online educational resources were out of reach to educators during the lockdown. Due to the lack of broadband connectivity and ICT access, many people could not use digital technology in their communities to access online educational materials and many students were unable to attend online classes during the lockdown period.
- **Lack of digital health care**: The Sub-Saharan African healthcare systems such as pharmacies, public and private hospitals do not have access to digital technologies that can assist them to identify vulnerable coronavirus cases. Many clinics and hospitals are still using paper-based written health records which makes it difficult to tackle the coronavirus.
- **Lack of digital public service:** The Sub-Saharan African government has limited innovations in the digital public services that can deliver at a large scale. The coronavirus pandemic has hastened many initiatives that focus on e-health and e-education as measures to tackle the pandemic. The use of e-learning platforms is among the many measures which was used across Africa. This platform is mainly sponsored by the government in collaboration with telecommunication companies to provide zero-rate online education resources. However, public, and private corporations with additional support from international development bodies should also be involved in these initiatives to scale up these efforts and provide the African society with high-quality digital education and health services.

SOLUTIONS

Proposed Digital Technologies Measures to Consider in Africa

The Sub-Saharan African countries need to adapt to the use of digital technologies to facilitate the continuous operation of the health systems and all economic sectors to prevent economic disruption or complete shutdown. Ben (2020) shows the various means by which digital technologies could be adopted as follows:

- **The use of smartphones:** Due to the ongoing infectious rate of COVID-19, there has not been adequate investment in ICT infrastructures and new hospital digitization in the healthcare sector of the Sub-Saharan African region. However, new start-ups and innovations using health technologies can assist community clinics with the diagnosis and logging of coronavirus cases via the use of smartphones. This will assist the Sub-Saharan Africa region to 'flatten the curve' and minimize the load on high-end specialized hospital care in emergency cases, whereby patients with unserious cases can recover from their respective homes after visiting the community clinics.
- **Access to e-commerce:** There has been a change in online purchase, whereby it now involves not just the purchase of luxury items such as electronics, but also the online purchase of everyday essential items such as groceries and personal items by online customers. Therefore, e-commerce has platforms that have grown exceptionally due to the coronavirus pandemic and many organizations have realized the value of digitization to operate their business. The adoption of e-commerce can be an essential tool that online users can use to order personalized goods especially when more people are forced to adapt to the trend of using digital technologies.

Also, customers can use virtual technology to experience the usefulness and details on the quality of their goods before purchase. Although pre-existing before the COVID-19 pandemic, e-commerce companies have amplified and enhanced their platforms to manage the well-organized delivery and supply of goods and services to stay-at-home customers during the pandemic. Essential goods such as food, medicine, and personalized good have been included in the items that can be delivered to consumers in need.

- **Adoption of fiber optic technology:** In an attempt to limit the spread of the pandemic, the government of many countries implemented lockdown measures to limit the spread of the virus. This caused many families to adopt bandwidth internet to facilitate their intention to work from home. Also, this situation has resulted in widespread internet usage and a shortage of internet bandwidth within households. Fiber-to-the-Home companies have implemented an increase in bandwidth which has double the speed or quota to assist their customers. Fiber optic technology encounters little or no major technology barriers to increasing speeds like 4G and 5G. Also, there has been a change in video entertainment, as community gaming servers were shut down due to the coronavirus pandemic in the Sub-Saharan Africa region (Ben, 2020). However, fast bandwidths have facilitated online video gaming services and increased multiplayer video gaming servers hosted in the Sub-Saharan Africa region.

- **Adoption of cashless economy:** The cashless economy is a mobile money payment system that allows users to make payments using internet-enabled digital devices such as Smartphones, Tablets, iPad, and Computers (Mieseigha and Ogbodo, 2013). Unlike cash payments which are not easy to trace because the users are anonymous, digital payments are believed to increase accountability, transparency, and tracking of online transactions, which in turn reduces the danger of corruption and theft (Oyewole et al., 2013).

In addition, due to the need to ensure social distancing measures during transactions, Sub-Saharan African countries need to fully adopt mobile monetary transactions via mobile phones, internet-enabled computers used mobile devices. Whilst some Sub-Saharan African countries such as Kenya, Tanzania, Uganda, Côte d'Ivoire, Egypt, Nigeria, and South Africa are slowly transitioning into the cashless payment method. Many other Sub-Saharan African countries are still struggling to adopt this system into their economy because of the lack of ICT infrastructure (Mieseigha and Ogbodo, 2013). Also, the adoption of a cashless economy could greatly assist the government of many Sub-Saharan African countries to enhance their economies through the collection of sufficient taxes which will contribute to the growth of their economies (*ibid*).

- **Internet adoption for online education:** The educational systems in the Sub-Saharan African region must adapt to online education platforms operated by high-speed bandwidth. Many schools or educational institutions still use traditional classroom-based learning instead of adopting digital learning. Educators can deliver online lectures on IoT and the cloud using internet-enabled smartphones to stream the lecture on the web to learners. This method could be used for remote learning during the COVID-19 lockdown.
- **Access to digital health care**: The use of digital technologies such as data science and artificial intelligence could be used to identify insights on the data of people susceptible to COVID-19 in public and private healthcare systems in Africa to avoid the spread of coronavirus.
- **Bridging the digital gap in the small and medium-sized enterprises (SMEs):** The government should assist SMEs with schemes that encourage the use of technologies in the Sub-Saharan African region. These schemes should be sponsored by the government and support financial inclusion while sustaining the development of new systems of e-commerce payments and financial resolution for entrepreneurs.

This study explored the use of digital technologies response to tackle the spread of the COVID-19 pandemic crisis in the Sub-Saharan African region. Another key discussion in the study is how the Sub-Saharan African countries have endeavored to address the issue of ongoing COVID-19 pandemic like many other countries in the globe using digital technologies response in the health systems as the main tool to disseminate information on preventive measures to curb the pandemic. Digital tools such as e-learning platforms, virtual reality, and online classes have been frequently used by educators and learners to overcome the lockdown measures caused by the pandemic in educational institutions of many countries.

Furthermore, the health sectors have adopted the use of digital technologies such as mobile phones, online and social media platforms, mobile applications, and computers software can be useful tools used to disseminate information to citizens of many Sub-Saharan African countries on the preventive measures of the COVID-19 pandemic.

RECOMMENDATIONS

There are some distinct implications to practice from this study. To limit the spread of the coronavirus, the government of the Sub-Saharan African countries needs to provide useful measures using digital technologies such as social media platforms to address the issues of disinformation about the cause and spread of the coronavirus. The government and ICT policymakers should also utilize digital technologies as an effective tool to disseminate and access information on future pandemics and infectious diseases.

To implement strict policies on effective management actions against the spread of the coronavirus, the governments and ICT policymakers should swiftly adopt digital technologies response applications in the public and private organizations that can assist in the proper planning, management, quarantine, and healthcare measures of the pandemic in the absence of face-to-face contact. The research suggests that policymakers should execute policies that can unite poor areas in unexpected situations such as the COVID-19 pandemic to limit socio-economic anxiety in the Sub-Saharan African region.

Finally, the Sub-Saharan African policymakers need to execute possible measures that can be used to revive their economies to avoid a huge amount of job loss during the recovering process of overcoming the pandemic. Also, the study suggests that more support should be issued out to large and small organizations to bridge the unemployment gap in the African Sub-Saharan.

FUTURE RESEARCH DIRECTION

Numerous preventive actions such as social distancing, stay-at-home measures, use of facemasks, constant washing of hands, and use of hand sanitizers were among the list of essentials executed by the government and health sectors of many Sub-Saharan African countries to minimize the spread of the pandemic. Due to the coronavirus, the government of the African Sub-Saharan region implemented lockdowns to sustain the pandemic which caused an economic recession that afflicted hardship on the citizens.

Remedial efforts made by the media, health sector, government, and non-governmental organizations were mostly via the utilization of digital technologies response to create awareness of the severity of the pandemic and reduce the resultant huge economic meltdown. Therefore, future research directions should focus on how to use digital technologies for campaign purposes, especially as many citizens of different countries are terrified of taking the vaccination due to the numerous death cases caused by blood clots that occurred from the vaccination intake. Therefore, digital technologies should be used to propagate the positive outcome of the vaccination intake to avoid the speculation of death and minimize fear amongst citizens living in the Sub-Saharan African region.

CONCLUSION

The chapter discussed the outbreak of the COVID-19 pandemic and how healthcare organizations were affected globally in 2020 before the advent of the vaccine which was developed to minimize the spread of the unexpected outbreak. Also, the outbreak has redefined how to address healthcare issues in many Sub-Saharan countries. The use of digital technologies has been adopted to spread and create awareness about the spread of the coronavirus which has been a major success in not only the healthcare sector but other sectors and government bodies.

Digital solutions such as using the internet, social media platforms, smartphones, open data, hackathons and events, useful links, and resources have been used to address the global challenges to minimize the spread of the COVID-19 pandemic in the Sub-Saharan African countries. Other awareness avenues include the creation of websites and emailing are essential solutions that were adopted to create awareness of the spread, prevent the spread, and the possible measures to minimize the contagious disease. This measure included the implementation of social distancing, the use of hand sanitizer, vaccination, the use of face masks and shields.

Although social media networks have the power to disseminate a large volume of information about the COVID-19 pandemic, the medium has been used to post fake news such as uncensored information about the pandemic due to the lack of online regulation. This has caused misinformation about the dangers of the coronavirus in the Sub-Saharan African region and many other countries causing negative outcome which has slowed down the management of the COVID-19 pandemic.

ACKNOWLEDGMENT

We would like to thank the University of Johannesburg for the library resources used for the write-up of this manuscript. The research work was conducted without funding support.

REFERENCES

Adepoju, P. (2020). Africa's COVID-19 health technologies' watershed moment. *The Lancet. Digital Health*, *2*(7), e346–e347. doi:10.1016/S2589-7500(20)30146-1

Akinyemi, O. O., Popoola, O. A., Fowotade, A., Adekanmbi, O., Cadmus, E. O., & Adebayo, A. (2021). A qualitative exploration of the health system response to COVID-19 pandemic applying the WHO health systems frame. A case: A case study of a Nigerian state. *Scientific African*, e00945-e00945.

Anadolu Agency. (2020). *Health, Africa, latest on coronavirus outbreak*. Available at: www.aa.com.tr

Armitage, R., & Nellums, L. B. (2020). Considering inequalities in the school closure response to COVID-19. *The Lancet. Global Health*, *8*(5), e644. doi:10.1016/S2214-109X(20)30116-9 PMID:32222161

Bakibinga-Gaswaga, E., Bakibinga, S., Bakibinga, D. B. M., & Bakibinga, P. (2020). Digital technologies in the COVID-19 responses in Sub-Saharan Africa: policies, problems and promises. *The Pan African Medical Journal, 35*(Suppl 2).

Baumgart, D. C. (2020). Digital advantage in the COVID-19 response: Perspective from Canada's largest integrated digitized healthcare system. *NPJ Digital Medicine*, *3*(1), 1–4. doi:10.103841746-020-00326-y PMID:32923691

Beaunoyer, E., Dupéré, S., & Guitton, M. J. (2020). COVID-19 and digital inequalities: Reciprocal impacts and mitigation strategies. *Computers in Human Behavior*, *111*, 106424. doi:10.1016/j.chb.2020.106424 PMID:32398890

Ben, R. (2020). *Did coronavirus kickstart the economy? An innovation, a viral tweet, the story begins there. 34 seconds that potentially changed the fortunes of Innovative Nairobi Craftsman, Stephen Odhiambo.* African innovations liquid telecom. Available at: https://www.liquidtelecom.com/insights/innovation-blog/Did_Coronavirus_just_kick_start_the_digital_economy

Bloom, G., Labrique, A., Hampshire, K., & Waldman, L. (2017). *Making mHealth Work for All.* doi:10.35648/20.500.12413/11781/ii286

Budd, J., Miller, B. S., Manning, E. M., Lampos, V., Zhuang, M., Edelstein, M., & McKendry, R. A. (2020). Digital technologies in the public-health response to COVID-19. *Nature Medicine, 26*(8), 1183–1192. doi:10.103841591-020-1011-4 PMID:32770165

Chitungo, I., Mhango, M., Mbunge, E., Dzobo, M., & Dzinamarira, T. (2021). Digital technologies and COVID-19: Reconsidering lockdown exit strategies for Africa. *The Pan African Medical Journal, 39*, 39. doi:10.11604/pamj.2021.39.93.29773 PMID:34466195

Communicating with Disaster Affected Communities (CDAC) Network. (2018). *Resources for those responding to COVID-19.* Available at www.cdacnetwork.org

Cronin, P., Ryan, F., & Coughlan, M. (2008). Undertaking a literature review: A step-by-step approach. *British Journal of Nursing (Mark Allen Publishing), 17*(1), 38–43. doi:10.12968/bjon.2008.17.1.28059 PMID:18399395

CSEA AFRICA. (2020). *Africa's digital technology response strategy to COVID-19.* Centre for the Study of the Economies of Africa.

Dehbi, Z. E. O., Sedrati, H., Chaqsare, S., Azami, A. I., Merzouki, M., Raji, M., ... Ghazal, H. (2021). Moroccan digital health response to the COVID-19 crisis. *Frontiers in Public Health*, 9. PMID:34485221

Dwivedi, Y. K., Hughes, D. L., Coombs, C., Constantiou, I., Duan, Y., Edwards, J. S., & Raman, R. (2020). Impact of COVID-19 pandemic on information management research and practice: Transforming education, work, and life. *International Journal of Information Management, 55*, 102211. doi:10.1016/j.ijinfomgt.2020.102211

Gabbiadini, A., Baldissarri, C., Durante, F., Valtorta, R. R., De Rosa, M., & Gallucci, M. (2020). Together apart: The mitigating role of digital communication technologies on negative affect during the COVID-19 outbreak in Italy. *Frontiers in Psychology, 11*, 2763. doi:10.3389/fpsyg.2020.554678 PMID:33192807

Gates, B. (2020). Responding to COVID-19: A Once-in-a-Century Pandemic? *The New England Journal of Medicine*, *382*(18), 1677–1679. doi:10.1056/NEJMp2003762 PMID:32109012

Geopoll. (2020a). *The financial impact of coronavirus in Sub-Saharan Africa.* Available at: https://f.hubspotusercontent30.net

Geopoll. (2020b). *Coronavirus in Sub-Sharan Africa: How Africans in 12 nations are responding to the COVID-19 outbreak.* Available at: https://cdn2.hubspot.net

Haman, M. (2020). The use of Twitter by state leaders and its impact on the public during the COVID-19 pandemic. *Heliyon*, *6*(11), 1–27. doi:10.1016/j.heliyon.2020.e05540 PMID:33294685

Hynes, D., & Richardson, H. (2009). What use is domestication theory to information systems research? In *Handbook of research on contemporary theoretical models in information systems* (pp. 482–494). IGI Global. doi:10.4018/978-1-60566-659-4.ch027

ICTworks. (2020). *10 Educational Technology Solutions for COVID-19 Out-of-School Children.* Wayan Vota. Available at: www.ictworks.org

International Labour Organization (ILO). (2020). *ILO Monitor: COVID-19 and the world of work* (4th ed.). International Labour Organization. Available at: http://www.ilo.org/global/topics/coronavirus/impacts-and-responds/WCMS_745963/lang--en/index.thm

Kalantaryan, S., & McMahon, S. (2020). *COVID-19 and Remittances in Africa.* EUR 30262 EN, Publications Office of the European Union. Available at https://ec.europa.eu/jrc

Katz, R.L., Callorda, F.M. & Jung, J. (2020, May 14). Can Digitization Mitigate COVID-19 Damages? Evidence from Developing Countries. *Evidence from Developing Countries.*

Knopke, V. (2013). Gender and Technology Education-theory and background. *Journal of Industrial Technology Design Teachers Association of Queensland*, *54*, 7–11.

Kuca, K. (2020). *The 2019 Novel Coronavirus (COVID-19) Outbreak in China and the world: A new lesson for public health system letters in drug design and discovery.* Academic Press.

Marinoni, G., Van't Land, H., & Jensen, T. (2020). *The impact of COVID-19 on higher education around the world.* IAU Global Survey Report. Available at www.iau.aiu.net

Marks, S. (2020). Ethiopian diaspora champions digital apps in the fight against COVID. *Voice of America News.*

McGowan, H. E. (2020). *How the coronavirus pandemic is accelerating the future of work.* Available at: https://www.forbes.com/sites/heathermcgowan/2020/03/23/the-coronavirus-pandemic-accelerates-the-future-of-work-and-provides-opportunity/?sh=43fe449b317f

Mhlanga, D., & Moloi, T. (2020). COVID-19 and the digital transformation of education: What are we learning on 4IR in South Africa? *Education Sciences, 10*(7), 180. doi:10.3390/educsci10070180

Mieseigha, E. G., & Ogbodo, U. K. (2013). An empirical analysis of the benefits of a cashless economy on Nigeria's economic development. *Research Journal of Finance and Accounting, 4*(17), 11–16.

Mpungose, C. B., & Khoza, S. B. (2020). *Digitalized curriculum to the rescue of a higher education institution.* African Identities.

Muhammad, F., Abdulkareem, J. H., & Chowdhury, A. A. (2017). Major public health problems in Nigeria: A review. *South East Asia Journal of Public Health, 7*(1), 6–11. doi:10.3329eajph.v7i1.34672

Mullet, D. R. (2018). A general critical discourse analysis framework for educational research. *Journal of Advanced Academics, 29*(2), 116–142. doi:10.1177/1932202X18758260

Olu, O., Muneene, D., Bataringaya, J. E., Nahimana, M. R., Ba, H., Turgeon, Y., & Dovlo, D. (2019). How can digital health technologies contribute to the sustainable attainment of universal health coverage in Africa? A perspective. *Frontiers in Public Health, 7*, 341. doi:10.3389/fpubh.2019.00341 PMID:31803706

Oluwole, V. (2021). *Top richest countries in Africa.* Business Insider Africa. Available at: https://africa.businessinsider.com/local/markets/top-20-richest-countries-in-africa/ndhb6cx

Oyewole, O. S., Gambo, J., Abba, M., & Onuh, M. E. (2013). Electronic payment system and economic growth: A review of transition to a cashless economy in Nigeria. *International Journal of Scientific Engineering and Technology, 2*(9), 913–918.

Ozili, P. K. (2020). COVID-19 in Africa: Socio-economic impact, policy response, and opportunities. *The International Journal of Sociology and Social Policy*. Advance online publication. doi:10.1108/IJSSP-05-2020-0171

Papadopoulos, T., Baltas, K. N., & Balta, M. E. (2020). The use of digital technologies by small and medium enterprises during COVID-19: Implications for theory and practice. *International Journal of Information Management, 55*, 102192. doi:10.1016/j.ijinfomgt.2020.102192 PMID:32836646

ResearchICTAfrica. (2020). *How Covid-19 exposes the defects in South Africa's digital economy*. Available at: https://researchictafrica.net/2020/03/26/how-covid-19-exposes-the-defects-in-south-africas-digital-economy/

Said, B., Hajar, E., & Amine, S. (2020). The COVID-19 outbreak: A catalyst for digitization in African countries. *The Journal of the Egyptian Public Health Association, 95*(1).

Silverstone, R. (2005). The sociology of mediation and communication. The SAGE handbook of sociology, 188-207.

Smith, M., & Marx, L. (1994). *Does Technology Drive History?: The Dilemma of Technological Determinism*. MIT Press.

Sumner, A., Hoy, C. & Oritz-Juarez, E. (2020). *Estimates of the impact of COVID-19 on Global Poverty.* World Institute for Development Economics Research (UNU-WIDER) (No. wp-2020-43).

Ting, D. S. W., Carin, L., Dzau, V., & Wong, T. Y. (2020). Digital technology and COVID-19. *Nature Medicine, 26*(4), 459–461. doi:10.103841591-020-0824-5 PMID:32284618

Van Dijk, J. (2020). The network society. *Sage (Atlanta, Ga.).*

Walsham, G. (2017). *Research methodologies for information systems in the development context: a tutorial. In The Digital Challenge: Information Technology in the Development Context. Information Technology in the Development context.* Routledge.

Walsham, G. (2020). Health information systems in developing countries: Some reflections on information for action. *Information Technology for Development, 26*(1), 194–200. doi:10.1080/02681102.2019.1586632

Whitelaw, S., Mamas, M. A., Topol, E., & Van Spall, H. G. (2020). *Application of digital technology in COVID-19 pandemic planning and response.* The Lancet Digital Health.

World Economic Outlook. (2018). *Groups and Aggregates Information.* World Economic Outlook. Available at: https://en.wikipedia.org/wiki/Developing_country#cite_note-107

World Health Organization. (2020). Coronavirus disease (COVID-19): Situation report. WHO.

Zu, Z. Y., Jiang, M. D., Xu, P. P., Chen, W., Ni, Q. Q., Lu, G. M., & Zhang, L. J. (2020). Coronavirus disease 2019 (COVID-19): A perspective from China. *Radiology, 296*(2), 200490. doi:10.1148/radiol.2020200490 PMID:32083985

ADDITIONAL READING

He, W., Zhang, Z. J., & Li, W. (2021). Information technology solutions, challenges, and suggestions for tackling the COVID-19 pandemic. *International Journal of Information Management, 57*, 102287. doi:10.1016/j.ijinfomgt.2020.102287 PMID:33318721

Kapoor, A., Guha, S., Das, M. K., Goswami, K. C., & Yadav, R. (2020). Digital healthcare: The only solution for better healthcare during the COVID-19 pandemic? *Indian Heart Journal, 72*(2), 61–64. doi:10.1016/j.ihj.2020.04.001 PMID:32534691

Mbunge, E. (2020). Integrating emerging technologies into COVID-19 contact tracing: Opportunities, challenges, and pitfalls. *Diabetes & Metabolic Syndrome, 14*(6), 1631–1636. doi:10.1016/j.dsx.2020.08.029 PMID:32892060

Vargo, D., Zhu, L., Benwell, B., & Yan, Z. (2021). Digital technology use during COVID-19 pandemic: A rapid review. *Human Behavior and Emerging Technologies, 3*(1), 13–24. doi:10.1002/hbe2.242

KEY TERMS AND DEFINITIONS

COVID-19: This is an infectious disease known as coronavirus that is caused by SARS-CoV-2 that triggers a respiratory tract infection and can cause death if vaccination is not taken.

Digital Technologies: These are digital tools, devices systems, and resources that can be used to store or process data. For example, smartphones, social media, online games, and multimedia.

Fibre Optic Technology: This refers to new technology that enables data transmission without including any electrical processing that may result in further transmission distances. This includes new devices such as optical couplers and optical switches that are supporting a recent trend known as all-optical networks.

Healthcare Sector: This includes businesses or institutions that provide medical services to patients, produce drugs or medical equipment, provide medical insurance.

Healthcare System: These are policies implemented in organizations that are designed to provide medical care for people. i.e., Hospitals, clinics, and community health centres.

Global Humanitarian Relief: This refers to material and logistic emergency aid given to victims of natural disasters, refugees, wars, famine, homeless, people that need assistance such as health assistance, food, shelter, warm clothing, and other essential relief that is essential for human existence in a short-term till long term assistance is granted by the government and other humanitarian institutions can provide permanent solutions.

Pandemic: This is the widespread pandemic of an infectious disease. i.e., multiple continents or global spread have affected a large number of people.

SORMAS: Surveillance, Outbreak Response Management, and Analysis System.

SPRP: Strategic Preparedness and Response Plan.

WHO: World Health Organization?

Chapter 5
Implementation of mHealth Interventions for Public Healthcare in East Africa:
Lessons Learnt

Patrick Ndayizigamiye
https://orcid.org/0000-0001-5721-6070
University of Johannesburg, South Africa

ABSTRACT

The potential of mobile technologies to address health-related challenges has been widely acknowledged. The objective of this chapter is to identify factors that led to the successful implementation of mobile health interventions for public healthcare in the East African Community (EAC) and lessons learnt from these implementations that could assist in devising successful mHealth interventions. Findings reveal that forging partnerships with key stakeholders, adapting mHealth interventions to the cultural context, leveraging local opportunities, involving users in the design phase of interventions, planning for sustainability from the design phase of mHealth interventions, having a policy framework and a monitoring system to guide mHealth activities are key factors that led to the success of these interventions.

INTRODUCTION

The use of mobile technologies to provide healthcare services or mHealth has received much attention in developing countries (Ndayizigamiye & Maharaj, 2016a; Ndayizigamiye & Maharaj, 2016b; Ndayizigamiye, 2016; Ndayizigamiye &

DOI: 10.4018/978-1-7998-8915-1.ch005

Maharaj, 2017; Ndayizigamiye, Hangulu & Akintola, 2017; Imaja, Ndayizigamiye & Maharaj, 2017; Ndayizigamiye & Maharaj, 2018; Ndayizigamiye, Soni, & Jere, 2018; Matiyabu & Ndayizigamiye, 2019; Soni, Ndayizigamiye, & Kante, 2019; Kante & Ndayizigamiye, 2020a; Kante & Ndayizigamiye, 2020b; Kante & Ndayizigamiye, 2021; Ndayizigamiye, Kante & Shingwenyana, 2020). The World Health Organisation (WHO) defines mHealth as "medical and public health practice supported by mobile devices, such as mobile phones, patient monitoring devices, personal digital assistants and other wireless devices" (WHO, 2011: 6). In Resource-Limited Countries (RLCs), there is a notable increase in the ownership of mobile cellphones (ITU, 2014) coupled with an expansion of mobile technology infrastructure (Aranda-Jan, Mohutsiwa-Dibe & LouakanoUTva, 2014). Thus, mHealth interventions can reach a large portion of the population from RLCs who would otherwise not have access to affordable healthcare. In this regard, mHealth interventions have often been hailed for being much more cost-effective compared to the conventional (non-ICT led) delivery of healthcare services. In addition, in RLCs, mHealth interventions have been identified as part of the solutions to the shortage of healthcare professionals in rural communities, lack of proximity of healthcare facilities and practicable roads that lead to such facilities (Schweitzer & Synowiec, 2012; Mishra & Singh, 2008). Hence, some mHealth interventions support Community Healthcare Workers (CHWs) in their quest to deliver healthcare services within communities either through SMS-based interventions or mobile applications loaded on smartphones. mHealth has also been used to strengthen healthcare systems by replacing inefficient paper-based data collection methods with mobile-enabled data collection systems (Aranda-Jan, et al., 2014) and in other cases to facilitate and enhance communication amongst healthcare professionals (Chang, et al., 2012) and training of healthcare professionals (Vélez, 2011; Chib, 2010; Knight & Holt, 2010). Other mHealth interventions are directly targeting the community through preventive and curative interventions. Preventive interventions include mHealth interventions for behavioural change to induce healthy lifestyles through education and awareness programs (Jamison, Karlan & Raffler, 2013), while curative interventions entail remote patients' diagnosis and treatment (DeRenzi, et al., 2012). mHealth has also been used to remotely monitor disease spread and epidemic outbreak, patients' health and patients' adherence to treatment (Sidney, et al., 2011; Chen, Fang, Chen & Dai, 2008). However, notwithstanding the potential and the demonstrated capabilities of mHealth to address healthcare issues in developing countries, there is a general agreement from the literature on the need for more evidence-based research to substantiate the call for scaling mHealth interventions (L'Engle, Plourde & Zan, 2017). Such evidence-based research is also needed to identify best practices that may lead to the successful uptake of mHealth interventions and yielded benefits. These best practices may assist implementers of mHealth to make informed decisions pertaining to introducing mHealth interventions into communities, and to avoid failures that have characterised several mHealth interventions that dissipated at the pilot stage. This paper provides a systematic review of mHealth interventions that demonstrated positive outcomes in the East African region. The paper highlights best practices that yielded positive outcomes in East Africa and lessons learnt therefrom. The aim is to present an evidence-based of what should be taken into consideration for the successful introduction of mHealth interventions within the context of developing countries.

OVERVIEW OF MHEALTH IMPLEMENTATIONS IN EAST AFRICA

In the context of East Africa, some mHealth interventions used text-based messages to bring an awareness of health-related issues such as HIV/AIDS (Jamison, Karlan & Raffler, 2013). These text-based interventions are opportunities to reach a wide audience at a low cost. Anonymised text-based messages also help preserve the privacy of respondents especially in cases where the respondents have to disclose sensitive information. mHealth has also been used for real-time data collection to support drug stock management in health facilities in East African countries (Githinji, et al., 2013; Barrington, et al., 2010). Some pilot projects in the region reveal that SMS-based interventions could be used for disease surveillance (Asiimwe, et al., 2011; Kamanga, et al., 2010) and for diagnostics and treatment support (DeRenzi, et al., 2012). Other mHealth interventions focused on the feasibility analysis of mHealth interventions (Ndayizigamiye & Maharaj, 2016; Ndayizigamiye, 2016). Although most of the implemented mHealth interventions in East Africa were in pilot phases, they demonstrated the potential to address healthcare issues. However, only a few of them described factors that led to the success of these interventions and lessons learnt therefrom. There is a need for more evidence-based research to suggest scaling up mHealth interventions (Aranda-Jan et al., 2014; Betjeman et al., 2013). Moreover, investigating factors that contribute to mHealth success and lessons learnt therefrom could inform the deployment of future mHealth interventions focusing on these success factors and hence, increasing the prospects of success for upcoming interventions. In 2014, the East African region contributed to "over 30% of the global innovative healthcare delivery programs" and Kenya ranked second after India for its innovative eHealth programs (Excelsior Group, 2014, p. 1). Thus, the East African region was chosen to be the focus of this paper because of its wide range of health IT programs and the innovation found in these programs.

METHODS

A systematic literature review was conducted using PubMed, Plos One databases and grey literature. The initial search criteria included any literature published in English that mentioned any mHealth intervention geared towards public healthcare in any of five countries in the East African Community (EAC). These countries are Burundi, Rwanda, Uganda, Kenya and Tanzania. Thus, the key search criteria were formulated as follows: "mobile + technology + health + Kenya + Burundi + Uganda + Tanzania + Rwanda". The search yielded 760 papers (PubMed [N=10]; Plos One[N=745]; Grey literature [N=5]). The papers' titles or abstracts had to imply the use of mobile technologies for public healthcare to qualify for further analysis. An initial screening based on the title and abstract revealed that only 42 records qualified for further analysis. Subsequently, 35 more records were excluded from the analysis due to duplication or lack of clear outcomes or lessons learnt from the mHealth implementation as depicted in Figure 1. Hence, the inclusion/exclusion criteria were that: (1) selected articles must be based on the implementation of an mHealth intervention geared towards public healthcare; (2) in the context of any country in the East African Community; and (3) must report the outcomes of the intervention with implicit or explicit lessons learnt.

Figure 1. Data screening process according to PRISMA guidelines

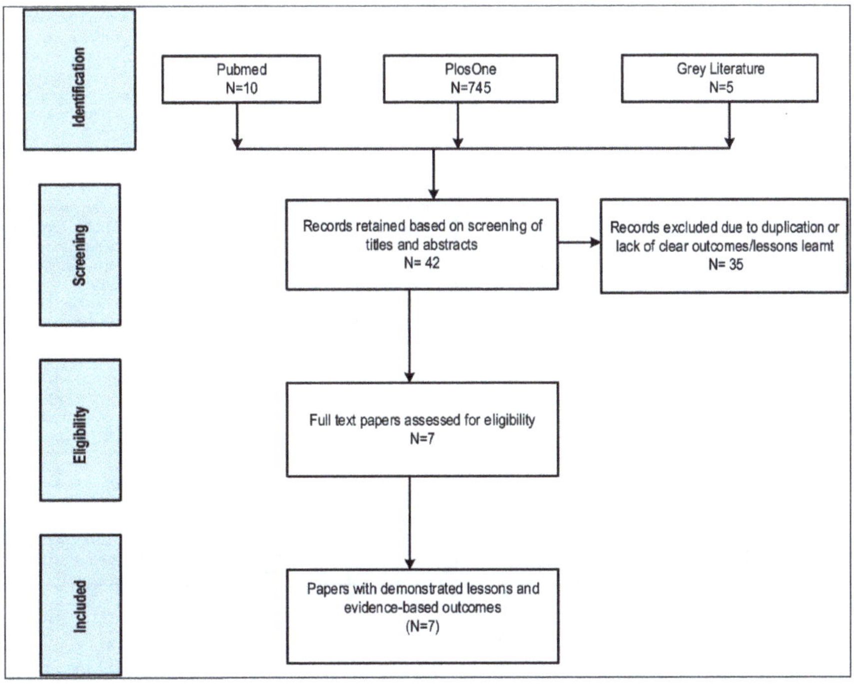

FINDINGS

Table 1. Description of selected papers

Author/Year	mHealth Intervention	Country	Purpose	Outcomes	Lessons Learnt
Burundi Ministry of health, 2014	Rapid SMS project	Rwanda	SMS based intervention designed to assist CHWs monitor maternal and infant's health status	Increase in attendance to antenatal care	Need to partner with key stakeholders. Involve users during the design phase of intervention. Need to provide incentives to users.
Chaos, 2008	Text to Change	Uganda	An SMS system (interactive quiz) designed to increase awareness of HIV/ AIDS	A 40% increase in the number of patients that reported for HIV testing in a six-week period	Need to collaborate with local partners. Design SMS messages in local languages.
Lester et al., 2010	WelTel1	Kenya	An SMS based intervention designed to stimulate HIV patients' adherence to ARV treatment	improvement in ART adherence	Need to leverage existing local opportunities. Need to forge partnerships with mobile health technology developers.
Lund et al., 2014	Wired mothers	Zanzibar (Tanzania)	SMS-based system designed to remind pregnant women to attend antenatal care and to seek skilled delivery care	Increase in attendance to antenatal care and seeking skilled delivery care	Scalability needs to be considered with scalability in mind. Partnership with stakeholders from the private sector is needed to ensure scalability. Adopt a phased approach to mHealth implementation. Diversify medium used to deploy the intervention to include voice messages. Consider gender issues. Needs a guiding policy framework and monitoring system to coordinate and guide mHealth activities.
DeRenzi et al., 2008	e-IMCI	Tanzania	A mobile phone-enabled application that guides a health worker through the Integrated Management of Childhood Illness (IMCI) treatment algorithm	More adherent to the IMCI guidelines compared to the traditional paper based one	Explore the tradeoff between having a fast and flexible system without compromising the core functionality of the system. Understand the barriers to continued use of the system.
Odeny et al., *2012*	Text messaging to improve adherence to post-operative clinic visits	Kenya	Text messaging to improve adherence to post-operative clinic visits	Increased rate of return to the clinics after 7 days after circumcision	Evaluate additional costs incurred by participants in the intervention. Compensate participants.
Mugo et al., 2016	Appointment reminders through text messages, phone calls and In-person reminder	Kenya	A multi-facetted intervention to increase the uptake of repeat HIV testing	Higher attendance to repeat HIV testing was associated with receiving appointment reminders	Design mHealth interventions in a way that they could be customized to suit participants' situations.

The screening process described in the above section led to seven papers that fit within the objective of this paper. Three of these papers discussed the outcomes of mHealth interventions in Kenya; two in Tanzania; one in Uganda; and one in Rwanda as depicted in Table 1 below:

Rapid SMS Project in Rwanda

Rapid SMS is an open-source platform used to build scalable SMS-based services.

It allows a two-way information flow and has been used to collect data, facilitate communication between remote parties and remote diagnostics, and track expectant mothers and newborn health, to name a few (RapidSMS, 2013). In 2010, Rwanda implemented the Rapid SMS for Community Health Workers (CHWs) to monitor the health status of expectant mothers, newborn babies, health risks, and infants' nutrition (Burundi Ministry of Health, 2014). The system was introduced to reduce expectant mothers' and newborns' deaths. Through the Rapid SMS system, CHWs received healthcare guidance. The system also helped healthcare centres to be more prepared to receive patients. The system also sent alert messages that could be channelled to ambulances, thus shortening the response time to emergencies.

Evidence from one of the districts in the Northern Province of Rwanda (Musanze district) where the system was rolled out, suggests that the system contributed to the increase in the number of expectant mothers attending antenatal care and a reduction in home births. In addition, newborns were given healthcare at an early stage (Burundi Ministry of Health, 2014). Thus, the system contributed to reducing maternal and neonatal mortality. In a 6-month period, the system was tracking 14,000 pregnancies.

There are notable factors that contributed to the success of the intervention (Burundi Ministry of Health, 2014). Firstly, only one mobile service provider was involved in the project. The service provider charged only 20% of the regular SMS rates during the pilot phase in the Musanze district. In addition, CHWs were consulted to determine the system's usefulness and its requirements. Moreover, incentives were given to the CHWs based on their performance during the pilot phase. Telecommunications infrastructure also played an important role in the success of the intervention as mobile telecommunications signals covered at least 95% of the Musanze district area.

Text to Change Implementation in Uganda

Text to Change (TTC) is an SMS-based intervention for HIV/AIDS awareness. The SMS system was piloted in 2008 in Mbarara (Uganda) to increase public awareness of AIDS and to encourage citizens to test and seek counselling for HIV/

AIDS (Chaos, 2008). The intervention sought to leverage the widespread use of text messaging functionality and to preserve the anonymity of the participants in the program. For three months, a multiple-choice quiz was sent to 15,000 mobile cellphone users residing in the rural area of Mbarara. The interactive quiz aimed to ascertain the participants' general knowledge about HIV transmission and the benefits associated with voluntary testing and counselling. Each response from the participants was recorded and the system responded with the right answer each time a participant provided a wrong answer. The quiz ended by encouraging participants to voluntarily test, seek HIV/AIDS counselling at their local health centres, and notified the participants about the location of their nearest testing centre.

Participants were given free airtime and those who reported to the health centres through the TTC program were provided with HIV testing and counselling free of charge. A 40% increase in the number of patients that reported for HIV testing was recorded in a six-week period since the implementation of the interactive SMS-based quiz. Through the participants' responses, it was discovered that the participants did not believe in the accuracy and anonymity of the HIV testing. Hence, this important finding was relayed to other healthcare stakeholders in the region to devise remedial actions.

The program identified that collaboration with local partners need to be strengthened by allowing local stakeholders to submit questions for the quiz. In addition, it was determined that the SMSes should be designed and delivered in the local languages so that non- English speakers can read the SMS messages. Through the intervention, the mobile telecommunication services provider was promoting its texting service which created a win-win situation between the mHealth implementers and the service provider. Due to the increase in the number of tests conducted through the intervention, the testing centre was able to seek more funding in order to extend its reach.

WelTel Kenya

In Kenya, the WelTel is an SMS-based intervention directed at HIV patients to improve adherence to ARV treatment and subsequently suppressing plasma HIV-1 RNA load. In three clinics in Kenya, patients on Anti-Retroviral Treatment (ART) received SMS-based support to enhance their adherence to the ART (Lester, Ritvo, Mills et al., 2010). The intervention targeted the clinics' patients aged over 18 years that had just initiated the ART for the first time, who had access to a mobile phone on a quasi-daily basis, and able to communicate through SMS. Those who did not own a phone but had shared access to a mobile device were also included in the intervention, and some of those who were illiterate were included if they could be assisted by someone close to them to read the SMS messages. Patients were randomly assigned to the intervention or to the control group (those who are not part of the SMS-based intervention). Unlike in the case of Text to Change in Uganda, airtime credit was not provided to the participants. Each Monday morning, clinical staff would send an SMS to the participants in the intervention group in the local language (Kiswahili) asking if they were fine or if they needed assistance. The participants were required to respond within 48 hours. The clinician would then call the patients who indicated that they have a problem or who did not respond within the stipulated timeframe (48 hours). Those who did not respond often cited logistical and cost factors or simply forgetting as the major reasons for not responding on time. All communications between healthcare workers and the patients were recorded. Follow-up visits were made at the 6th and 12th months of the intervention whereby participants were asked about the number of pills that they missed in the past 30 days. Those that reported that they had taken at least 95% of the provided pills were classified as adherents. Between May 2007 and October 2008, the outcomes of the intervention revealed that patients that were part of the intervention reported an improvement in ART adherence (of over 95%) at both follow-up visits and viral suppression (<400 copies per mL) at 12 months compared to those who were not part of the intervention (Lester, Ritvo, Mills et al., 2010). A plasma HIV-1 RNA load of 400 copies per mL or less (at the 12th month visit) indicated that the virus was suppressed, otherwise, the virus was not suppressed (i.e. failure).

The study demonstrated that leveraging existing local opportunities could yield positive results. Before the study commenced, Kenya was already leveraging mobile technology through the mobile money transfer platform, M-PESA. Thus, the Kenyan population was already acquainted with mobile technology innovation, which could have facilitated the uptake of the intervention. An evaluation of the implementation also suggests that the efficiency and scalability of the programme could be enhanced through partnerships (public or private) with mobile health technology developers.

Wired Mothers Intervention in Zanzibar

The 'Wired Mothers' is an mHealth intervention that linked pregnant women to their primary health care provider throughout their pregnancy, childbirth and the postpartum period. The intervention used mobile technology to send appointment reminders and educational information via SMS. The intervention was carried out in 24 healthcare facilities of six districts of Zanzibar (Lund, Nielsen, Hemed, et al., 2014). The intervention included 1,311 pregnant women who were part of the mobile-based intervention against 1,239 who received standard care. Both women were recruited during their first antenatal care visit at the healthcare facilities and were monitored up to 42 days after giving birth. Automated SMS messages were sent to the women who enrolled for the intervention to remind them to attend antenatal care and to seek skilled delivery care. These two components (antenatal care and skilled delivery care) are essential components needed to reduce maternal mortality and improve perinatal survival. The intervention was also an avenue to provide health education to pregnant women. Women in the intervention group were required to provide a phone number (either their own or any other that they could be reached on). An individual timeline was created (through specialised software) and text messages were sent automatically to the participants informing them about the stage of their pregnancy and other healthcare information related to their pregnancy, in their local language (Kiswahili). Through the partnership with Ministry of Health in Zanzibar, a voucher system (airtime credits) that allowed participants to communicate directly to a midwife was introduced. In case of an emergency, the system allowed the midwife to quickly refer the patient to a hospital.

The intervention led to an increase in attendance to antenatal care as 44% of women in the intervention group attended four or more antenatal sessions compared to 31% of women who received standard care. In addition, 60% of women in the intervention group delivered with the assistance of a skilled healthcare professional compared to 47% in the other group that only received standard care (Lund, Nielsen, Hemed, et al., 2014). However, notable increase in skilled delivery attendance was recorded in urban areas but not in rural areas. Moreover, perinatal mortality rate was lower in the intervention group (19%) compared to the other group (36%). In 2012, a decision was taken by the Ministry of Health in Zanzibar to scale the intervention to the national level. The following were identified as the major principles upon which the scalability of the intervention should be based. Firstly, scalability has to be considered with sustainability in mind. To ensure sustainability, partnership with stakeholders from the private sector is necessary and also the intervention should be implemented in phases. In addition, voice messages (with the possibility of a toll-free number) should also be considered for the intervention to reach a wider audience.

A post-implementation evaluation of the intervention suggests that mobile health interventions should take special consideration of the needs of rural women. In the specific context of the intervention, a suggestion was made to include mobile banking systems as part of the intervention's implementation strategy. Furthermore, it was suggested that a policy framework be implemented accompanied by a monitoring system to coordinate and guide mHealth activities in low and middle-income countries. Such a framework would ensure that there are concerted efforts toward achieving the set national health priorities.

e-IMCI Implementation in Tanzania

e-IMCI is a mobile phone-enabled application that guides a health worker through the Integrated Management of Childhood Illness (IMCI) treatment algorithm

(DeRenzi, Lesh, Parikh et al., 2008). The intervention was motivated by the need to reduce the time required to follow through the IMCI chart booklet, to reduce the expenses related to training clinicians on the use of the paper-based IMCI chart and to encourage clinicians to consistently follow through the protocols outlined in the IMCI. e-IMCI is the electronic version of the paper-based IMCI and runs on a Personal Digital Assistant (PDA). In one of the clinics in the Mtwara region of Tanzania where the intervention was piloted, clinicians identified that e-IMCI enables a health worker to go through the IMCI treatment algorithm much faster compared to the paper-based version. This is a significant factor as the paper-based one was often not utilised properly due to the time and effort required to follow through all the diagnostic protocols. Thus, in most cases, clinicians relied on their own memory or experience to diagnose patients. In addition, the paper-based IMIC did not take into account some factors, which compelled clinicians to override it. The initial assessment of the electronic version (e-IMCI) revealed that clinicians were more adherent to the IMCI guidelines compared to the traditional paper-based one. The electronic version also gave some flexibility to the clinicians in terms of choosing drugs and the use of approximate measures to certain investigations. The time required to be acquainted with the electronic version was less than 20 minutes, and four clinicians who evaluated the electronic system unanimously agreed that the system was faster and easier to use compared to the chart booklet. One key recommendation from the study is to explore the tradeoff between having a fast and flexible system without compromising the core functionality of the system and to understand the barriers to the continued use of a system.

Text Messaging to Improve Adherence to Post-operative Clinic Visits in Kenya

Male circumcision has been identified as one of the interventions that could curb the surge in HIV infections (WHO, 2007). The World Health Organisation (WHO) recommends that newly circumcised men should present themselves to their respective clinics seven days after the procedure for routine checkups to avert any adverse effects (WHO, 2011). However, previous reports highlight that a large portion of newly circumcised men fail to report to their clinics within one week after they are circumcised (Lissouba, Taljaard, Rech et al., 2010). Hence, in Nyanza province of Kenya, an SMS-based intervention was introduced in an attempt to stimulate men to return to their clinics for a checkup, seven days after circumcision. At the time of the intervention, the province had the highest HIV infection rate and lowest male circumcision rate in the country (MoH, 2007; KNBS, 2010). Participants in the intervention were recruited based on their age (18 years old older), phone ownership, having undergone circumcision on the day of screening, and willing to respond to a questionnaire that was administered 42 days after circumcision (Odeny, Bailey, Bukusi, et al., 2012). Between September 2010 and April 2011, 1,200 men were randomly assigned to the intervention group (i.e. receiving text messages) or control group (not receiving text messages). Participants were asked to register on the system by sending a text message to a number linked to an automated system. All participants were compensated for their airtime credits used to send the SMS to the value of $0.25. Daily text messages were sent to the participants in the intervention within seven days after circumcision. The intervention led to an increased rate of return to the clinics seven days after circumcision, from 59.7% to 65.4% (Odeny, Bailey, Bukusi, et al., 2012). In addition, transport costs influenced the return visits as men who spent $1.25 or less were more likely to return to the clinic compared to those who spent more than $1.25. Thus, mHealth interventions need to take into account additional costs that the recipients may incur in the short and long run.

Effect of a Combination of Text Messages, Phone Calls, and In-Person Appointment Reminders on Uptake of Repeat HIV Testing in Kenya

According to Kenya HIV Estimates Report (2014), Kenya has a rate of approximately 100,000 HIV infections annually. It was estimated that 40% of these infections are transmitted by individuals who contracted the disease within a month (acute stage) or within six months (early stage) (Powers et al., 2011). This is mainly due to the fact that viral loads are very high during this period coupled with high-risk sexual behaviour within 6 months after being infected (Serna-Bolea et al., 2010; Pettifor et al., 2011; Yeatman et al., 2015). Diagnosing acute HIV infection can reduce subsequent transmission of the disease (Cohen et al., 2013; Smith et al., 2013). In 2013, an intervention that combined the use of text messages, phone calls, and In-Person appointment reminders was devised to encourage repeat HIV testing in Kenya. Participants were tested for HIV and those who tested negative were advised to come back to the clinic for a repeat test, while those who tested positive were requested to do further tests and to attend counselling sessions. Participants were randomly assigned to either a standard appointment or an enhanced appointment. Participants in the standard appointment group were issued envelopes that contained instructions to return to the clinic two weeks after the first HIV test. In the enhanced appointment group, participants were given the same instructions as the first group and were also called or sent SMSes or a field worker would visit those who do not own a phone. SMS-based text messages were sent in the Kiswahili language. This intervention led to a 40% increase in the uptake of repeat HIV tests. Higher attendance to repeat HIV testing was associated with receiving appointment reminders. In addition, the intervention showed that the effect of in-person reminders was similar to phone reminders. It was also found that younger patients and patients with multiple partners were less likely to attend the repeat test. There was also a strong association between visit attendance and the study site (clinics where the intervention was carried out). One clear factor that contributed to the success of the intervention is that it was customized to the participants' circumstances. Those who owned cellphones were either called or sent SMSes, while those who did not or were unreachable through their phones were paid a visit by a healthcare worker.

DISCUSSION

Seven studies were included in this review. The findings reveal that establishing partnerships with public or private entities is one of the factors contributing to the success of mHealth interventions as exemplified by the Rwandan Rapid SMS system implementation, the TTC intervention, and the Wired Mothers intervention. Previous studies have also shown the importance of public-private partnerships in the implementation of mHealth interventions (VanderKop, et al., 2012; Chang, et al., 2011; Barrington, et al., 2010). Such partnerships may also extend to collaborations between institutions of higher learning in developed and developing countries, research institutions, non-profit organisations, public and private hospitals (Aranda-Jan, et al., 2014 quoted in Ndayizigamiye, 2016). As in the case of the mHealth intervention that used appointment reminders through text messages, phone calls, in-person reminders, and the WelTel intervention in Kenya, other authors also concur that adapting mHealth interventions to the local context and language is part of the determinants for the success of mHealth interventions (Odigie, et al., 2012; Zurovac, et al., 2012; Shao et al, 2015). Lester, et al. (2010) argue that providing adequate incentives is one of the factors that lead to a high response rate to mHealth projects. In the Rwandan case of Rapid SMS adoption, performance-based incentives were put in place to increase Community Based Health Workers adoption and ownership of the system (Burundi Ministry of Health, 2014).

CONCLUSION

The aim of the systematic literature was to present an evidence-based impact assessment of mobile health interventions for public healthcare in the East African region with specific emphasis on factors leading to the success of the interventions. Although the literature presented in this review refer to interventions that were still in pilot phases, these initial observations provide valuable insights that could assist future mobile health interventions. This review demonstrated that the success of mHealth interventions is driven by an array of factors that involve many actors within the mHealth ecosystem. Thus, there is a need for an environmental scanning to identify current and future stakeholders during the planning phase of any mHealth intervention. Such stakeholders need to be involved in the design of the intervention to mitigate the risks of rejecting the intervention at the implementation phase. However, more evidence-based outcomes and lessons learnt from scaled interventions are needed in order to have a better perspective of what works or does not work in larger, perhaps countrywide or regional settings.

In the context of the current Covid-19, many healthcare services are using mHealth in the prevention and treatment of the airborne disease or to build resilient healthcare systems. Thus, it is anticipated that the lessons learnt depicted in this study will help stakeholders in the fight against the pandemic to design successful mHealth interventions to ensure continuity of care even amid pandemics or other events that may hamper the normal provision of care.

LIMITATION

This review focused on papers published in PubMed, Plos One databases and grey literature. Thus, the authors recognise that the review may not be comprehensive as there could be other papers relating to mHealth interventions in the East Africa region that could have been published in other databases. However, the review search included papers that were published within a 16-year span to gather as many papers as possible that fit within the inclusion criteria.

REFERENCES

Aranda-Jan, C., Mohutsiwa-Dibe, N., & Louakanova, S. (2014). Systematic review on what works, what does not work and why of implementation of mobile health (mHealth) projects in Africa. *BioMed Central Public Health*, *14*(1), 188–203. doi:10.1186/1471-2458-14-188 PMID:24555733

Asiimwe, C., Gelvin, D., Lee, E., Amor, Y. B., Quinto, E., Katureebe, C., Sundaram, L., Bell, D., & Berg, M. (2011). Use of an innovative, affordable, and open-source short message service-based tool to monitor malaria in remote areas of Uganda. *The American Journal of Tropical Medicine and Hygiene*, *85*(1), 26–33. doi:10.4269/ajtmh.2011.10-0528 PMID:21734120

Barrington, J., Wereko-Brobby, O., Ward, P., Mwafongo, W., & Kungulwe, S. (2010). SMS for Life: A pilot project to improve anti-malarial drug supply management in rural Tanzania using standard technology. *Malaria Journal*, *9*(1), 1–9. doi:10.1186/1475-2875-9-298 PMID:20979633

Burundi Ministry of Health. (2014). *Kira-Mama project*. Retrieved June 09 2016 from https://unicefstories.files.wordpress.com/2014/05/burundi-final-english-300ppi.pdf

Chang, A. Y., Littman-Quinn, R., Ketshogileng, D., Chandra, A., Rijken, T., Ghose, S., Kyer, A., Seymour, A. K., & Kovarik, C. L. (2012). Smartphone-based mobile learning with physician trainees in Botswana. *International Journal of Mobile and Blended Learning*, *4*(1), 1–14. doi:10.4018/jmbl.2012040101

Chaos. (2008). *Text to Change (TTC)*. Retrieved February 23 2018 from http://images.aarogya.com/aids/pdf/unandzain.pdf

Chen, Z., Fang, L., Chen, L., & Dai, H. (2008). Comparison of an SMS text messaging and phone reminder to improve attendance at a health promotion centres: A randomized controlled trial. *Journal of Zhejiang University. Science. B.*, *9*(1), 34–38. doi:10.1631/jzus.B071464 PMID:18196610

Chib, A. (2010). The Aceh Besar midwives with mobile phones project: Design and evaluation perspectives using the information and communication technologies for healthcare development model. *Journal of Computer-Mediated Communication*, *15*(1), 500–525. doi:10.1111/j.1083-6101.2010.01515.x

Cohen, M. S., Smith, M. K., Muessig, K. E., Hallett, T. B., Powers, K. A., & Kashuba, A. D. (2013). Antiretroviral treatment of HIV-1 prevents transmission of HIV-1: Where do we go from here? *Lancet*, *382*(9903), 1515–1524. doi:10.1016/S0140-6736(13)61998-4 PMID:24152938

DeRenzi, B., Birnbaum, B., Findlater, L., Mangilima, J., Payne, J., Parikh, T., Borriello, G., & Lesh, N. (2012). Improving community health worker performance through automated SMS. *Proceedings for the Fifth International Conference on Information and Communication Technologies and Development (ICTD2012)*, 25-34. 10.1145/2160673.2160677

DeRenzi, B., Lesh, N., Parikh, T., Sims, C., Maokla, W., Chemba, M., Hamisi, Y., Mitchell, M., & Borriello, G. (2008). E-IMCI: Improving pediatric health care in low-income countries. In *Proceedings of the SIGCHI conference on human factors in computing systems* (pp. 753-762). New York: ACM. 10.1145/1357054.1357174

Githinji, S., Kigen, S., Memusi, D., Nyandigisi, A., Mbithi, A. M., Wamari, A., Muturi, A. N., Jagoe, G., Barrington, J., Snow, R. W., & Zurovac, D. (2013). Reducing stock-outs of life saving malaria commodities using mobile phone text-messaging: SMS for life study in Kenya. *PLoS One*, *8*(1), 1–8. doi:10.1371/journal.pone.0054066 PMID:23349786

Imaja, I. M., Ndayizigamiye, P., & Maharaj, M. (2017). A design of a mobile health intervention for the prevention and treatment of Cholera in South Kivu in the Democratic Republic of Congo. In *2017 IEEE Global Humanitarian Technology Conference (GHTC)* (pp. 1-5). IEEE. 10.1109/GHTC.2017.8239251

ITU. (2014). *ICT Facts and Figures*. Retrieved May 16, 2016 from https://www.itu.int/en/ITU-D/Statistics/Documents/facts/ICTFactsFigures2014-e.pdf

Jamison, J., Karlan, D., & Raffler, P. (2013). Mixed Method Evaluation of a Passive mHealth Sexual Information Texting Service in Uganda. *Information Technologies and International Development*, *9*(3), 1–19.

Kamanga, A., Moono, P., Stresman, G., Mharakurwa, S., & Shiff, C. (2010). Rural health centres, communities and malaria case detection in Zambia using mobile telephones: A means to detect potential reservoirs of infection in unstable transmission conditions. *Malaria Journal*, *9*(1), 1–7. doi:10.1186/1475-2875-9-96 PMID:20398318

Kante, M., & Ndayizigamiye, P. (2020a). A systematic mapping of the adoption of Internet of Things to provide healthcare services in developing countries. In P. Ndayizigamiye, G. Barlow-Jones, R. Brink, S. Bvuma, R. Minty, & S. Mhlongo (Eds.), *Perspectives on ICT4D and Socio-Economic Growth Opportunities in Developing Countries* (pp. 99–126). IGI Global. doi:10.4018/978-1-7998-2983-6.ch004

Kante, M., & Ndayizigamiye, P. (2020b). An analysis of the current status of Internet of Medical Things policies in developing countries. *NPG. Neurologie, Psychiatrie, Gériatrie*, *20*(119), 259–265. doi:10.1016/j.npg.2020.03.002

Kante, M., & Ndayizigamiye, P. (2021). Internet of Medical Things, Policies and Geriatrics: An Analysis of the National Digital Health Strategy for South Africa 2019-2024 from the Policy Triangle Framework Perspective. *Scientific African*, e00759.

Knight, D., & Holt, A. (2010). Internet and mobile technologies in healthcare service delivery: A case study exploring elements within their use and potential use in midwifery service delivery. Proceedings of Postgraduate Day 2010, 53-54.

L'Engle, K., Plourde, K. F., & Zan, T. (2017). *Evidence-based adaptation and scale-up of a mobile phone health information service*. Retrieved November 25, 2018, from https://mhealth.amegroups.com/article/view/14104/14325

Lester, R. T., Ritvo, P., Mills, E. J., Kariri, A., Karanja, S., Chung, M. H., Jack, W., Habyarimana, J., Sadatsafavi, M., Najafzadeh, M., Marra, C. A., Estambale, B., Ngugi, E., Ball, T. B., Thabane, L., Gelmon, L. J., Kimani, J., Ackers, M., & Plummer, F. A. (2010). Effects of a mobile phone short message service on antiretroviral treatment adherence in Kenya (WelTel Kenya1): A randomised trial. *Lancet*, *376*(9755), 1838–1845. doi:10.1016/S0140-6736(10)61997-6 PMID:21071074

Lissouba, P., Taljaard, D., Rech, D., Doyle, S., Shabangu, D., Nhlapo, C., Otchere-Darko, J., Mashigo, T., Matson, C., Lewis, D., Billy, S., & Auvert, B. (2010). A Model for the Roll-Out of Comprehensive Adult Male Circumcision Services in African Low-Income Settings of High HIV Incidence: The ANRS 12126 Bophelo Pele Project. *PLoS Medicine*, *7*(7), e1000309. doi:10.1371/journal.pmed.1000309 PMID:20652013

Lund, S., Nielsen, B. B., Hemed, M., Boas, I. M., Said, A., Said, K., Makungu, M. H., & Rasch, V. (2014). Mobile phones improve antenatal care attendance in Zanzibar: A cluster randomized controlled trial. *BMC Pregnancy and Childbirth*, *14*(29), 1–10. doi:10.1186/1471-2393-14-29 PMID:24438517

Matiyabu, I. I., & Ndayizigamiye, P. (2019). The potential use of Social Media for Healthcare Advocacy in the Democratic Republic of Congo. *Proceedings of 4th International Conference, 12*, 105-111.

Mishra, S., & Singh, I. (2008). *mHealth: A Developing Country Perspective*. Retrieved June, 14, 2016 from http://www.ehealth-connection.org/files/conf-materials/mHealth_%20A%20Developing%20Country%20Perspective_0.pdf

Ndayizigamiye, P. (2016). *Potential adoption of mobile health technologies for public healthcare in Burundi* (Doctoral dissertation).

Ndayizigamiye, P., Hangulu, L., & Akintola, O. (2017). A design of a mobile health intervention to enhance home-carers' disposal of medical waste in South Africa. In *2017 IEEE Global Humanitarian Technology Conference (GHTC)* (pp. 1-6). IEEE. 10.1109/GHTC.2017.8239241

Ndayizigamiye, P., Kante, M., & Shingwenyana, S. (2020). An adoption model of mHealth applications that promote physical activity. *Cogent Psychology*, *7*(1), 1764703. doi:10.1080/23311908.2020.1764703

Ndayizigamiye, P., & Maharaj, M. (2016a). Mobile health adoption in Burundi: A UTAUT perspective. In *2016 IEEE Global Humanitarian Technology Conference (GHTC)* (pp. 613-623). IEEE. 10.1109/GHTC.2016.7857342

Ndayizigamiye, P., & Maharaj, M. (2016b). *Applying bridges framework to investigate challenges to the adoption of mHealth in Burundi. In 2016 IST-Africa Week Conference*. IEEE.

Ndayizigamiye, P., & Maharaj, M. (2017). Determinants of mobile health adoption in Burundi. *The African Journal of Information Systems*, *9*(3), 1–23.

Ndayizigamiye, P., & Maharaj, M. (2018). *A Systematic review of mHealth interventions for public healthcare in East Africa in AMCIS 2018 proceedings*. AIS.

Ndayizigamiye, P., Soni, T. C., & Jere, N. (2018). *Factors Motivating the Adoption of Self-Healthcare Monitoring Mobile Applications by the South African Youth. In 2018 IST-Africa Week Conference (IST-Africa)*. IEEE.

Odeny, T. A., Bailey, R. C., Bukusi, E. A., Simoni, J. M., Tapia, K. A., Yuhas, K., Holmes, K. K., & McClelland, R. S. (2012). Text messaging to improve attendance at post-operative clinic visits after adult male circumcision for HIV prevention: A randomized controlled trial. *PLoS One*, *7*(9), e43832. doi:10.1371/journal.pone.0043832 PMID:22957034

Pettifor, A., MacPhail, C., Corneli, A., Sibeko, J., Kamanga, G., Rosenberg, N., Miller, W. C., Hoffman, I., Rees, H., & Cohen, M. S. (2011). Continued high risk sexual behavior following diagnosis with acute HIV infection in South Africa and Malawi: Implications for prevention. *AIDS and Behavior*, *15*(6), 1243–1250. doi:10.100710461-010-9839-0 PMID:20978833

Powers, K. A., Ghani, A. C., Miller, W. C., Hoffman, I. F., Pettifor, A. E., Kamanga, G., Martinson, F. E., & Cohen, M. S. (2011). The role of acute and early HIV infection in the spread of HIV and implications for transmission prevention strategies in Lilongwe, Malawi: A modelling study. *Lancet*, *378*(9787), 256–268. doi:10.1016/S0140-6736(11)60842-8 PMID:21684591

Rapid S. M. S. (2013). Retrieved February 09 2018 from https://www.rapidsms.org/

Schweitzer, J., & Synowiec, C. (2012). The economics of eHealth and mHealth. *Journal of Health Communication*, *17*(1), 73–81. doi:10.1080/10810730.2011.649158 PMID:22548602

Serna-Bolea, C., Munoz, J., Almeida, J. M., Nhacolo, A., Letang, E., Nhampossa, T., Ferreira, E., Alonso, P., & Naniche, D. (2010). High prevalence of symptomatic acute HIV infection in an outpatient ward in southern Mozambique: Identification and follow-up. *AIDS (London, England)*, *24*(4), 603–608. doi:10.1097/QAD.0b013e328335cda3 PMID:20019574

Sidney, K., Antony, J., Rodrigues, R., Arumugam, K., Krishnamurthy, S., D'souza, G., De Costa, A., & Shet, A. (2011). Supporting patient adherence to antiretrovirals using mobile phone reminders: Patient responses from South India. *AIDS Care*, *24*(5), 612–617. doi:10.1080/09540121.2011.630357 PMID:22150088

Smith, M. K., Rutstein, S. E., Powers, K. A., Fidler, S., Miller, W. C., Eron, J. J. Jr, & Cohen, M. S. (2013). The detection and management of early HIV infection: A clinical and public health emergency.). *Journal of Acquired Immune Deficiency Syndromes*, *63*(2), 187–199. doi:10.1097/QAI.0b013e31829871e0 PMID:23764635

Soni, T. C., Ndayizigamiye, P., & Kante, M. (2019). Determinants of the Adoption of Self-healthcare Monitoring Mobile Applications. *Fortieth International Conference on Information Systems (ICIS)*, Munich, Germany.

Vélez, O. (2011). *Design and usability testing of an mHealth application for midwives in rural Ghana*. Retrieved October 15 2015 from https://academiccommons.columbia.edu/catalog/ac:137838

WHO/UNAIDS. (2007). New Data on Male Circumcision and HIV Prevention: Policy and Programme Implications In WHO/UNAIDS Technical Consultation on Male Circumcision and HIV Prevention: Research Implications for Policy and Programming. Geneva: WHO Press.

WHO/UNAIDS/JHPIEGO. (2009). *Manual for Male Circumcision under Local Anaesthesia*. Retrieved July 8, 2011 from http://www.malecircumcision.org/about/documents/MC_manual_local_anaesthesia.pdf

Yeatman, S. E., Hoffman, R. M., Chilungo, A., Lungu, S. R., Namadingo, H. C., Chimwaza, A. F., & Trinitapoly, J. A. (2015). Brief Report: Health-Seeking Behavior and Symptoms Associated with Early HIV Infection: Results from a Population-Based Cohort in Southern Malawi. *Journal of Acquired Immune Deficiency Syndromes*, *69*(1), 126–130. doi:10.1097/QAI.0000000000000536 PMID:25942464

KEY TERMS AND DEFINITIONS

East Africa: East Africa, is the eastern sub-region of the African continent. It comprises 19 countries: Burundi, Comoros, Djibouti, Ethiopia, Eritrea, Kenya, Madagascar, Malawi, Mauritius, Mozambique, Réunion, Rwanda, Seychelles, Somalia, Somaliland, Tanzania, Uganda, Zambia, and Zimbabwe.

mHealth: mHealth (mobile health) is a general term for the use of mobile phones and other wireless technology in medical care.

Public Healthcare: A field that seeks to improve lives and the health of communities through the prevention and treatment of disease and the promotion of healthy behaviors such as healthy eating and exercise.

Systematic Literature Review: A systematic literature review (SLR) identifies, selects, and critically appraises research in order to answer a clearly formulated question.

Chapter 6
The Impact of mHealth on Supply Chain Management of Medical Supplies in Village Clinics:
A Case of Cstock mHealth in Malawi

Mwai Chipeta
Mangochi District Hospital, Malawi

Donald Flywell Malanga
https://orcid.org/0000-0001-9681-6503
University of Livingstonia, Malawi

ABSTRACT

This chapter reports the results of a study that evaluated the impact of an mHealth system named Cstock on the supply chain management of medical supplies in village clinics of Mangochi district in Malawi. The study found that Cstock was used for requesting health products, supply, and resupply from healthcare facilities. In terms of quality, it was reported that the system was fast, easy to learn, and rarely displayed error reports. Cstock mHealth also yielded positive impacts through time and cost savings, improved communication, and availability of essential medical stocks at all levels of the supply chain and improved data visibility for decision-making. However, poor network coverage, lack of power source for charging phone batteries, absence of monetary incentives, lack of technical support compromised the effective utilisation of the system. The chapter offers insights to policy makers, implementers, and research practitioners on how to build resilience in the management of medical supply chain in a primary healthcare setting through the use of innovative mHealth technology.

DOI: 10.4018/978-1-7998-8915-1.ch006

INTRODUCTION

Globally, it is recognised that malaria, pneumonia, malnutrition, and diarrheal diseases are the leading causes of childhood morbidity and mortality. In fact, about 70% of these early childhood diseases and deaths can be prevented or treated with access to simple and affordable interventions (WHO, 2011). This situation has become more prevalent in the sub-Saharan African countries, due to limited or no access to health services in rural communities and other factors such as cost of healthcare, geographical location of healthcare facilities, and long distances people have to travel to access healthcare services (Nyaga, 2021). However, with approximately 5.9 billion mobile phone users globally, opportunities for mobile phone technologies to play an important role in the delivery of health services, especially in developing countries are increasingly being recognised (GSMA, 2021; Kallander et al., 2013).

Mobile health (mHealth) describes the use of mobile phones, and other portable electronic devices with software applications to provide health services and/or manage patient information (Malanga, 2017). Previous studies demonstrate the positive impact of mHealth applications on improving child and maternal health outcomes in developing countries (Nyemba-Mudenda & Chigona, 2018; Malanga & Chigona, 2018). Key areas of health systems' improvements as a result of mHealth interventions include adherence to treatment/medication, appointment compliance, data collection and monitoring, point of care services, health promotion and education (Shiferaw et al., 2018). Besides, mHealth applications can also support community health workers (CHWs) to deliver effective community health management services to children whose present symptoms of diarrhoea, pneumonia, and malaria are prevalent particularly in underserved rural locations in low-income countries (Shiferaw et al., 2018).

Despite this evidence, studies also suggest many challenges that affect the adoption and scaling or maintenance of existing mHealth interventions. These challenges include lack of sustainable financing, weak organisation structure, poor ICT infrastructure, lack of technical capacity, lack of interoperability and integration, and security and privacy concerns. However, there is limited evidence on the impact of mHealth applications on supply chain management of medical supplies in low-resourced settings in developing countries. Previous studies (Nyemba-Mudenda & Chigona, 2018; Binyaruka & Borghi, 2017; Njoroge et al, 2017) have looked at mHealth adoption at generic level with little or no attention to the role of mHealth in supply chain management of medical supplies, particularly in developing countries like Malawi.

PROBLEM STATEMENT

Having reliable and available health commodities is fundamental to diagnosing and treating illnesses in primary healthcare settings. Health commodities include medicines, vaccines, diagnostic consumables and other health supplies (Binyaruka & Borghi, 2017). In Malawi like other developing countries, mHealth is increasingly being adopted to manage health commodity supplies in primary healthcare settings (Nyemba-Mudenda & Chigona, 2018). This is aimed at improving data visibility, decision-making, and reducing instances of shortages of essential health commodities.

To this effect, in 2016, the Malawi government through the Ministry of Health and other development partners deployed a Cstock mHealth logistic management system in at least 18 out of 28 districts of the country (Malanga, 2017; Shieshia et al, 2014). The objective of this mHealth intervention was to ensure effective supply chain management of essential medical supplies, especially in primary healthcare settings, where transport infrastructure remains a problem(Shieshia et al, 2014). However, since its deployment, there are few studies that have evaluated whether this mHealth intervention is a success or a failure.

Prior studies on Cstock mHealth system so far have looked at feasibility, implementation and acceptability of the technology using health indicators as theoretical foundations (SC4CCM, 2018; Friderichs, Foh, & Gathinji, 2014; Shieshia et al, 2014). Due to the complex nature of information technology (IT) implementation such as mHealth, using health indicators to conduct impact evaluation has been criticized as being limited. Some scholars have suggested the integration of information system metrics to potentially achieve a holistic approach to measure the impact of IT such as mHealth on healthcare systems (Pankomera, & van Greunen, 2018). Thus, the cited studies aforementioned have shown the negligible impact of Cstock mHealth on supply chain management of medical supplies particularly in primary healthcare settings.

Besides, most mHealth interventions in developing countries are implemented as pilot projects and driven by international donor funding (Malanga, 2017; Malanga & Chigona, 2018). As such, their impact evaluations have been criticized by information system researchers and other scholars for being biased toward donors and lacking theoretical grounding (Pankomera, & van Greunen, 2018). Based on this limited evidence, this study sought to evaluate the impact of Cstock mHealth on supply chain management of medical supplies in village clinics of Mangochi district in Malawi.

The study was conducted with the aim of providing policy recommendations on how mHealth technology can be improved to strengthen health care systems resilience in a primary healthcare setting of Malawi. To address this main objective, the following specific objectives were formulated:

- To identify the level of use of Cstock mHealth,
- To establish users' view of the quality of Cstock mHealth,
- To determine the users' satisfaction with Cstock mHealth,
- To examine the net impacts of Cstock mHealth.

To achieve the specific objectives, the study adopted the Information System Success model (McLean & DeLone, 2016), as the guiding theoretical lens of this study. The model is also commonly known as "McLean and DeLone model". The reason for selecting this model was that it captures all the constructs or variables that were in line with the specific objectives of this study such as usage, quality, satisfaction, and impacts. The rest of the chapter is arranged according to the following sections: Literature review, contextual setting, analytical framework, methodology, results and discussion, and conclusion and recommendations.

LITERATURE REVIEW

Defining Information and Communication for Development

The proliferation of ICTs in both developed and developing worlds has demanded political, academic and socio-economic attention (Olah &Kyobe, 2017). As a result, the field of Information and Communication for development (ICT4D) has become a venture for academic researchers in the world. ICT4D entails the use of ICT to support socio-economic growth, well-being and political transformation, particularly in developing countries. ICT4D covers digital technologies that support the process of communication, gathering, processing and dissemination of information (Nyemba-Mudenda, &Chigona, 2017). As a field of study, ICT4D research streams involves developing and implementing technology-enabled products and services to achieve targeted development goals in a developing country. A critical discourse within the ICT4D space is the emphasis on technology-enabled devices as tools for development.

Defining Mobile Technology

Mobile technology refers to mobile phones, smartphones, Portable Assistant Devices (PDAs) that facilitate the performance of tasks (Osah & Kyobe, 2017). The rapid and ubiquitous innovations in mobile technologies in several ICT4D landscapes has led to the creation of a separate stream of study known as mobile for development (m4D) that is not yet established but growing significantly (Donner & Escobari, 2010). As such, mobile technology provides linkages to people, information sources, health services, economic markets and public services such as health (Malanga & Banda,

2021a). However, many developing countries are characterised by the poorly wired network infrastructure and unreliable electrical power supply. Thus, in these settings, mobile phones are preferred due to their battery life span, their affordability, and the fact that they allow people to be connected from remote locations.

A recent report by GSMA (2021) suggests that as of 2021, the number of mobile subscribers has now reached 5.2 billion representing 67% of the total world population with a penetration rate of 71%. It is also estimated that the mobile phones penetration rate is expected to grow by 2.1% which will translate to 5.9 billion subscribers by 2025. At a continental level, the number of mobile phone mobile subscribers varies across regions. Europe ranks the highest, then North America and Sub-Sahara Africa rank the least with a penetration rate of 46%.

Furthermore, in 2020, literature indicated that about 420 million subscribers (44%) were from the Sub-Saharan African region to which Malawi belongs (GSMA, 2021). It is projected that the region will continue to experience a faster increase in mobile phones penetration rates than any other region. For instance, it is estimated that by 2025, more than half a billion people in Su-Saharan Africa will have subscribed to a mobile phone. This is evidence that mobile phones are becoming an important ICT tool even in remote and rural areas of developing countries. Their ubiquitous power, the rapid development of mobile technology, low cost and ease of use qualify them as appropriate and adaptable tools to bridge the digital divide (Nyemba-Mudenda & Chigona, 2018)

Conceptualising mHealth

Mobile Health (mHealth) care can bring about a revolution in healthcare in developing nations. This technology is well suited for healthcare delivery where accessibility is a key barrier (Vital Wave Consulting, 2009). The investment in mHealth also reduces spending on stationery, travel, and time and thus meets the challenge of shortage of human resources (World Health Organisation [WHO], 2011).

mHealth is the provision of health services and information through mobile technologies such as mobile phones and Personal Digital Assistants (Malanga, 2017; WHO,2011). In addition, mHealth enables health workers to access various data content and services through mobile devices such as mobile phones, smartphones, Potable Digital Assistants, laptops and other wireless media (Vital Wave Consulting, 2009). Therefore, mHealth seems to be a viable solution to deal with human resources shortages and poor accessibility of health services in rural and underserved areas in developing countries.

Potential Role of mHealth

There is a range of categories where mHealth applications could be used to deliver health services, especially in developing countries. The use of diagnostic and treatment support are critical in improving the healthcare of the people. mHealth intervention such as RapidSMS (Rapid short message service), can be used by health facilities to support interactions among health workers and with the patients (WHO, 2011). In Colombia, the CellPhone GuideView systems broke down complex diagnostic and treatment procedures into simple and steps for health workers using an authoring tool in which text, pictures audio and video were embedded to help health workers understand diagnostic and treatment procedures. Community health workers (CHWs) were able to transmit images, data and audio to remote experts for further advice(Vital Wave Consulting, 2009).

mHealth also helps to connect health workers with relevant sources of information through mobile devices and thus empowering them. mHealth applications provide the support needed by health workers to perform their duties effectively and self-sufficiently. In addition, mHealth provides a clinical decision support system that enables both patients and health workers to receive medical advice using technology rather than rely on face-to-face interactions (VWC, 2009).

mHealth applications can help to track and manage supplies of medicines and other essential commodities, help prevent stock-outs and facilitate the inventory and maintenance of medical equipment. mHealth also helps to monitor patients remotely using mHealth applications. This has opened new ways of treating outpatients in areas where access to hospital beds and health facilities is limited (Malanga, 2017). For example, an mHealth intervention delivered short message services (SMS) to community-based peer health workers in rural Uganda, supporting antiretroviral treatment of HIV patients. This mHealth intervention reported improvement in peer health workers morale and confidence and peer health worker-patients relationships.

In addition, mHealth educate, empower and engage individuals on health issues. Through the use of SMS, community members can communicate directly with community health workers. SMS campaigns for health education, promotion, awareness can help to disseminate information and prevention messages directly to patients. Mobile phones have also helped CHWs to communicate directly with one another and provide peer support. CHWs also use mHealth to receive updated information on drugs stocks, patient-attendance records, and other relevant health information (WHO, 2011).

Moreover, mHealth can help to track the outbreak of communicable diseases before they turn into pandemics. In areas where outbreaks of disease occur, CHWs can use mHealth to track medicine stocks and report observed cases(Malanga & Chigona, 2018). CHWS can also minimise the impact of disease outbreaks by disseminating educational information about disease prevention and handling. In Uganda, an mHealth intervention called *Integrated Community for Case Management* (ICCM), CHWs used mobile phones to send emergency alerts and requisition of medical supplies to support ICCM activities in treating Pneumonia, diarrhoea, and malaria. Similar mHealth applications are being used for disease and epidemic outbreak tracking in Rwanda, India and Peru(Vital Wave Consulting, 2009).

The Use of mHealth in Developing Countries

The rapid growth of mobile phone technology in recent years has encouraged developing countries to use mHealth to solve a wide range of challenges in the health sector. Text messaging, voice calls, cameras, automated sensing video messaging, and the internet are some of the mobile technologies that are utilised in mHealth to improve access and quality of information services (Nyemba-mudenda, 2015; Nyemba-Mudenda & Chigona, 2018). In both developed and developing worlds, mHealth interventions have been deployed and used for chronic disease monitoring and tracking, the delivery of medical test results, disease and emergence tracking, access to health records for remote diagnosis, patient-provider communication, data collection, and health information communication (WHO, 2011).

Recent studies suggest that the commonly used mobile phone for mHealth in developing countries are short text messages (SMSs). SMS is readily available in basic phones, therefore, tends to be convenient and affordable compared to other applications(Kruse et al., 2019). Concerning Sub-Saharan Africa (SSA), studies have suggested that within the past decade, over 500 mHealth projects have been implemented. mHealth has been deployed in rural areas to improve and reduce the costs of patient monitoring, medical adherence, and healthcare worker communication (Betjeman, Soghoian & Foran, 2013). mHealth has also been used for the emergence and disaster response, store, analyse, standardize and share patient information.

The pervasiveness of mobile phones is used to spread health information for education and awareness. SMSs are commonly used for this purpose because they are cost-effective and efficient for providing outreach services, covering a wide range of health issues (Kruse et al., 2019). Mass communication through the use of SMS alerts is also an effective way in targeting disadvantaged communities, especially in rural areas where there is a shortage of healthcare workers, clinics; and the limited access to health information services prevent people from making informed decisions about their healthcare (Nyaga, 2021).

Mobile phones are also used by community health workers (CHWs) to collect data from the field. This has reduced data errors and improved the quality of up-to-date information required for decision-making. mHealth interventions for remote diagnosis and treatment adherence by primary health workers enhance efficiency and cost reduction in services delivery. Remote monitoring, awareness campaigns for health promotion through mHealth interventions have led to timely dissemination of health information. This has potentially improved the ability to treat, track, diagnose disease and provide more accurate public health information for decision-making in developing countries (Njoroge et al, 2017).

Challenges to mHealth Adoption in Developing Countries

Despite the proliferation of mHealth projects in African countries and other least developed countries, the potential impact of mHealth is largely untapped (Kaium et al., 2019). This is due to socio-technical, socio-economic, cultural and regulatory barriers. In their review of mHealth research in developing countries, Njoroge et al (2017) found that the design, implementation and adoption of mHealth in developing countries are met with myriad challenges. These included mHealth applications not aligned with the local environment of developing countries. The study also revealed that poor network connectivity, low level of literacy, privacy and data security, institutional and legal framework, incentives, and culture are also barriers that hinder the adoption of mHealth (Munyua, Rotich, & Kimwele, 2015).

CONTEXTUAL SETTING

Malawi is one of the landlocked countries in Sub-saharan Africa. It shares borders with Tanzania, Zambia, and Mozambique (National Statistics Office, 2018). Its total population is estimated at 17.2 Million of which 87% lives in rural areas. Agriculture remains the economic backbone of the country (World Bank, 2021). About 43% of the population lives below the poverty line. Challenges related to healthcare includes access to timely and quality healthcare; poor infrastructure; shortage of skilled healthcare workers; chronic child malnutrition; maternal mortality rates; and HIV/AIDS prevalence remain high (UNDP, 2020). The average life expectancy is estimated at 46.3 years, adult literacy at 64%, GDP per Capita is USD 667, and the proportion of underweight children under-five-year-old is 22% (UNICEF Malawi, 2020).

Healthcare System of Malawi

Malawi's Ministry of Health (MoH) is responsible for developing, reviewing and enforcing health and related policies for the health sector, regulating the health sector including the private sector as well as providing technical supervision, monitoring, and evaluation of health interventions (Malawi National Health Policy, 2017). The

Ministry of Health categorised the level of health delivery systems into (i) primary healthcare; (ii)secondary healthcare/district hospital; and (iii) tertiary healthcare/ central hospitals (UNDP, 2020). Primary healthcare is organized to meet the needs of primary health care services. It includes health posts, maternity units, village clinics, dispensaries, health centres, rural hospitals, and community health centres (Malawi National Health Policy, 2017). Secondary healthcare provides specialized services to patients referred from the primary healthcare level. Tertiary healthcare consists of highly specialized services for specific diseases with a specific group of patients. The three-tier level healthcare delivery systems are linked to each other through a robust referral system that has been established within the Ministry of Health (UNDP, 2020).

ICTs Landscape in Malawi

To reduce some of the challenges facing the country, the Malawi government recognizes the role that ICTs play in socio-economic development (Makoza, 2013). To this end, the Ministry of Information drafted the ICT policy which was enacted into law in 2013(ICT Policy, 2013). Following the enactment of the ICT Policy, the government has implemented a number of initiatives. For instance, the government has created many websites to inform the public and its services and has further digitised many of its operations. The Malawi government also developed an Electronic Health (e-Health) Strategy for 2011-2016 as a roadmap for the implementation of ICT projects in the health sector. Some of the ICT projects that have been deployed in the public health sector include the implementation of Health Management Information Systems (HMIS).

The Malawi Communication Regulatory Authority [MACRA] (2015) reports that the mobile phone penetration rate is estimated at 45% while internet penetration is 6.5%. The proportion of individuals that own computer devices is 26.6%. of which 13.9% are people from rural areas, while 36.1% are from urban areas (Malanga, 2022; Malanga & Chigona, 2018). There are gender disparities when it comes to ICT ownership in the country. About 3.9% of women own a desktop computer, 34.2% of women own a mobile phone. Whereas just .2% of women have access to the Internet compared to their male counterparts (Malanga, 2022). This is clear evidence that mobile devices have taken over fixed phone and computer devices ownership in the country (Malanga & Banda, 2021b).

mHealth Development Initiatives

Recently, the Malawi government through the Ministry of Health (MoH), has shown commitment to employing a number of mHealth initiatives in the country to solve some of the health challenges facing Malawians (MACRA, 2015). This is despite having one of the lowest mobile penetration rates (45%) in Africa. These mHealth interventions tend to target rural areas and focus on nutrition, supply chain management, HIV/AIDs and Maternal, Neonatal, and Child Health (MNCH) (Pankomera & van Greunen, 2018). Besides, most of these mHealth projects are implemented in primary healthcare settings through Apps, SMS, and Hotlines. They are driven by non-Governmental organizations (NGOs), and of which, 56% rely on donor funding. Some of the projects have proved to be successful in increasing maternal and child health knowledge, follow-up visits, attendance visits, and others.

Despite such significant benefits, studies have also revealed that both technical and human factors hinder the successful adoption of mHealth applications in the country. These include poor infrastructure, lack of financial resources, lack of interoperability standards; poor ICT governance; lack of buy-in from both users and government; and lack of coordination (Pankomera & Va Greunen, 2018; Malanga, 2017b).

ANALYTICAL FRAMEWORK

There are various models and theories that are used to measure the impact of information systems at the individual, organisation, and national level. Examples of such models and theories include the Diffusion of Innovation; Technology Acceptance (TAM) Model, Unified Theory of Acceptance and Use of Technology (UTAUT) Model, Decomposed Theory of Planned Behavioural (DTPB), Information Systems Success Model, among others (Chawinga & Zinn, 2016). However, this study adopted the Information Systems Success Model developed in 1992, and further revised in 2003 and 2016 (DeLone & McLean, 2016). It is also simply known as DeLone and McLean Model. The DeLone and McLean model (2016) proposes six dimensions that provide a comprehensive measure of Information System (IS) success namely: systems quality, information quality, service quality, systems use, user satisfaction, and net impacts.

- **Systems Quality**: This is a technical level where IS researchers focus on the desirable characteristics of information systems. Examples include ease of use, systems flexibility, ease of learning, response time, reliability, systems features of intuitiveness (DeLone &McLean, 2016).
- **Information Quality**: This is a desirable characteristic of an information system output. Examples include relevance, accuracy, security, understandability, usability, and timeliness (DeLone & McLean, 2016). This implies that for mHealth to make positive impacts, it has to have these information quality features.

- **Service Quality**: This refers to the quality of the support that system users receive from the information system organisation or IS department. Examples include responsiveness, accuracy, reliability, technical competence, empathy of the staff (DeLone &McLean, 2016). In the context of mHealth, there is a need to have a fully-fledged department to oversee the implementation and sustainability of mHealth at primary, secondary (district), and tertiary healthcare levels. There is also a need to have competent and responsive ICT staff to manage and administer mHealth systems.
- **Systems Use**: It is the extent to which and the manner users and customers utilise the capabilities of an information system. It measures the amount of use, the frequency of use, nature of use, the purpose of use, and the extent of the appropriate use of an information system (DeLone &McLean, 2016). For mHealth systems to yield positive impact, users need to know their roles in the system, the purpose of using the system and frequency of use, nature of use, and relevance of the systems to their job and overall objective of the organisation.
- **User Satisfaction**: Refers to the user's level of satisfaction with reports, support services and overall use of the system. In the context of mHealth, this may imply users satisfaction with the quality of reports the mHealth application produces an overall effective and efficient use of the mHealth system.
- **Net Impact**: Refers to the extent to which an information system is contributing to the success of an individual user, group, organization, industry, nation or state. This could be for improved decision-making, improved productivity, cost reductions, increased sales, improved performance, improved image, recognition, promotion, and others (DeLone &McLean, 2003). Figure 1 depicts the elements of the DeLone and McLean Model and their relationships.

Figure 1. DeLone and McLean Model (2016)

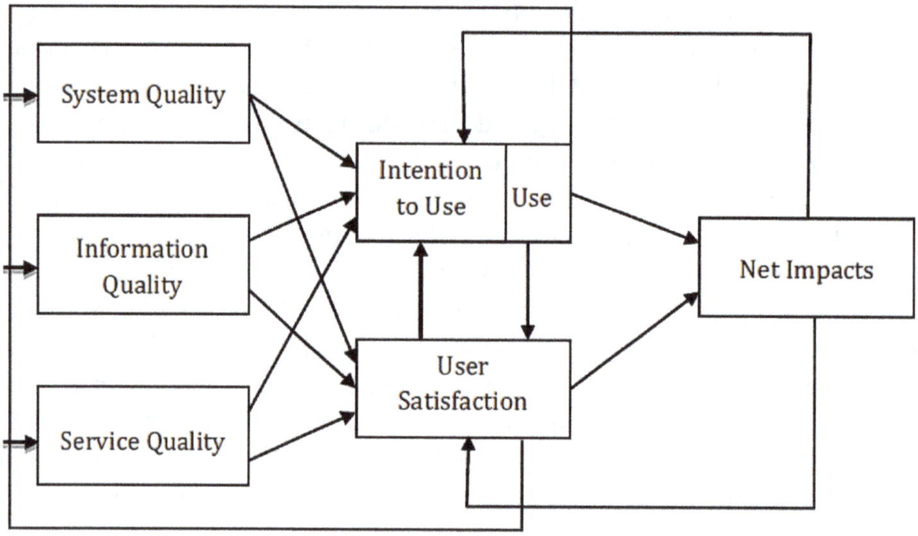

DeLone and McLean (2016) caution that the practical application of this model is dependent on the organisational context. At the same time, the selection of success dimensions and specific metrics are dependent on the nature and purpose of the systems being evaluated. This model was selected as suitable to underpin the current study based on its flexibility. In addition, a literature review on IS success has reported that DeLone and McLean model is one of the standard models used to measure IS success and has been cited in more than 10 thousand highly ranked IS journals (Nguyen, Nguyen, & Cao, 2015).

METHODOLOGY

This section introduces the research methodology that was used to conduct this study. The section briefly describes the research design, empirical case description, data collection procedures and methods of data analysis adopted in the study.

Research Design

Research design is a conceptual structure within which research is conducted. It constitutes a blueprint for the collection, measurement and analysis of data (Kothari, 2004). This study adopted a cross-sectional survey design. This type of survey design deals with opinions of individuals that are collected at one point in time. The reasons for employing survey design were that it is popular and allows the collection of a large amount of data from a sizeable population (Creswell, 2014). This study adopted a quantitative research method (Saunders et al. 2016).

The study targeted community health workers (CHWs) also known as health surveillance Assistants (HSAs) in Malawi, clinicians, pharmacists, and other stakeholders who directly or indirectly interacted with the Cstock mHealth system in Mangochi district of the Eastern region of Malawi. About 120 survey questionnaires were distributed to research participants randomly selected in 15 health centres in Mangochi district. However, only 112 usable questionnaires were returned for data analysis representing a response rate of 86.2%.

Empirical Case Description: Cstock mHealth

Cstock mHealth is a rapid Short Message Service (SMS) and web-based reporting and resupply system that is used by HSAs to report stock data through mobile phones. Cstock mHealth calculates healthcare supply quantities needed by HSA and sends this information to a health facility staff. The health facility staff receives this information and picks and packs the requested supplies. He/she then notifies the HSAs about when (time and date) the medical supplies (Shieshia et al, 2014).

The Cstock mHealth web-based dashboard is simple, easy to generate reports that show stock levels, reporting rates, and send alerts for central and district level managers. The dashboard enables district and central managers to see data sent by HSAs. The district and central level managers can then use this information to make decisions. Figure 2, provides a brief illustration of how data and supplies flow in a Cstock mHealth application.

Currently, the literature indicates that Cstock mHealth is actively implemented in 14 out of 29 districts of Malawi (SC4CCM, 2018). The project is funded by Melinda and Gates Foundation in partnership with the Malawi Ministry of Health. Based on the wide implementation of Cstock mHealth intervention in the country, it is then imperative to evaluate its impact in managing the availability of medical supplies in a primary healthcare setting of Malawi.

Figure 2. Cstock Data and Product Flow
(SC4CCM, 2018)

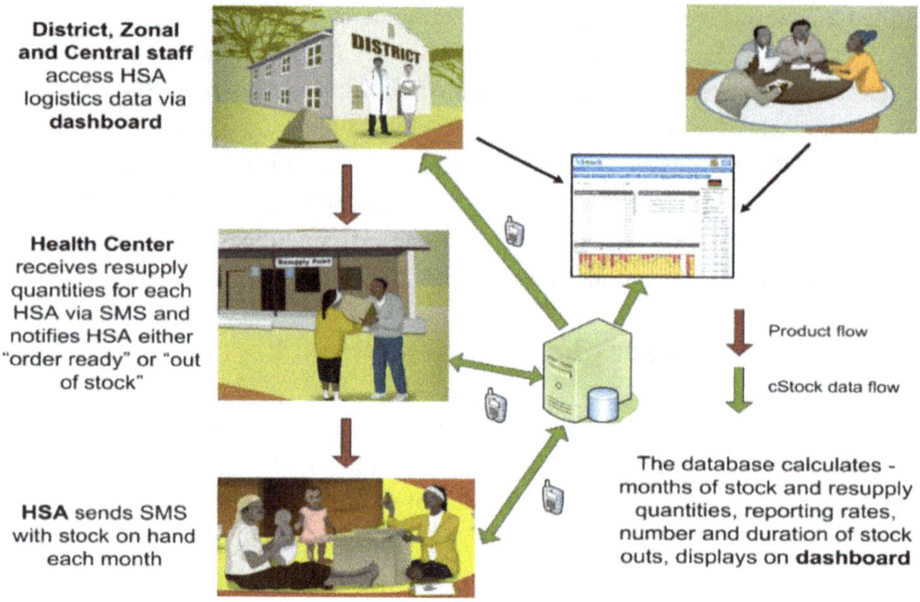

Data Collection Procedure and Analysis

Permission to conduct the study was sought from the University of Livingstonia Research Ethics Committee before data collection commenced. This study was part of a dissertation towards partial fulfilment for the award of BSc degree in Public Health at the University of Livingstonia in Malawi. Permission to conduct the study was also obtained from the Mangochi district health office. All participants were informed in advance that participation in the study was voluntary, and they were free to withdraw from the study at any time before the exercise of administering the questionnaires began (Creswell, 2014; Malanga & Chigona, 2018). The researchers personally collected the data from the field. The IBM Statistical Package for Social Sciences (IBM SPSS) Version 25 was used to analyse data. Descriptive statistics such as tables, graphs, pie charts were used to present and interpret data.

RESULTS AND DISCUSSION

This section reports the findings of the study with the aim of evaluating the impact of mHealth on supply chain management of medicines in village clinics of Malawi.

The section is arranged according to the following sub-sections: demographic profile of respondents, the use of Cstock mHealth, users' views on the quality of Cstock mHealth, users' satisfaction with Cstock mHealth, and net impact of Cstock mHealth.

Demographic Profile of Participants

The demographic profile of respondents is reported based on age, level of education, access to Csctok mHealth, mode of delivery for Cstock mHealth, and gender. The demographic profile of the participants is presented in Table 1.

Table 1. Demographic profile of respondents

Variable(s)		F(N=112	%
Age	20-25	28	25.0
	26-30	61	54.5
	31-35	12	10.7
	36-40	6	5.4
	41+	5	4.5
Mobile Phone Used to access Cstock mHealth	Basic phone	56	50.0
	Featured Phone	30	26.8
	Smartphone	21	18.8
	Tablet	5	4.5
Level of Education	J.C.E	48	42.9
	M.S.C.E	36	32.1
	Professional Certificate	9	8.0
	Diploma	12	10.7
	Degree	7	6.3
Gender	Male	78	69.6
	Female	34	30.4
Mode of delivery for Cstock mHealth	Short Text Messages (SMS)	103	92.0
	Voice call	7	6.3
	Video call	2	1.8

From Table 1, the findings indicate that the majority of respondents who participated in the survey were aged between 26-30 (54.5%) and 20-25 (25.0%) while few (10.7%) of the respondents were aged between 31-35.

With respect to education, at least half (42.9%) of the respondents who participated in the study were Junior certificate education (J.C.E) holders, (32.1%) were holders of Malawi School Certificate of Education (M.S.C.E), few of them were holders of degrees(6.3%). This was not surprising because most health workers found in rural communities in Malawi are HSAs, who are mainly holders of JCE and MSCE qualifications. Their major role is to provide primary health services and community case management in health posts and village clinics of the country (Shieshia et al, 2014).

The study also found that at least half of the respondents (50.0%) owned a basic phone that was connected to the Cstock mHealth, 26.8% of the respondents owned featured phones, and 18.8% owned smartphones. In Malawi, the smartphone penetration rate is still low as they are expensive for most average workers in the country. However, when it comes to basic and feature phones, most general workers like HSAs can afford them because they are cheap compared to smartphones and mobile tablets (Malanga &Banda, 2021b; MACRA, 2015).

In terms of gender, most of the respondents who participated in the study were males (69.8%), while female participants were only 30.4%. The results were not surprising in the context of Malawi, as like in other developing countries, gender imbalance in employment remains a systemic problem in Malawi (Malanga, 2020). Moreover, it was also established that respondents were using SMS (92.0%) to deliver health information through Cstock mHealth, while only 6.3% of respondents used voice calls. This finding confirmed previous studies that reported that mHealth in developing countries is mainly delivered through SMSs compared to video or voice calls (Kruse et al., 2019; Nyemba-Mudenda &Chigona, 2018; Munyua et al., 2015).

Usage of Cstock mHealth

The first objective of the study was to understand the usage of Cstock mHealth. Within McLean and DeLone model, usage is defined as the degree and manner in which employees and customers utilise the capabilities of an information system (McLean & DeLone, 2016). Although, there are many indicators for measuring information system usage, in this study only users' role, the purpose of use, and the frequency of use of Cstock mHealth were investigated.

Users Role/Designation in Cstock mHealth

The success of an information system depends on its usage by its target users and users roles, among other attributes (Chawinga et al.,2020). As presented in Figure 3, the results show that most users of Cstock mHealth were health surveillance assistants (HSAs) (79.5%) and very few HSAs supervisors (9.8%). The findings were in line with previous studies that have reported that the Cstock mHealth logistic management system is meant to be used by community health workers to deliver effective community case management to children who present symptoms of diarrhoea, pneumonia, and malaria, particularly in rural areas in developing countries (Shiferaw et al., 2018; SC4CCM, 2018).

Figure 3. Users role/designation in Cstock mHealth

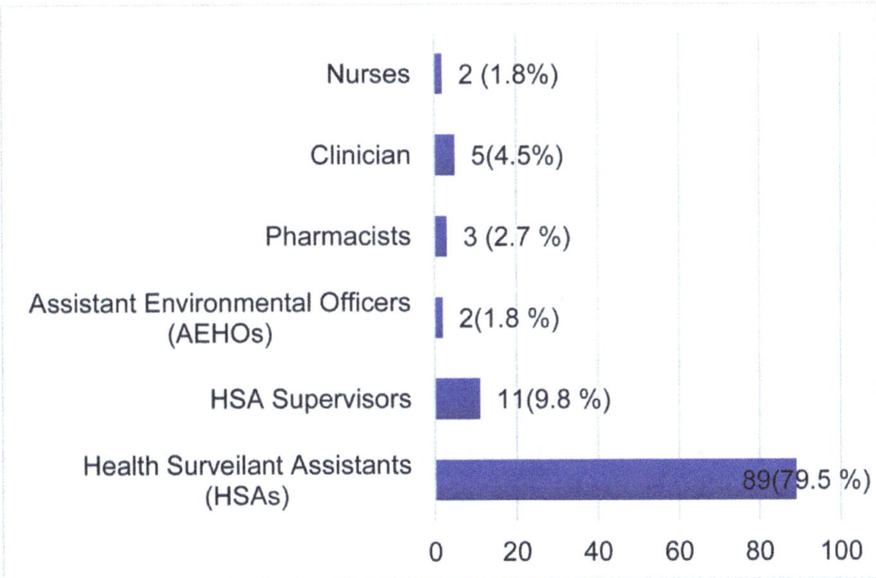

Purpose of Using Cstock mHealth

One of the indicators used to measure the usage level of an information system is the purpose for which the system is used. As presented in Table 5, the study revealed that Cstock mHealth was used for checking medical stockouts (87.5%), for identifying medical supplies to supply (75.0%), reporting medical supplies (69.6%), reporting receipts of medical supplies (63.4%), and requesting medical supplies (59.8%). This is in line with a study by Shieshia et al. (2014) that reported that the main usage of Cstock mHealth was to deliver community case management in rural areas is to request health products for supply and resupply from the health facility, and report the receipt of the health commodities supplied from health facilities.

Table 2. Purpose of using Cstock mHealth

Purpose	F(N=112)	%
For general health information	49	43.8
For seeking technical support	37	33.0
For checking medical stockouts	98	87.5
For emergencies	33	29.5
For reporting medical supplies	78	69.6
For meetings	24	21.4
Follow-up for non-reporting HSAs	46	41.1
For requesting medical supplies	67	59.8
For identification of medical quantities to supply	84	75.0
For reporting receipt of medical supplies	71	63.4

Note: Multiple responses were allowed

Frequency of Use of Cstock mHealth

Further, the respondents indicated the frequency of using Cstock mHealth. As presented in Figure 4, the study revealed that 54.5% of respondents used the system on monthly basis, while 28.6% used the system daily. This was in line with previous studies that reported that most SMS mHealth systems like Cstock are basically used on a monthly basis. This is because the end of each month is when most CHWs and other stakeholders get involved in sending or receiving reports, supply and re-supply of medical stocks.

Figure 4. Frequency of use for Cstock mHealth

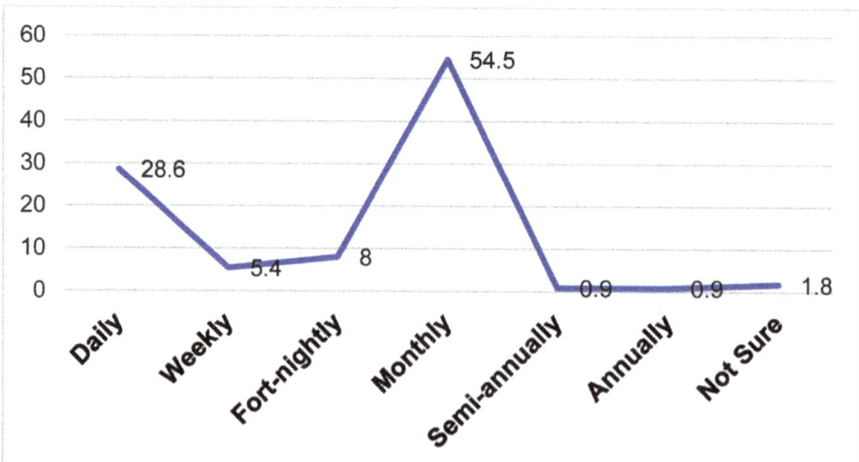

Users' Views on Quality of Cstock mHealth

The second objective of the study was also to determine users' views on the quality of Cstock mHealth. Three qualities were investigated: system quality, information quality, and service quality.

System Quality of Cstock mHealth

System quality denotes the desirable characteristics of an information system. The salient examples include ease of use, system flexibility, system reliability, response times, among others (McLean & DeLone, 2016). A system's performance in these aspects can either encourage or discourage users to use the system. As can be seen in Table 3, the study showed that respondents viewed the Cstock mHealth as easy to use (52,7%), easy to learn (60.0%), flexible (43.2%), and a bit reliable (34.5%). However, it was also noted that other respondents stated that Cstock mHealth was sometimes not responsive (44.2%), and the mobile network for accessing the system was not good (54.3%).

Mobile network challenge in Malawi is not a new phenomenon. Previous studies (Malanga & Banda, 2021b; Malanga & Banda, 2021a; Malanga & Chigona, 2018) have reported that in Malawi the quality of mobile networks is poor especially in rural communities. Most of the CHWs who are users of Cstock mHealth are posted to work in rural communities, where access to a mobile network is a challenge. This makes it difficult for HSAs and other stakeholders to utilise Cstock mHealth effectively. Therefore, it is recommended that government should work collaboratively with mobile operators to improve the quality of mobile networks in rural areas of Malawi for mHealth interventions such as Cstock mHealth to be effective.

Table 3. System quality of Cstock mHealth

Cstock mHealth System Quality İndicator (s)	Strongly Disagree	Disagree	Neutral	Agree	Strongly Agree
	%	%	%	%	%
Cstock mHealth is easy to use	3.7	3.6	14.5	29.1	52.7
Cstock mHealth is easy to learn	0.8	2.9	14.8	21.8	60.0
Cstock mHealth is flexible	24.5	8.6	3.4	43.2	20.3
Cstock mHealth is reliable	5.5	10.9	16.4	32.7	34.5
Cstock mHealth is responsive	44.2	5.3	12.1	30.4	8.0
The network for accessing Cstock mHealth is good	54.3	29.6	1.1	1.8	16.3

Information Quality of Cstock mHealth

Information quality of the system refers to the desirable characteristics of the outputs of a system. These may include management of reports and web pages, relevance, currency, completeness, the accuracy of information (McLean & DeLone, 2016). These aspects of information quality can also either encourage or inhibit users to adopt an information system. As indicated in Table 4, this study found that Cstock mHealth provided relevant (49.2%), accurate(35.7%), timely information(48.1%), and in clear format (40.9%). Other respondents mentioned that the Cstock information system security was a problem. This means that while the Cstock mHealth system meets at least all the standards of information quality, security remains a challenge that should be addressed in order to gain trust from users of the Cstock mHealth.

Table 4. System quality of Cstock mHealth

Cstock mHealth İnformation Quality İndicator (s)	Strongly Disagree	Disagree	Neutral	Agree	Stongly Agree
	%	%	%	%	%
Cstock mHealth provides relevant information	*30.5*	*7.0*	*1.0*	*12.3*	*49.2*
Cstock mHealth provides accurate information	*4.1*	*12.2*	*14.7*	*35.7*	*33.3*
Cstock mHealth provides timely information	*11.1*	*1.9*	*11.3*	*27.8*	*48.1*
Cstock mHealth provides secure information	*45.6*	*23.4*	*1.9*	*21.9*	*7.2*
Cstock mHealth provides usable information	*29.3*	*0.7*	*2.1*	*55.1*	*12.8*
Cstock mHealth provides information in a clear format	*13.4*	*11.4*	*7.0*	*27.3*	*40.9*

Service Quality of Cstock mHealth

Service quality refers to the quality of support that system users receive from the information system organisation and ICT support personnel. Some examples of service quality include responsiveness, accuracy, reliability, technical competence, and empathy of an organisation's ICT personnel. In this study as depicted in Table 5, about 63.0% of research participants indicated that technical staff are not competent, while 51.3% of respondents indicated that they are not reliable.

Respondents(65.6%), also mentioned that the power blackouts affected phone battery charging, while 62.5% and 46.8% of respondents stated that the ICT support staff was not emphatic and responsive respectively. The findings were not surprising considering that Cstock mHealth system does not have technical support both at the district health and primary health facility levels.

Table 5. System quality of Cstock mHealth

Cstock mHealth Service Quality İndicator (s)	Strongly Disagree	Disagree	Neutral	Agree	Stongly Agree
	%	%	%	%	%
Cstock mHealth technical staff are competent	21.4	63.0	1.9	5.7	8.0
Cstock mHealth technical staff are reliable for support	51.3	27.2	7.6	9.6	4.3
Cstock mHealth technical staff are empathetic	62.5	24.7	5.6	2.9	9.9
Cstock mHealth technical staff provides accurate technical support	55.4	13.0	1.4	24.9	5.3
Cstock mHealth technical staff are responsive	46.8	29.3	3.6	13.5	6.8
Electricity is always available to charge our phone batteries	65.6	19.4	3.2	10.7	1.1

User Satisfaction with Cstock mHealth

McLean and DeLone model (2016) postulate that for an information system to have positive impact, users must be satisfied with the systems' reports, website, and support services. Therefore, one of the objectives of this study was to establish the users' satisfaction with using Cstock mHealth. Figure 4 shows that a substantial number of Cstock mHealth users were satisfied with the system (45.5% or 51) and 19.6%(22) were fully satisfied. This implies that more than half of the respondents were satisfied with the system. McLean and DeLone model posits that user satisfaction is a critical factor for measuring whether the system is a success or a failure (McLean &DeLone, 2016). With respect to the present study, previously users were using a manual system (paper-based) to deliver health data on medical supplies. This activity was time-consuming, tedious, and subject to many erroneous reports. Therefore, it was expected that the users would be fully satisfied (100%) with the present Cstock mHealth system. However, this was not the case. This means that the health administrators should address the challenges identified pertaining to the usage and some of the quality attributes of the Cstock mHealth system.

Figure 5. User satisfaction with Cstock mHealth

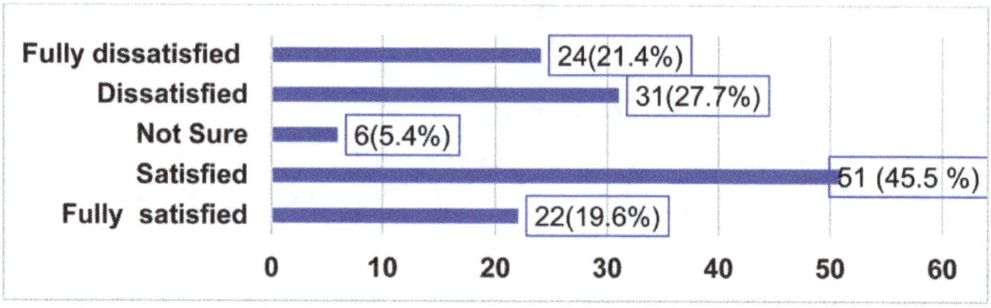

The Net Impact of Cstock mHealth

Last but not least, another question that was posed to research participants was related to identifying the impact of Cstock mHealth. McLean and DeLone (2016) view net impact as the extent to which information system is contributing to the success of individuals, groups, organisations, industries, and nations. These include cost reductions, improved profits, improved productivity, increased sales, creation of jobs, improved decision-making, among others. However, McLean and DeLone (2016) warned researchers that the selection of net impact indicators depends on the organisational context and type of information system in use.

In this study, as Table 6 indicates, the net impact were investigated to determine the extent to which the Cstock mHealth was contributing to the success of the supply chain management of medical supplies in village clinics.

Table 6. System quality of Cstock mHealth

Net Impact (s) of Cstock mHealth	F (N=112)	%
Improved health communication	46	41.1
Provided real-time data	91	81.3
Improved decision-making using timely available data	56	50.0
Reduced medical supply pilferage	69	61.6
Improved supportive supervision	53	47.3
Improved data visibility	42	37.5
Improved data quality reporting	88	78.6
Saved time and cost	49	43.8
Improved my job performance	64	57.1

Note: Multiple responses were allowed

The study found that to some extent Cstock mHealth improved the success of supply chain management of medical supplies at community levels in Malawi. Respondents(81.3%) mentioned that Cstock mHealth improved real data collection and monitoring, data reporting (78.6%), reduced medical pilferage (61.5%) which was one of the problems with the previous manual reporting system(SC4CCM, 2018).

CONCLUSION AND RECOMMENDATION

Using McLean and DeLone model (2016) as an analytical framework, the study evaluated the impact of mHealth on supply chain management of medical supplies in village clinics of Mangochi district of Malawi. The study found that most of the users of Cstock mHealth were Health surveillance assistants (HSAs), with few HSA supervisors, pharmacists, clinicians, and environmental assistant officers. The study also showed that most of the users of the Cstock mHealth system were using basic phones and much of the system transactions were delivered largely via small messages texts (SMS). Most of the users owned low-cost and affordable mobile phones with basic and features.

The study found that Cstock mHealth was used for checking medical stockouts, identifying medical supplies to supply, reporting medical supplies, and reporting receipt of medical supplies. With respect to the quality of the system, the study found that Cstock mHealth was easy to use, flexible, reliable sometimes, and easy to learn. Worth noting, it was found that the system offered accurate, timely, relevant information in a clear format. However, the study revealed that the service quality of Cstock mHealth was poor due to lack of technical, competent staff, poor mobile network, intermittent power supply to charge phone batteries, and ICT support staff were not responsive. Consequently, this had an effect on the level of users' satisfaction with Cstock mHealth.

Nevertheless, the study revealed that Cstock mHealth contributed positively to the supply chain management of essential medical supplies at primary healthcare setting in Malawi. The study confirmed most of the net impact attributes based on the McLean and DeLone model (2016). This was evident as most of the sampled participants indicated that Cstock mHealth improved real data collection and monitoring, improved data reporting, reduced medical pilferage, which had remained a systemic problem during the manual reporting system. In conclusion, the study found that to a greater extent Cstock mHealth yielded positive impact to the supply chain management of medical supplies in health facilities of the rural community. The findings have both theoretical and policy implications.

The use of McLean and DeLone model and its salient attributes have provided a theoretical and analytical description of the impact of mHealth technology on strengthening health systems in developing country contexts, such as Malawi. This study also makes a unique empirical contribution to policy direction. This is because the study has demonstrated the role that mHealth plays in strengthening the supply chain management of essential medical supplies in a primary healthcare setting. Consequently, this reduces supply chain logistical challenges and enhances transparency and accountability in the utilisation of essential health products.

The study also unearthed the current limitations of Cstock mHealth. For instance, the failure of the Ministry of Health (MoH) to decentralise the Cstock mHealth system so that technical support services can be handled at both primary and district health facility levels. This calls for a concerted effort among policymakers and other stakeholders to use these findings to address the challenges highlighted including intermittent power supply, poor quality of mobile network and lack of training. Addressing these challenges would potentially make the Cstock mHealth system more effective and efficient to yield positive health outcomes in short, medium, and long terms.

Despite the empirical contribution of the study, the following limitations were noted, that warrant further research. The study employed a descriptive survey design, which has its own weakness. Therefore, future research may adopt mixed methods research to gain more insights into the study phenomena. Second, the study targeted only Mangochi district health facility in Malawi. In this regard, future studies should be replicated to other district health facilities in the country, where Cstock mHealth has been rolled out. This would ensure a comprehensive understanding of the study phenomenon and possibly for the generalisation of research findings. Furthermore, the study did not measure all information system success attributes as suggested by McLean and DeLone model (2016). Therefore, future studies should test and utilise all the attributes and validate them statistically to enhance the theoretical model's suitability to the mHealth domain and developing countries context.

REFERENCES

Betjeman, T. J., Soghoian, S. E., & Foran, M. P. (2013). mHealth in Sub-Saharan Africa. *International Journal of Telemedicine and Applications, 2013*, 1–7. Advance online publication. doi:10.1155/2013/482324 PMID:24369460

Binyaruka, P., & Borghi, J. (2017). Improving quality of care through payment for performance: Examining effects on the availability and stock-out of essential medical commodities in Tanzania. *Tropical Medicine & International Health, 22*(1), 92–102. doi:10.1111/tmi.12809 PMID:27928874

Chawinga, W. D., Chawinga, C., Kapondera, S. K., Chipeta, G. T., Majawa, F., & Nyasulu, C. (2020). Towards e-judicial services in Malawi: Implications for justice delivery. *The Electronic Journal on Information Systems in Developing Countries, 86*(2), e12121. doi:10.1002/isd2.12121

Chawinga, W. D., & Zinn, S. (2016). Use of Web 2.0 by students in the Faculty of Information Science and Communications at Mzuzu University, Malawi. *South African Journal of Information Management, 18*(1), 1–15. doi:10.4102ajim.v18i1.694

Creswell, J. W. (2014). *Qualitative, Quantitative and Mixed Methods Approaches* (4th ed.). SAGE Publication.

DeLone, W. H., & McLean, E. R. (2016). Information Systems Success Measurement. *Foundations and Trends in Information Systems, 2*(1), 1–116. doi:10.1561/2900000005

Donner, J., & Escobari, M. X. (2010). A review of evidence on mobile use by micro and small enterprises in developing countries. *Journal of International Development, 22*(5), 641–658. doi:10.1002/jid.1717

Friderichs, G., Foh, K., & Gathinji, C. M. (2014). *mHealth Country Feasibility Report Malawi*. https://www.gsma.com/mobilefordevelopment/programme/mhealth/gsma-country-feasibility-report-malawi-2014

GSMA. (2021). *Mobile Economy*. https://data.gsmaintelligence.com/api-web/v2/research-file-download?id=60621126&file=250621-Mobile-Economy-2021.pdf

Kaium, M. A., Bao, Y., Alam, M. Z., Hasan, N., & Hoque, M. R. (2019). Understanding the insight of factors affecting mHealth adoption: A systematic review. *International Journal of Research in Business and Social Science, 8*(6), 181-200.

Källander, K., Tibenderana, J. K., Akpogheneta, O. J., Strachan, D. L., Hill, Z., ten Asbroek, A. H. A., Conteh, L., Kirkwood, B. R., & Meek, S. R. (2013). Mobile health (mHealth) approaches and lessons for increased performance and retention of community health workers in low-and middle-income countries: A review. *Journal of Medical Internet Research, 15*(1), e17. doi:10.2196/jmir.2130 PMID:23353680

Kothari, C. R. (2004). *Research Methodology: Methods and Techniques (3rd ed.)*. New Age International Publishers.

Kruse, C., Betancourt, J., Ortiz, S., Luna, S. M. V., Bamrah, I. K., & Segovia, N. (2019). Barriers to the use of mobile health in improving health outcomes in developing countries: Systematic review. *Journal of Medical Internet Research, 21*(10), e13263. doi:10.2196/13263 PMID:31593543

Malanga, D. F. (2017). Implementation of Mobile Health Initiatives in Malawi: Current Status, Issues, and Challenges. Health Information Systems and Advancement of Medical Practice in Developing Countries, 115-128. doi:10.4018/978-1-5225-2262-1.ch007

Malanga, D. F. (2017b). *Assessing information literacy skills: A survey of undergraduate education students at the University of Livingstonia in Malawi.* https://digitalcommons.unl.edu/libphilprac/1806/

Malanga, D. F. (2020). *Tackling Gender-Based Cyber Violence against Women and Girls in Malawi amidst the Covid-19 Pandemic.* African Declarations on Internet Rights and Freedoms & APC, 1-12. https://africaninternetrights.org/sites/default/files/Donald_Flywell-1.pdf

Malanga, D. F. (2022). The Prevalence of Online Violence Against Female Students at a Private University in Malawi. In Handbook of Research on Digital Violence and Discrimination Studies (pp. 451-465). doi:10.4018/978-1-7998-9187-1.ch019

Malanga, D. F., & Banda, M. (2021). *ICT Use and Livelihoods of Women Microenterprises in Malawi.* arXiv preprint arXiv:2108.09807.

Malanga, D. F., & Banda, M. J. (2021b). *The use of mobile phones by women microenterprises in Malawi: a sustainable livelihoods perspective.* Global Knowledge, Memory and Communication. doi:10.1108/GKMC-09-2020-0143

Malanga, D. F., & Chigona, W. (2018). Mobile Health Initiatives in Malawi: Understanding Impact, Funding Model and Challenges. *International Journal of Privacy and Health Information Management*, *6*(1), 49–60. doi:10.4018/IJPHIM.2018010104

Malawi Communications Regulatory Authority. (2015). *National Survey on Access and Usage of ICT Services in Malawi.* http://www.macra.org.mw/wp-content/uploads/2016/01/MACRA-Survey-Report-National-Household-and-Individual-access-to-and-usage-of-ICT.pdf

Malawi National Health Policy. (2017). https://npc.mw/wp-content/uploads/2020/07/national-health-policy.pdf

Munyua, S., Rotich, G., & Kimwele, M. (2015). Factors affecting the adoption of mhealth in maternal health care in nakuru provincial general hospital. *Int J Sci Technol Res*, *2015*, 4.

NationalICT Policy. (2013). https://www.itu.int/en/ITU-D/Cybersecurity/Documents/National_Strategies_Repository/Malawi_2013_Malawi_ICT_Policy.pdf

National Statistics Office. (2015). *Survey on Access and Usage of ICT services in Malawi.* https://www.yumpu.com/en/document/view/55017822/national-survey-on-access-to-andusage-of-ict-services-in-malawi-2015

Nguyen, T. D., Nguyen, T. M., & Cao, T. H. (2015). Information systems success: a literature review. In *International Conference on Future Data and Security Engineering* (pp. 242-256). Springer. 10.1007/978-3-319-26135-5_18

Njoroge, M., Zurovac, D., Ogara, E. A. A., Chuma, J., & Kirigia, D. (2017). Assessing the feasibility of eHealth and mHealth: A systematic review and analysis of initiatives implemented in Kenya. *BMC Research Notes, 10*(1), 90. doi:10.118613104-017-2416-0 PMID:28183341

Nyaga, G. N. (2021). *mHealth Impact on Demand-Capacity Mismatch in Accessing Health Services in Africa.* https://research.wpcarey.asu.edu/carisca/wp-content/uploads/2021/07/Session-1-Gilbert-Nyaga-mHealth.pdf

Nyemba-Mudenda, M., & Chigona, W. (2018). mHealth outcomes for pregnant mothers in Malawi: A capability perspective. *Information Technology for Development, 24*(2), 245–278. doi:10.1080/02681102.2017.1397594

Osah, O., & Kyobe, M. (2017). Predicting user continuance intention towards M-pesa in Kenya. *African Journal of Economic and Management Studies, 8*(1), 36–50. doi:10.1108/AJEMS-03-2017-148

Pankomera, R., & van Greunen, D. (2018). A model for implementing sustainable mHealth applications in a resource-constrained setting: A case of Malawi. *The Electronic Journal on Information Systems in Developing Countries, 84*(2), e12019. doi:10.1002/isd2.12019

SC4CCM. (2018). *Emerging Lessons of Cstock.* http://sc4ccm.jsi.com/emerging-lessons/cstock/

Saunders, M., Lewis, P., & Thornhill, A. (2016). *Research Methods for Business Students* (7th ed.). Apprentice Hall.

Shieshia, M., Noel, M., Andersson, S., Felling, B., Alva, S., Agarwal, S., Lefevre, A., Misomali, A., Chimphanga, B., Nsona, H., & Chandani, Y. (2014). Strengthening community health supply chain performance through an integrated approach: Using mHealth technology and multilevel teams in Malawi. *Journal of Global Health, 4*(2). Advance online publication. doi:10.7189/jogh.04.020406 PMID:25520796

Shiferaw, S., Workneh, A., Yirgu, R., Dinant, G. J., & Spigt, M. (2018). Designing mHealth for maternity services in primary health facilities in a low-income setting–lessons from a partially successful implementation. *BMC Medical Informatics and Decision Making*, *18*(1), 1–14. doi:10.118612911-018-0704-9 PMID:29301576

UNICEF Malawi. (2020). *Annual Report*. https://www.unicef.org/malawi/media/4981/file/UNICEF%20Malawi%20Annual%20Report%202020.pdf

United Nations Development Programme (UNDP). (2020). http://www.mw.undp.org/

World Health Organization (WHO). (2011). mHealth: New horizons for health through mobile technologies. Global Observatory for eHealth Series, 3.

KEY TERMS AND DEFINITIONS

Cstock mHealth: Is a rapid Short Message Service (SMS) and web-based reporting and resupply system that is used by community health workers to report stock data through mobile phones.

Healthcare Supply Chain Management: Involves obtaining health resources, managing health supplies, and delivering them to health providers and patients.

Information and Communication for Development (ICT4D): Is the practice of utilising ICT to support socio-ecomic growth and well-being of poor and marginalised people in developing communities.

Information and Communication Technology: Consists of hardware, software, networks, and media for collection, storage, processing, transmission, and presentation of information (voice, data, text, images).

mHealth: Refers to the provision of health services and information through mobile technologies such as mobile phones, Personal Digital Assistants, and mobile tablets.

Mobile Technology: Refers to mobile phones, smartphones, Portable Assistant Devices (PDAs) that facilitate the performance of tasks.

Primary Healthcare: Is the first level of contact for individuals, family, and the community with the national health system in addressing main health problems, providing health promotion, rehabilitative, and curative health services.

Chapter 7
Reliability of Performance Factors for Evaluating Electronic Health Information Systems

Margaret Nagwovuma
Makerere University, Uganda

Agnes Nakakawa
Makerere University, Uganda

Gilbert Maiga
Makerere University, Uganda

Emmanuel Eilu
https://orcid.org/0000-0002-2482-0535
Uganda Christian University, Uganda

ABSTRACT

This chapter investigates the reliability of performance factors for evaluating electronic health information systems. The chapter posits that assessing information system functions performance like electronic health information systems (EHIS) has been an issue for information systems executives who continue to seek evidence for returns on information technology investments. Apparently, there is no fit-it-all standard performance evaluation approach designed for evaluating EHIS because choosing between indicators is dependent on values and objectives that informed the evaluation. In this chapter, different approaches for information systems performance evaluation and EHIS evaluation were assessed to establish factors that should be incorporated in performance evaluation. Findings reveal that net benefits, quality of system, quality of information, system use, quality of service, organisational factors, personnel factors, user satisfaction can be used as the measurements of the resilience of EHIS.

DOI: 10.4018/978-1-7998-8915-1.ch007

INTRODUCTION

The International Telecommunication Union (ITU) defines an electronic health system (eHealth) as a computerised medical record used to capture, store, and share information amongst healthcare providers within an organisation, supporting the delivery of healthcare services to patients. Over the decade, there has been a growing number of eHealth initiatives in developing countries, most of which are donor-funded. The presence of ICTs and technological innovations has given health services providers the means to diagnose, prevent disease, treat problems and illnesses, and facilitate the provision of health services. Benefits of eHealth include ease of access to health information, reduction in medical errors, efficiency in healthcare delivery, improvement and support for medical training and research facilitation, and improvement of management and supervision for health services. In addition, eHealth technologies can improve communication between health institutions, medication management and ordering and follow-up and detect patient care and progress. However, it is vital to show that the current growth for eHealth is driven by consumer preferences, technical capabilities, health system policy and economic considerations.

ICT in the Health Sector

eHealth initiatives in developing countries support a wide range of ICT applications ranging from computer-based health systems to mobile health systems supported by e-infrastructures, internet and other worldwide systems of integrated advanced high-performance networking. According to the global survey on eHealth conducted by the WHO in 2015, 57 out of 125 (about 46%) of the low- and middle-income countries have a National Electronic Health (EHR) system (Silvestre, 2018). These EHR systems were set up to improve the quality and efficiency of healthcare in these countries (Schopf et al., 2019). A study by Moucheraud et al. (2017) on the sustainability of health information systems based on a qualitative study in Southern Africa acknowledges the significance of Health information systems in developing countries as central to strong health systems in Malawi, Zambia and Zimbabwe. The study points out the importance of these systems to improve on the following; disease surveillance, quality improvement, program management and strategic use of information. In this study, eHealth initiatives are referred to as Electronic Health Information Systems (EHIS). According to McHaney et al. (2019), these are "electronic systems used by healthcare facilities to collect, store, manage and share patient's electronic health or medical records for patient care research and quality management". (Khubone, Tlou, and Mashamba-Thompson, 2020) defines EHIS as

" systems that support healthcare workers in providing health care services to an individual client to enable data exchange among service providers".

Blaya et al. (2010) identified and classified eHealth initiatives systems in developing countries into eight significant categories, i.e. electronic health record, laboratory information management systems, pharmacy Information Systems (IS), patient registration or scheduling systems, monitoring, evaluation, and patient tracking systems, clinical decision support systems (DSS), patient reminder systems and research/data collection systems. Electronic health records are created using ICTs about a person; thus, they can be modified by different medical personnel or staff (Kiberu, Mars, and Scott, 2017). Laboratory IS are used to report any patient's laboratory results to healthcare personnel and administrators (Kasusse et al., 2014). Pharmacy Information systems are used to track medication for patients using computerised data entry. Patient registration IS being used to manage patients through different stages of healthcare at a medical facility (Hindemark, 2013). Monitoring, evaluation and patient tracking IS are used to collect and report information about a patient, monitor and follow-up on patient's status, for example, use of the Health Management Information System (HMIS) and Mobile Tracking (mTrac) system in Uganda. Clinical DSS are used to improve decision making using IS to make patient-specific recommendations. Patient reminder IS being used to remind a patient to perform a particular task, like taking medication at a particular time. Lastly, research/ data collection IS being used to collect data for research-based purposes.

However, these initiatives experience several challenges such as technology and operational, social and cultural, native environment, legal, policymaking and financial challenges (Khalifehsoltani & Gerami, 2010). In this regard, evaluations are conducted to facilitate key personnel in eHealth (i.e. Information System and or Technology Information System and or Technology (IS/T) for health) to improve their efficiency and effectiveness in operations (Bethlehem.edu). Information System and or Technology (IS/T) Evaluation is defined as a decision-making technique that facilitates organisations to benchmark and establishes costs, benefits, risks and implications of investing in IS/T systems and infrastructures (Arviansyah & Hillergersberg, 2015). Evaluation of Electronic Health Information Systems (EHIS) helps ascertain the extent to which desired objectives are met. Evaluation of EHIS can either be summative or formative (Chen et al., 2011).

It is important to note that most EHIS implementations in developing countries are acquired as ready products and implemented, donor-funded with stipulated timelines, some are replicated (Kiberu et al., 2017). In addition, it is not easy to justify the investment made for these initiatives to plan for their sustainability or continuity in a bid to solicit funding. Thus, if summative evaluation is conducted periodically, it would play a pivotal role to realise improvement in the performance of EHIS about the set objectives to guide decision making on available systems and plan for new initiatives.

On the other hand, as organisations increasingly depend on Information Systems to attain their desired goals and objectives, evaluating the performance is deemed essential and a critical issue for IS executives to handle (Saunders and Jones, 2015). Evaluation is sustained before and after comparing any intervention in terms of ascertaining improvement, while performance focuses on particular results targeted by different interventions (Barr, 2013). A working definition of performance evaluation of EHIS was adopted from the work of Cassandra (2020) as a formal and dynamic process facilitated by organisations to provide feedback on EHIS performance at a point in time. Those results are documented for further action. Saunders and Jones (2015) showed an urgent need to refine IS performance measures. Consequently, performance evaluations vary in structure and format depending on the organisation. These may include rating scales, self-assessment checklists, formal observations or performance tasks (Cassandra, 2020).

However, choosing between these indicators or measures is largely dependent on the values and objectives driving the evaluation. Even though evaluating the effectiveness of an electronic health information system (EHIS) is observed as one of the main issues in health information systems research, there is a need for well-defined outcome measures to compare results from different research studies. In this case, success measures are highly needed as requirements to evaluate the health information system, policies and procedures. However, it is unlikely to be found such a desirable measure to be found (Eivazzadeh, 2019). Fortunately for us, research provides taxonomies of success variables that can be used in different circumstances. Overall, the success of a health information system can be evaluated in three ways, namely; Quality of information provided to the stakeholders, the effect or impact of the health information system on stakeholder's actions or decisions and lastly, the effect or impact of the health information system on the organisational level costs and benefits (Ahrq, 2019; Ammenwerth et al., 2003). In this regard, different approaches have been developed to evaluate EHIS.

Donors and funders of eHealth are advised to sponsor evaluations as part of eHealth implementations to ensure that future investments in eHealth are focused on achieving the desired intentions (Blaya et al., 2010). Furthermore, to ensure proper implementation, continuity and sustainability of these multimillion-dollar initiatives in developing countries, there is a need to evaluate the performance of eHealth in these countries (Omaswa, 2016). Blaya et al. (2010) add that to realise more benefits of eHealth in developing countries, long term follow-up rigorous evaluations are required by independent evaluators.

eHealth Evaluation Challenge

Whereas several developing countries have adopted eHealth, evaluating eHealth initiatives in these countries has been a great challenge (Ammenwerth et al., 2003; Blaya et al., 2010; Lau & Kuziemsky, 2016). For example, a report published by the WHO (2010) recognised the ability of eHealth to transform the health system in many African countries (Molefi, 2010). Conversely, out of the 52 eHealth projects studied in East, South, West, North, Central Africa, and also the Indian Ocean Islands of Mauritius and Madagascar, the same report pointed out that the overall success of these eHealth projects was uncertain as a result of the limited documentation and proper evaluation of the projects.

In the study conducted by Shuvo et al. (2015), it was reported that 70% of African countries have an eHealth implementation, and less than 10% have evaluated these implementations. Nabukenya and Ashaba (2019) also acknowledged that evaluating the outcome and impact attributed to eHealth initiatives in a country like Uganda had not been a key activity with most of the eHealth implementers. Only 50% of the eHealth implementers carried out eHealth evaluation to a great extent (Nabukenya & Ashaba, 2019). In another study conducted to assess the feasibility of eHealth projects studied, only 28 (41%) reported having evaluated the project under implementation (Njoroge et al., 2017). Nabukenya and Ashabe (2019) attributed the limited level of evaluating eHealth initiatives in Uganda to the fact that the country did not have guidelines on impact evaluation for eHealth implementation. However, Vis et al. (2020) add that it may be difficult to effectively evaluate the performance of eHealth initiatives due to the diverse and rapidly evolving nature of the technological properties and the amalgamative nature of eHealth. This is about the interconnectedness of eHealth with behaviour, cultural and organisational aspects of healthcare delivery; thus a need to explore available performance evaluation approaches.

eHealth Evaluation Approaches

Several approaches have been developed to evaluate eHealth initiatives; these include; Performance of Routine Information Systems (PRISM) (Aqil et al., 2009); Human Organisation and Technology-fit (HOT-Fit) (Yusof et al., 2008), Infoway benefits evaluation framework (source: Lau et al., 2007); Clinical, Human, Organisation, Education, Administrative, Technical and Social (CHEATS) (Shaw, 2002); Health Information Technology Research-based Evaluation Framework (HITREF) (Sockolow, 2012); and an evaluation framework for Laboratory Information Systems (TTP-LIS) (Yusof & Arifin, 2016).

However, back in 2008, the ITU stressed that there is no universally-acknowledged methodology for evaluating eHealth solutions, either in industrialised countries or in the developing world. Moreover, in 2020, Bonten (2020) observed that eHealth researchers find it difficult to determine the most suitable evaluation approach to evaluate novel eHealth. Thus, prompting the need to explore available Information System (IS) performance evaluation measures since EHIS are a category of IS within the health sector.

Information System Performance Evaluation Factors

Sulaiman (1996) derived taxonomy of 7 categories of Information System performance evaluation measures. These include; operational, Service performance, system development, personnel, managerial, strategic and financial performance factors. The first category is operational performance factors, defined as "measurable aspects of outcomes" that affect information systems within an organization (Azim et al., 2015). Operational factors include; **quality of system, quality of information, system utility and user satisfacti**on (Sulaiman, 1996). Details of each of these four factors are as follows. The role of quality of system is to measure the desired functionality and effectiveness characteristics of EHIS and interactivity (Zaidi, 2017). Quality of system factors includes; Reliability, Technical support, Information Sharing, Ease of use, Learning/research, EHIS accessibility, Responsiveness, Data Accuracy, Data currency, EHIS security, Flexibility of EHIS, Response time, Performance efficiency, Completeness of functionality, EHIS availability, Knowledge transfer, Cost-effectiveness, Perceived usefulness, Maintainability, Awareness and Portability (ISO, 2011; Sulaiman, 1996; Zaidi, 2017). **Quality of Information** is concerned by the worth of information produced by the system/technology (Yusof et al., 2008). Information produced by EHIS includes; patient records, reports, images and prescriptions. Thus, it is crucial to identify the measures of information quality (Zaidi, 2017; Yusof et al., 2008; DeLone and McLean, 2003). Quality of information includes Legibility, Usefulness, Reliability, Timeliness, Importance, Relevance, Understandability and Geo-enablement (Ebener et al., 2018; Sulaiman, 1996).

System utility is one sub-criterion under operational factors considered for successful IS implementations in organisations (Liang et al., 2007). Sulaimain (1996) referred to system utility as the attitude or willingness to use the Information Systems (IS). Aspects of system utility include; Amount of Use, Frequency of Use, Nature and purpose of use, Motivation and acceptance, Knowledge, and Belief and expectations (DeLone and McLean, 2003; Liang et al., 2007; Sulaiman, 1996; Yusof et al., 2008; Zaidi, 2017). **User Satisfaction** is the last sub-criterion under operational factors. User satisfaction is a predominant construct under the Delone and McLean Information System success model (2003), used to evaluate EHIS. User satisfaction is defined as the overall evaluation of a user's experience in using the system and the potential impact (Yusof et al., 2008). Therefore, it can be related to the user's perceived usefulness and attitudes towards EHIS, which are influenced by his/her characteristics. User satisfaction includes satisfaction with specific functions, overall satisfaction, perceived usefulness, enjoyment, software satisfaction and decision making (DeLone and McLean, 2003; Yusof et al., 2008; Zaidi, 2017).

The second category of IS performance factors is Service performance. Predominantly referred to as quality of service under the Delone and McLean Information System success model (2003), it is concerned with support availed by the service provider of EHIS technology regardless of whether the service is delivered internally or outsourced (Yusof et al., 2008). When services are delivered in time, the IS department makes effective, timely and resourceful decisions, in turn improving on internal organisational efficiency (Zaidi, 2017). Aspects of service performance include; Responsiveness, Assurance, Flexibility of services, Empathy, Cost Reductions, EHIS Training and Service Provider Quality (Chang and King, 2005; DeLone and McLean, 2003; Yusof et al., 2008; Zaidi, 2017).

The third category of performance factors is system development. It promotes an organised approach to system design, development and documentation throughout the organisation. Sulaiman (1996) points out that although system development performance evaluation has not been one top 5 five priorities to be measured, efforts should be put in place to consider it whenever evaluating IS performance is to be done. Aspects of System development include; Developed and completed within time, Developed and completed within budget, Consideration of user needs, Availability of EHIS documentation, Active help desk, Timely responses, Compliance to standards, Developed by skilled personnel and User involvement (ISO, 2011; Sulaiman, 1996). Out of seven, the fourth category of IS performance evaluation factors is personnel. In every organisation, personnel are required to develop, operate and maintain an information system; thus, their interests as stakeholders should be addressed. Therefore, organisations should keep their personnel technically competent to achieve the desired system goals, primarily through adequate training. Personnel factors include; Technical capabilities, Training and Career satisfaction (Sulaiman, 1996).

Managerial performance factors are the fifth category of IS performance evaluation factors, must be measured because managers are in charge of running the organisation; thus, their support is needed to ensure the IS perform as it was designed to do (Sulaiman, 1996). Managerial factors include; senior management attitude and user's manager's attitude. The sixth category of IS performance evaluation factors is the strategic factors. Strategically, comprehensive approaches are needed to help businesses/organisations achieve their goals (Tapera, 2014). Strategic factors include; Competitive advantage, Increase in profit and market share and Information system importance.

Lastly, the seventh category of IS performance evaluation factors is financial factors. These are used to compute the value of the EHIS concerning costs and benefits. Alternatively, they can be referred to as factors that are used to evaluate alternatives concerning financial measures (Igi-global, 2021). Sulaiman highlighted different aspects of financial factors such as using cost-benefit analysis, Information economics, Profit contribution, Budget performance, Return on investment, Return on management, cost of maintaining the system, distribution of cost by industry, matching objective, projects and technique, Critical success factors, art criticism, professional review and quasi-legal (adversary), among others.

The Information System Functional Scorecard (ISFS) model is another model for evaluating the performance of IS; it is based on IS' role to support organisational performance and business process effectiveness (Chang and King, 2005). The model considers three dimensions, i.e., system performance, information effectiveness and service performance. System performance assesses different quality aspects of information systems and impacts of IS on the user's operations like; ease of use, reliability, system features, effect on internal processes, effect on external constituents on the job, among others. Information effectiveness assesses the quality of information produced from the available information systems in relation to the Intrinsic quality of information, contextual quality of information, presentation, accessibility, reliability, flexibility and usefulness, among others. Lastly, service performance assesses the quality and flexibility a user attains based on the services availed by the IS function, right from system development to help desk services. Service performance is measured based on responsiveness, reliability, service provider quality, empathy, training, flexibility, cost/benefit of services, among others.

The product quality model, i.e. ISO/IEC 25010:2011, is used as a basis for assessing the properties of software products. The model considers eight quality characteristics. These include; Functional suitability, Performance efficiency, Compatibility, Usability, Reliability, Security, Maintainability and Portability (ISO, 2011). Kanaan and Shahizan (2016) urge that the updated Delone and McLean Information System success model (2003) is widely used by IS researchers for understanding, organising and assessing IS success in different domains like eHealth. The Delone and Mclean IS success model is comprised of 6 significant variables, i.e., information quality, system quality, service quality, use, user satisfaction and net benefits. Yusof et al. (2008) extended the Delone and McLean Information System success model (2003) with the Technology Task Fit model and developed the HOTfit framework. HOTfit is comprised of the following categories or groupings, i.e., Human (use and user satisfaction), Technology (information quality, system quality, and service quality), Organisation and Net benefits.

Lastly, EHIS potential and performance that elevated using geospatial data and technologies. Ebener et al. (2018) developed a framework of 9 factors to guide the geo-enabling of EHIS. The nine factors are; i) a vision, strategy, and plan for geo-enabling the HIS; (ii) An IS governance structure covering geospatial data and technologies; (iii) A minimum technical capacity to manage and use geospatial data and technologies (iv)Defined geospatial data specifications, standards and protocols, (v) Master lists for the core geographic objects (e.g., health facilities, villages, administrative and reporting divisions) and a common geo-registry, (vi) Appropriate geospatial technologies, (vii) Map production and use, (viii) Policies supporting and enforcing all of the above as well as geospatial data accessibility; and (ix) resources for sustainability. Using these nine factors, available EHIS's performance can be improved to guide decision-makers in planning, allocation and distribution of resources, identification of disadvantaged areas and supporting a more comprehensive array of multi-disciplinary research, among others (Aghajani, Farnia and Velayati, 2017).

Research shows that several approaches have been developed eHealth initiatives' performance (Aqil, Lippeveld, & Hozumi, 2009; Sockolow, Bowles, & Rogers, 2015; Yusof & Arifin, 2016; Vis et al., 2020). However, they do not capture eHealth's diverse aspects and amalgamative nature in a particular contextual setting. Many approaches majorly focus on the technological aspect of eHealth and put little or no consideration on aspects such as behaviour, cultural and organisational aspects of the initiative in a particular kind of setting (Lee, 2016; Vis et al., 2016; Ashaba and Nabukenya, 2020). There is no "fit it all" standard performance evaluation approach designed for evaluating eHealth (Bonten et al., 2020; Vis et al., 2020). Thus, this study attempts to extend the key modules of the HOTfit framework to build a robust approach to evaluate the performance of EHIS in the developing country's context, as elaborated in the following subsection. In summary, the following factors for EHIS performance evaluations have been identified based on the HOTfit framework and other approaches, these include; Quality of information, Quality of System, System Use, User satisfaction, Personnel, Organisation (structure and environment) and Quality of Service. These factors were used to identify a better approach for evaluating the performance of EHIS, as explained below.

- **Quality of System**: Quality of system is defined as a measure of the extent to which the system is technically sound (Narasimhaiah et al., 2010). Governments have adopted EHIS to improve service delivery in the health sector, both web-based and mobile applications. In this regard, it becomes essential to identify aspects required to measure system quality from existing studies (DeLone & McLean, 2003; Maryati Mohd Yusof et al., 2008). These include; Reliability, Technical support, Information Sharing, Ease of use, Learning/research, EHIS accessibility, Responsiveness, Data Accuracy, Data currency, EHIS security, Flexibility of EHIS, Response time, Performance efficiency, Completeness of functionality, EHIS availability, Knowledge transfer, Cost-effectiveness, Perceived usefulness, Maintainability, Awareness and Portability. Sulaiman (1996) recommends that as part of information system performance, System development is a measure of evaluation for IS Performance. System development promotes an organised approach to system design, development and documentation throughout the organisation. Thus, it is prudent to identify its measures, i.e., Developed and completed within time, Developed and completed within budget, Consideration of user needs, Availability of EHIS documentation, Active help desk, Timely responses, Compliance to standards, Developed by skilled personnel and User involvement (Sulaiman, 1996).

- **Quality of information**: The quality of information produced by an information system/technology is used to measure its operational performance (Maryati Mohd Yusof et al., 2008). EHIS produces information used as a basis for system development and enables users to execute their tasks (Sulaiman, 1996). Ebener, Roth, and Khetrapal (2018) urges that it is also vital to improve the performance of EHIS by using spatial data and technologies to improve healthcare delivery. Spatial data is simply a quality of information. Therefore, quality of information is measured by; Legibility, Usefulness, Reliability, Timeliness, Importance, Relevance, Understandability and Geo-enablement.
- **Quality of Service**: conversely, IS/IT departments operate as service units for various users in an organisation, and organisational achievement depends on how well the IS services are delivered. Service quality can be measured through Responsiveness, Assurance, Flexibility of services, Empathy, Cost Reductions, EHIS Training and Service Provider Quality (Zaidi, 2017; Yusof et al., 2008; Chang and King, 2005; DeLone and McLean, 2003). **System Use**: System use is measured by Amount of Use, Frequency of Use, Nature and purpose of use, Motivation and acceptance, Knowledge, and Belief and expectations (DeLone and McLean, 2003; Sulaiman, 1996; (Liang et al., 2007); Yusof et al., 2008; Zaidi, 2017).
- **User Satisfaction**: Measure of user satisfaction include: satisfaction with specific functions, overall satisfaction, perceived usefulness, enjoyment, software satisfaction and decision making (DeLone and McLean, 2003; Yusof et al., 2008; Zaidi, 2017). **Personnel Factors**: Personnel factors are measured with; Technical capabilities, Personnel training, Career satisfaction and Business knowledge (Sulaiman, 1996; DeLone and McLean, 2003; (Liang et al., 2007).
- **Organisation**: Yusof et al. (2008) extended the D & M IS model (2003) with organisational factors pertinent to IS evaluation in the healthcare domain. Organisational factors enable healthcare institutions to achieve their targets or purpose using an electronic health information system. These factors can be evaluated based on structure and environment. In Yusof's study, organisational

factors are measured by structure and environment. Environment factors include; Financing Source, Government / Regulatory authorities, Politics, Localisation, Competition, Inter-organisational relationship, Population served and External communication. Nevertheless, for this study, only the financing source, localisation and external communication were considered. Structure factors include; Nature (type, size), Culture, Planning and control systems, Strategy, Management, Clinical process, Autonomy, Communication, Top management support, medical staff sponsorship and teamwork. However, for this study, culture, strategy, management, top management support and teamwork were considered.

- **Net Benefits**: Electronic health information systems benefit a number of stakeholders and agencies, both public and private. Net benefits measure the difference between positive and negative impacts of eHealth among different stakeholders and organisations. The benefits can be at both individual and organisational levels. At the individual level, it is associated with performance, user task change, and improved productivity. Furthermore, at the organisational level, net benefits are defined as the impact of information on organisational performance, especially healthcare delivery. The measures of Net benefits include; Efficiency, Communication, Effectiveness and Decision making (DeLone & McLean, 2003; Kiberu et al., 2014; Yusof et al., 2008).

It is evident that there are no factors defined to systematically evaluate the performance of EHIS to inform and support decision making for policy and practice (Vis et al., 2020). Therefore, it is prudent to explore factors for the performance evaluation of EHIS in developing countries. It was based on this evidence that a study was carried out in Uganda guided by the following questions; a) What are the factors for performance evaluation for EHIS? b) What is the reliability of the identified factors? In the context of Uganda, this study sought to identify and examine the reliability of those factors for performance evaluation for EHIS. The objective of this chapter is achieved in the following subsections; section 2 as the materials and methods, section 3 as the presentation of results, section 4 as the discussion of results, and lastly, section 5 as the conclusion.

MATERIALS AND METHODS

A survey was conducted in Uganda as a case of a developing country. Within Uganda a sample of 15 out of 146 districts (EC, 2020) were selected for the study i.e., Gulu, Kampala, Lira, Apac, Mbarara, Jinja, Namayingo, Iganga, Busia, Mubende, Oyam,

Nakaseke, Mityana, Luweero and Otuke. These districts were selected because they are connected to the National Internet Backbone Infrastructure (NIBI) and had electronic health system projects running in some health centres. The total number of districts on the NIBI is only 26. In addition, some districts are close (urban) to the NIBI, and others are a little distant (rural) from it.

The nature of EHIS to consider in the study were not clearly established because, on a daily basis, key EHIS users would interact with one or more systems depending on his/her role in the health sector. The respondents' organisations included Ministries, District health offices, Religious Medical Bureaus, Health Implementing Partners, Health Facilitating Partners, ICT regulators, Health facilities. Lastly, private providers for EHIS, among others. Category on respondents included; Biostatistician, Data Managers, DHO, Health Information Officer, HMIS Focal Point Person, ICT Personnel, M&E Officer, Medical Director, Medical Records Officer, Clinical officers and Other categories. Stratified sampling was used to categorise users of EHIS in both rural and urban settings. Purposively sampling was later used to select respondents who knew the subject matter. Quantitative techniques in the form of structured questions were used to obtain quantitative data, and qualitative techniques in the form of interview guides were used to gather qualitative data. Quantitative data were analysed using Stata 15.0 software and partial least squares – structured equation modelling (PLS-SEM). In this paper, only quantitative results are presented. Cronbach alpha & Fornell-Lacker criteria were used as techniques to test the reliability of the results. The composite reliability criterion is always recommended as an alternative due to its common failure to uphold the tau-equivalency assumption of Cronbach alpha. Confidentiality of respondents was maintained irrespective of their positions. Lastly, the validity and reliability of the study were sought through introduction letters and making appointments with respondents.

PRESENTATION OF RESULTS

Results from the survey are presented in the following subsections, i.e., responses and gender (3.1) and reliability testing (3.2).

- **Responses Levels and Gender**: Total responses from 15 districts are 180 (92%) of 195 questionnaires distributed. Results from analysis revealed that; 15.1% of the respondents are from Gulu district while 13.5% are from Kampala, 10.3% are from Lira, 8.7% are from Apac, 8.1% are from Mbarara, 7.6% are from Jinja, 6.5% are from Namayingo, 6% are from Iganga, 6% are from Busia, 3.8% are from Mubende, 3.8% are from Oyam, 3.2% are from

Nakaseke, 2.7% are from Mityana, 2.7% are from Luwero and 2.2% are from Otuke. 60% of the respondents were male, while 40% were female.

- **Reliability Testing**: Both content and composite reliability for the performance evaluation factors were tested by piloting the questionnaire. Content reliability was established by calculating Cronbach's Alpha Coefficient to determine its reliability and validity using stata 15.0. In making a reliability analysis, the reliability coefficients that are suitable in obtaining the reliability of the scale and the structure of the empirical study must be calculated and examined. The sample size is also essential to determine the reliability level of the scale. Cronbach's alpha reliability estimate is a measure of internal consistency, that is, how closely related a set of items are as a group. Table 3.1 summarises the reliability of scale (alpha) measures.

Table 1. Reliability of the Factors

Construct	Cronbach's Alpha Value
Net Benefits	0.791
Quality of System	0.927
Quality of Information	0.914
System Use	0.824
Quality of Service	0.821
Organisational factors	0.848
Personnel factors	0.805
User Satisfaction	0.235

Table 1 shows that most of the constructs met the required level of Cronbach's Alpha, i.e., 0.60, which is the acceptable level with the exception of user satisfaction. The net benefits construct scored 0.791 on the Cronbach Alpha scale, and hence it is above the recommended threshold of 0.6; and hence the entire construct is considered internally consistent and adopted for measurement of the resilience of EHIS. The quality of system construct scored a Cronbach Alpha value of 0.927, which is above the acceptable threshold of 0.6; hence the construct is adopted for measurement of EHIS. The quality of information construct scored 0.914 on the Cronbach Alpha scale; it proved to be internally consistent and subsequently adopted as a reliable measurement of EHIS. The construct on system use scored 0.824 on the Cronbach Alpha scale and is hence deemed a reliable construct for the measurement of EHIS and adopted. Quality of service construct scored measured 0.821 on the Cronbach Alpha scale and therefore meet the threshold for internal consistency and are adopted for the measurement of EHIS. Organisational factor construct scored 0.848 on the Cronbach Alpha scale and was therefore adopted for EHIS measurement as it meets the recommended criterion of 0.6 for construct internal consistency. Personnel factors have a Cronbach Alpha value of 0.805 hence meeting the minimum requirements for determining the internal consistency of a construct; hence it was adopted for EHIS measurement. User satisfaction scored 0.235 on the Cronbach Alpha; hence it was not accepted for EHIS measurement.

Composite reliability also referred to as construct reliability, is a measure of internal consistency in scale items and can be depicted as the total amount of true score variance relative to the total scale score variance (Brunner & SÜβ, 2005). It is also an "indicator of the shared variance among the observed variables used as an indicator of a latent construct" (Fornell & Larcker, 1981). Netemeyer et al. (2003) state in Scaling Procedures: Issues and Applications that it is "reasonable" for a narrowly defined construct with five to eight items to meet a minimum threshold of 0.80. This was calculated using PLS-SEM as shown in figure 1.

Figure 1. Reliability of constructs (Composite reliability scores)

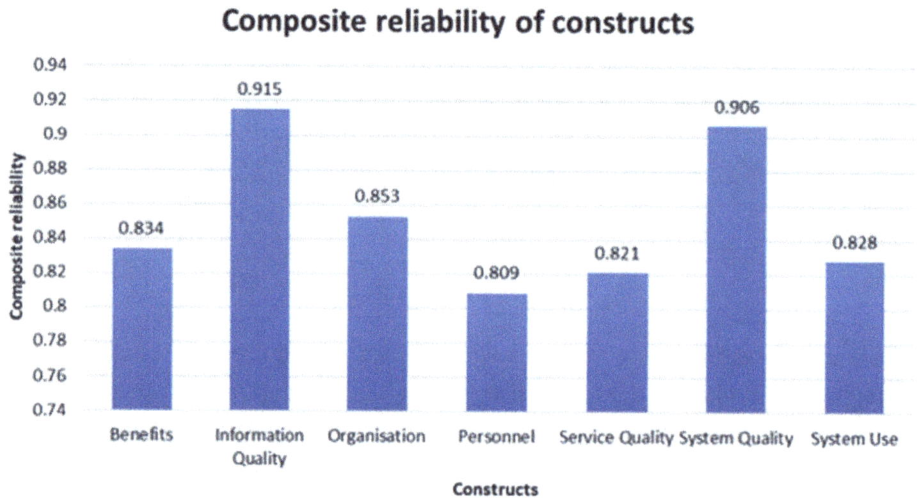

Figure 1 shows that the constructs are considered to have achieved internal consistency when the composite reliability level of each construct was calculated using the Fornell-Larcker criterion, they exceeded the threshold of 0.8 (Netemeyer et al., 2003). The ability of the constructs to meet this level of reliability indicates the replicability of the results obtained as part of this study under similar circumstances using reliable data collection instruments. Hence, the findings are reliable and reproducible.

DISCUSSION OF RESULTS

The study's objective was to identify factors for evaluating the performance of electronic health information systems and examine their reliability. Thus, questionnaires were distributed to 195 respondents from Gulu district, Kampala, Lira, Apac, Mbarara, Jinja, Namayingo, Iganga, Busia, Mubende, Oyam, Nakaseke, Mityana, Luwero, and Otuke. The response rate of 92% (180) was received, and it is in line with Fincham (2008), who states that the response rate of >60% must be the goal of every researcher. In this regard, the study attracted more responses. Especially in developing country's research, it is important to highlight how different groups contribute and are distributed with different services in the society (Stephens, Lewis, and Reddy, 2018). The reliability test of the questionnaire scales was carried out using Cronbach alpha. The Alpha coefficient method (Cronbach, 1951; Taber, 2018) is a suitable method that can be used for Likert scale items (e.g., 1-3, 1-4, 1-5) and is not limited to the true-false or correct-incorrect format. At the same time, Taber (2018) and Nunnally (1988) posits that an alpha value of 0.60 and 0.70 or above is considered to be the criteria for considering internal consistency of the new scales and the established scales, respectively. In the study to model digital library success using the Delone and Mclean Information success model, the Cronbach alpha for quality of information, quality of service and quality of system scored 0.831, 0.784, 0.788, respectively. In this study, the net benefits construct scored 0.791, quality of system construct scored a value of 0.927, quality of information construct scored 0.914, construct on system use scored 0.824, quality of service construct scored measured 0.821, Organisational factor construct scored 0.848, Personnel factors have a Cronbach Alpha value of 0.805, and the User satisfaction construct scored 0.235, and maybe the reason being the construct could not have much influence in this study. Most of the constructs passed the Cronbach alpha test with coefficients above 0.7. The results indicated internal consistency among indicators (Alzahrani et al., 2017). Regarding composite reliability, the net benefits construct scored 0.834, quality of system construct scored a value of 0.906, quality of information construct scored 0.915, construct on system use score o.828, quality of service construct score measured 0.821, organisational factors construct scored 0.853, personnel factors have a Cronbach alpha of 0.809.

The composite reliability scores were generally the same or slightly higher for the Cronbach Alpha scores except for the quality of system construct, with the differences ranging from 0 for the quality of service construct to 0.043 for the net benefits construct. This comparison is consistent with the results of Peterson and Kim (2013), who found that an analysis of 2,524 pairs of coefficient alpha and composite reliability values revealed a difference that was insignificant for practical applications. Al-Mamary et al. (2014) point out that, to date, information systems use modern technologies to present users with easy-to-understand information. In addition, given the proper support, users can use information systems effectively. The relevance of results for use, organisation and personnel are supported by Erixon (2012), who demonstrates that as information systems are integrated as part of daily activities to improve service delivery in organisations, organisations turn to key IS providers such as technical personnel to manage these resources. Lastly, Gustafsson et al. (2018) support the findings by highlighting that to date, organisations and practitioners that have adopted ICTs have achieved better communication, improved decision-making levels and become more effective and efficient. Hence, results from reliability indicated consistency among all factors and their relevance for evaluating the performance of Electronic Health Information Systems.

CONCLUSION

In summary, the following factors for EHIS performance evaluations have been identified; these include; Quality of information, Quality of System, System Use, Personnel, Organisation and Quality of Service. The reliability results indicated all these factors had Cronbach alpha score above 0.7. In addition, the results for composite reliability analysis revealed that all the constructs had a composite reliability score above 0.8. This proved that there is internal consistency among factors for evaluating the performance of electronic health information systems. Limitations of the study included; EHIS reporting systems, deployment level of EHIS, which excluded clinicians in Uganda who stop at data input in manual registers, timely delivery of study results and failure to navigate the western region due to lack of access to an experienced research assistant. The way forward is to test the validity of those identified factors for performance evaluation, which would, in turn, guide the design of a fit-for-all performance evaluation approach for EHIS in a developing country's context.

REFERENCES

Aghajani, J., Farnia, P., & Velayati, A. A. (2017). Impact of geographical information system on public health sciences. *Biomedical and Biotechnology Research Journal*, *1*(2), 94. doi:10.4103/bbrj.bbrj_34_17

Ahrq. (2019). *2019 National Healthcare Quality and Disparities Report*. https://www.ahrq.gov/research/findings/nhqrdr/nhqdr19/index.html

Al-Mamary, Y. H., Shamsuddin, A., & Aziati, N. (2014). The relationship between system quality, information quality, and organizational performance. *International Journal of Knowledge and Research in Management & E-Commerce, 4*, 7-10. https://www.researchgate.net/profile/Yaser-Hasan-Salem-Al-Mamary-d-yasr-hsn-almmry/publication/269463861_The_Relationship_between_System_Quality_Information_Quality_and_Organizational_Performance/links/5530f5380cf27acb0de8b002/The-Relationship-between-Sys

Alzahrani, A. I., Mahmud, I., Ramayah, T., Alfarraj, O., & Alalwan, N. (2017). *Modelling digital library success using the DeLone and McLean information system success model*. doi:10.1177/0961000617726123

Ammenwerth, E., Gräber, S., Herrmann, G., Bürkle, T., & König, J. (2003). *Evaluation of health information systems—problems and challenges*. doi:10.1016/S1386-5056(03)00131-X

Aqil, A., Lippeveld, T., & Hozumi, D. (2009). PRISM framework: A paradigm shift for designing, strengthening and evaluating routine health information systems. *Health Policy and Planning, 24*(3), 217–228. Advance online publication. doi:10.1093/heapol/czp010 PMID:19304786

Arviansyah, S. T., & Hillergersberg, J. V. (2015). Development and assessment of an instrument to measure equivocal situation and its causes in IS / IT project evaluation. *CES1*. doi:10.12821/ijispm030302

Azim, M. D., Ahmed, H., & Khan, A. S. (2015). Operational performance and profitability: An empirical study on the Bangladeshi Ceramic companies. *Researchgate.Net, 3*(1), 63–73. https://www.researchgate.net/profile/Md-Azim-2/publication/323414631_OPERATIONAL_PERFORMANCE_AND_PROFITABILITY_AN_EMPIRICAL_STUDY_ON_THE_BANGLADESHI_CERAMIC_COMPANIES/links/5b910e20a6fdcce8a4ca27f7/OPERATIONAL-PERFORMANCE-AND-PROFITABILITY-AN-EMPIRICAL-STUDY-ON-THE-BANGLADESHI-CERAMIC-COMPANIES.pdf

Blaya, J. A., Fraser, H. S. F., & Holt, B. (2010). E-health technologies show promise in developing countries. *Health Affairs, 29*(2), 244–251. Advance online publication. doi:10.1377/hlthaff.2009.0894 PMID:20348068

Bonten, T. N., Rauwerdink, A., Wyatt, J. C., Kasteleyn, M. J., Witkamp, L., Riper, H., Gemert-Pijnen, L. J., van, Cresswell, K., Sheikh, A., Schijven, M. P., & Chavannes, N. H. (2020). Online Guide for Electronic Health Evaluation Approaches: Systematic Scoping Review and Concept Mapping Study. *Journal of Medical Internet Research, 22*(8), e17774. Advance online publication. doi:10.2196/17774 PMID:32784173

Brunner, M., & SÜβ, H.-M. (2005). Analyzing the reliability of multidimensional measures: An example from intelligence research. *Journals.Sagepub. Com, 65*(2), 227–240. doi:10.1177/0013164404268669

Cassandra, W. (2020). *Employee Performance Evaluation: Definition, Benefits and How To Prepare*. https://www.indeed.com/career-advice/career-development/employee-performance-evaluation

Chang, J. C. J., & King, W. R. (2005). Measuring the performance of information systems: A functional scorecard. Journal of Management Information Systems. doi:10.1080/07421222.2003.11045833

Chen, S., Osman, N. M., Nunes, J. M. B., & Peng, G. C. (2011). Information systems evaluation methodologies. *Proceedings of the IADIS International Workshop on Information Systems Research Trends, Approaches and Methodologies*.

Cronbach, L. J. (1951). Coefficient alpha and the internal structure of tests. *Psychometrika, 16*(3), 297–334. doi:10.1007/BF02310555

DeLone, W. H., & McLean, E. R. (2003). The DeLone and McLean model of information systems success: A ten-year update. *Journal of Management Information Systems, 19*(4), 9–30. doi:10.1080/07421222.2003.11045748

Ebener, S., Roth, S., & Khetrapal, S. (2018). *Building Capacity for Geo-Enabling Health Information Systems: Supporting Equitable Health Services and Well-Being For ALL*. Academic Press.

EC. (2020). *Electoral Commission Statistics*. https://www.ec.or.ug/electoral-commission-statistics

Eivazzadeh, S. (2019). *Evaluating Success Factors of Health Information Systems*. Academic Press.

Erixon, C. (2012). *Information System Providers and Business Relationships: A Study on the Impact of Connections*. https://www.diva-portal.org/smash/record.jsf?pid=diva2:523537

Fincham, J. E. (2008). Response rates and responsiveness for surveys, standards, and the Journal. *American Journal of Pharmaceutical Education, 72*(2), 43. doi:10.5688/aj720243 PMID:18483608

Fornell, C., & Larcker, D. F. (1981). Evaluating Structural Equation Models with Unobservable Variables and Measurement Error. *JMR, Journal of Marketing Research, 18*(1), 39–50. doi:10.1177/002224378101800104

Gustafsson, M., Norlinder, J., & Rehn, M. (2018). *Using an ICT System to Increase Efficiency and Effectiveness in Patient-Practitioner Communication*. www.it.uu.se

Hindemark, F. (2013). *E-Health at Outpatient Clinics in Uganda*. https://www.diva-portal.org/smash/get/diva2:680178/FULLTEXT01.pdf

IGI-Global. (2021). *What is Financial Factors*. https://www.igi-global.com/dictionary/financial-factors/39752

ISO. (2011). *Product Quality Model*. ISO/IEC 25010:2011. https://www.iso.org/standard/35733.html

Kanaan, A. G., & Hassan, S. B., & Shahzad, A. (2016). A Conceptual Model for E-Government Success Factors in Developing Countries. *International Journal of Scientific and Research Publications, 6*(12), 39–44.

Kasusse, M., Rosette, M., Burke, E., Mwangi, C., Batamwita, R., Tumwesigye, N., & Aisu, S. (2014). Understanding ICT behaviors among health workers in sub-Saharan Africa: A cross-sectional study for laboratory persons in Uganda. *IJSSH, 8*(2), 258-261. https://citeseerx.ist.psu.edu/viewdoc/download?doi=10.1.1.975.6541&rep=rep1&type=pdf

Khalifehsoltani, S. N., & Gerami, M. R. (2010). E-health challenges, opportunities and experiences of developing countries. *International Conference on E-Education, e-Business, e-Management and e-Learning*, 264-268. 10.1109/IC4E.2010.119

Khubone, T., Tlou, B., & Mashamba-Thompson, T. P. (2020). Electronic Health Information Systems to Improve Disease Diagnosis and Management at Point-of-Care in Low and Middle Income Countries: A Narrative Review. *Diagnostics (Basel), 10*(5), 327. Advance online publication. doi:10.3390/diagnostics10050327 PMID:32443856

Kiberu, V. M., Mars, M., & Scott, R. E. (2017). Barriers and opportunities to implementation of sustainable e-Health programmes in Uganda: A literature review. African Journal of Primary Health Care and Family Medicine. doi:10.4102/phcfm.v9i1.1277

Kiberu, V. M., Matovu, J. K., Makumbi, F., Kyozira, C., Mukooyo, E., & Wanyenze, R. K. (2014). Strengthening district-based health reporting through the district health management information software system: The Ugandan experience. *BMC Medical Informatics and Decision Making*, *14*(1), 40. doi:10.1186/1472-6947-14-40 PMID:24886567

Lau, F., Hagens, S., & Muttitt, S. (2007). *A proposed benefits evaluation framework for health information systems in Canada*. Healthcare Quarterly.

Lau, F., & Kuziemsky, C. (2016). *Handbook of eHealth Evaluation: An Evidence-based Approach*. http://venus.library.uvic.ca/handle/1828/7814

Liang, T., Huang, C., Yeh, Y., & Lin, B. (2007). Adoption of mobile technology in business: A fit-viability model. *Industrial Management & Data Systems*, *107*(8), 1154–1169. doi:10.1108/02635570710822796

McHaney, R. W., Reychev, I., Azuri, J., McHaney, M. E., & Moshonov, R. (2019). *Impacts of Information Technology on Patient Care and Empowerment*. IGI Global. https://books.google.com/books?hl=en&lr=&id=kmqtDwAAQBAJ&oi=fnd&pg=PR1&dq=Roger+W.+McHaney+(Kansas+State+University,+USA),+Iris+Reychev+(Ariel+University,+Israel),+Joseph+Azuri+(Maccabi+Healthcare+Services,+Israel),+Mark+E.+McHaney+(U.S.+Air+Force,+USA)+a

Molefi, M. (2010). *An Assessment of eHealth Projects and Initiatives in Africa*. https://scholar.google.com/scholar?hl=en&as_sdt=0%2C5&q=10.%09Molefi+M.+An+Assessment+of+eHealth+Projects+and+Initiatives+in+Africa.+World+Heal+Organ+Geneva%2C+Switz.+2010.&btnG=

Moucheraud, C., Schwitters, A., Boudreaux, C., Giles, D., Kilmarx, P. H., Ntolo, N., Bangani, Z., St Louis, M. E., & Bossert, T. J. (2017). Sustainability of health information systems: A three-country qualitative study in southern Africa. *BMC Health Services Research*, *17*(1). Advance online publication. doi:10.118612913-016-1971-8 PMID:28073361

Nabukenya, J., & Ashaba, J. (2019). *Evaluation of eHealth Implementations in Uganda: Investigating Practices, Challenges and Insights*. https://europepmc.org/article/ppr/ppr147961

Netemeyer, R. G., Bearden, W. O., & Sharma, S. (2003). *Scaling procedures: Issues and applications*. Sage Publications. doi:10.4135/9781412985772

Njoroge, M., Zurovac, D., Ogara, E. A. A., Chuma, J., & Kirigia, D. (2017). Assessing the feasibility of eHealth and mHealth: A systematic review and analysis of initiatives implemented in Kenya. *BMC Research Notes*, *10*(1), 90. Advance online publication. doi:10.118613104-017-2416-0 PMID:28183341

Nunnally, J. C. (1988). *Psychometric Theory*. McGraw-Hill Book Company. http://www.sciepub.com/reference/131748

Omaswa, C. (2016). *Ministry of Health: Uganda National eHealth policy*. Academic Press.

Peterson, R. A., & Kim, Y. (2013). On the relationship between coefficient alpha and composite reliability. *The Journal of Applied Psychology*, *98*(1), 194–198. doi:10.1037/a0030767 PMID:23127213

Saunders, C. S., & Jones, J. W. (2015). Measuring Performance of the Information Systems Function. *Journal of Management Information Systems*. Advance online publication. doi:10.1080/07421222.1992.11517939

Schopf, T. R., Nedrebø, B., Hufthammer, K. O., Daphu, I. K., & Lærum, H. (2019). How well is the electronic health record supporting the clinical tasks of hospital physicians? A survey of physicians at three Norwegian hospitals. *BMC Health Services Research*, *19*(1), 934. doi:10.118612913-019-4763-0 PMID:31801518

Shaw, N. T. (2002). "CHEATS": A generic information communication technology (ICT) evaluation framework. *Computers in Biology and Medicine*, *32*(3), 209–220. Advance online publication. doi:10.1016/S0010-4825(02)00016-1 PMID:11922936

Shuvo, T. A., Islam, R., Hossain, S., Evans, J. L., Khatun, F., Ahmed, T., Gazi, R., & Adams, A. M. (2015). Innovation and Entrepreneurship in Health Dovepress eHealth innovations in LMICs of Africa and Asia: A literature review exploring factors affecting implementation, scale-up, and sustainability. *Innovation and Entrepreneurship in Health*, *2*, 95–106. doi:10.2147/IEH.S88809

Silvestre, E. (2018). *How Electronic Health Records Strengthen the Health Systems of Low- and Middle-Income Countries: Learning from Eswatini and Mexico*. Academic Press.

Sockolow, P. S., Bowles, K. H., & Rogers, M. (2015). Health Information Technology Evaluation Framework (HITREF) Comprehensiveness as Assessed in Electronic Point-of-Care Documentation Systems Evaluations. *Studies in Health Technology and Informatics*. Advance online publication. doi:10.3233/978-1-61499-564-7-406 PMID:26262081

Stephens, A., Lewis, E. D., & Reddy, S. (2018). Towards an inclusive systemic evaluation for the SDGs: Gender equality, environments and marginalized voices (GEMs). *Journals.Sagepub. Com*, *24*(2), 220–236. doi:10.1177/1356389018766093

Sulaiman, A. (1996). *A Review Of Information Systems Performance Evaluation Measures*. Academic Press.

Taber, K. S. (2018). The Use of Cronbach's Alpha When Developing and Reporting Research Instruments in Science Education. *Research in Science Education*, *48*(6), 1273–1296. doi:10.100711165-016-9602-2

Tapera, J. (2014). The importance of strategic management to business organizations. *Research Journal of Social Sciences and Management*. https://www.academia.edu/download/60296058/THEIMPORTANCEOFSTRATEGICMANAGEMENTTOBUSINESSORGANIZATION20190814-60656-fu9ked.pdf

Vis, C., Bührmann, L., Riper, H., & Ossebaard, H. C. (2020). Health technology assessment frameworks for eHealth: A systematic review. *International Journal of Technology Assessment in Health Care Cite This Article*, *36*(3), 204–216. doi:10.1017/S026646232000015X PMID:32297588

Yusof, M. M., & Arifin, A. (2016, November). Towards an evaluation framework for Laboratory Information Systems. *Journal of Infection and Public Health*, *9*(6), 766–773. Advance online publication. doi:10.1016/j.jiph.2016.08.014

Yusof, M. M., Kuljis, J., Papazafeiropoulou, A., & Stergioulas, L. K. (2008). An evaluation framework for Health Information Systems: Human, organization and technology-fit factors (HOT-fit). *International Journal of Medical Informatics*, *77*(6), 386–398. doi:10.1016/j.ijmedinf.2007.08.011 PMID:17964851

Yusof, M. M., Papazafeiropoulou, A., Paul, R. J., & Stergioulas, L. K. (2008, June). Investigating evaluation frameworks for health information systems. *International Journal of Medical Informatics*, *77*(6), 377–385. Advance online publication. doi:10.1016/j.ijmedinf.2007.08.004 PMID:17904898

Zaidi, S. (2017). *E-government services effectiveness evaluation framework (E-GEEF): A case study of Indian e-tax service*. http://repository.londonmet.ac.uk/id/eprint/1254

Chapter 8
Impediments to the Adoption of mHealth Interventions in Burundi

Patrick Ndayizigamiye
https://orcid.org/0000-0001-5721-6070
University of Johannesburg, South Africa

ABSTRACT

This chapter investigates the impediments to mHealth adoption in Burundi. A survey was conducted with 212 healthcare professionals from 48 primary healthcare centres in Burundi. The findings reveal that although there is a high acceptance of mHealth capabilities from the primary healthcare workers, a host of factors mitigate against the implementation of mHealth interventions in Burundi. Amongst these are lack of skills to develop mHealth applications, high cost of mobile devices, low rate of cellphone and other mobile devices penetration, unreliable network coverage in rural areas, and a high cost of network connection. These factors have a low effect size on the acceptance of mHealth capabilities by primary healthcare workers in Burundi. Partnerships between Burundi's Ministry of Health and mobile service providers, extensive consultation with potential users of mHealth systems, and a performance-based system are further factors that need to be considered for the successful implementation of mHealth projects in Burundi.

INTRODUCTION

Many studies have recognized the potential of mHealth capabilities to address healthcare issues in developing countries (Seidenberg et al., 2012; Bellina and Missoni,

DOI: 10.4018/978-1-7998-8915-1.ch008

2009; Colven et al., 2011; Ndayizigamiye, 2016;Ndayizigamiye & Maharaj, 2016a; Ndayizigamiye & Maharaj, 2016b;Ndayizigamiye & Maharaj, 2017; Ndayizigamiye, Hangulu & Akintola, 2017; Imaja, Ndayizigamiye & Maharaj, 2017; Ndayizigamiye & Maharaj, 2018; Matiyabu & Ndayizigamiye, 2019; Ndayizigamiye, Soni, & Jere, 2018; Soni, Ndayizigamiye, & Kante, 2019; Kante & Ndayizigamiye, 2020a; Kante & Ndayizigamiye, 2020b; Ndayizigamiye, Kante & Shingwenyana, 2020; Kante & Ndayizigamiye, 2021). Although the outcomes of some mHealth interventions have been assessed as positive (Andreatta et al., 2011; Adedeji et al., 2011; Wakadha et al., 2013), Wave (2009) emphasizes the need for designing scalable mHealth interventions. The emphasis has shifted from just having experimental and pilot projects, to having mHealth interventions that have a larger impact countrywide. Scalable mHealth interventions can also assist in building resilience within healthcare systems especially in developing settings that often experience adverse conditions that hamper the deployment of healthcare services. Indeed, many mHealth interventions have focused on the continuity of care in developing countries amid a shortage of healthcare professionals and limited access to healthcare in remote areas (Wave, 2009).

In 2014, the East African region contributed "over 30% of the global innovative healthcare delivery programs" with Kenya ranked second after India for its innovative eHealth programs (Excelsior, 2014:1). However, Burundi has lagged in terms of mHealth adoption compared to other East African Community (EAC) member states.

This chapter investigates the impediments to mHealth adoption that need to be taken into consideration for successful mHealth interventions to address healthcare challenges in Burundi and enable the attainment of the country's national health goals.

COUNTRY'S PROFILE

Burundi was classified as the fourth poorest country in the world (ADBG, 2011). It is believed that 69% of people living in rural areas are poor while the poverty level in urban areas sat at 34% (ADBG, 2011). In 2014, the ratio of doctors to inhabitants was 1:19,231, far below the World Health Organization's (WHO) recommended ratio of 1:10,000. For nurses, the ratio was 1:11,349 which is far less than the 1:3,000 WHO's recommended ratio (Burundian Ministry of Health, 2014). Furthermore, qualified doctors and nurses were unequally distributed across the country with 50% of doctors and 21% of qualified nurses based in the capital city Bujumbura. In 2006, The Government of Burundi (GoB) introduced free healthcare services for infants and mothers, but still the country is far from achieving the Sustainable Development Goals in terms of access to healthcare (Burundian Ministry of Health, 2014). In 2010, the maternal mortality rate was still very high with 800 deaths per 100,000 births (UNICEF, 2013) (see Figure 1), ranking it the fifth-highest for maternal mortality in the world (after Chad, Somalia, Sierra Leone and the Democratic Republic of Congo).

Figure 1. Trend in Maternal mortality (deaths per 100,000 live births): 1990-2015

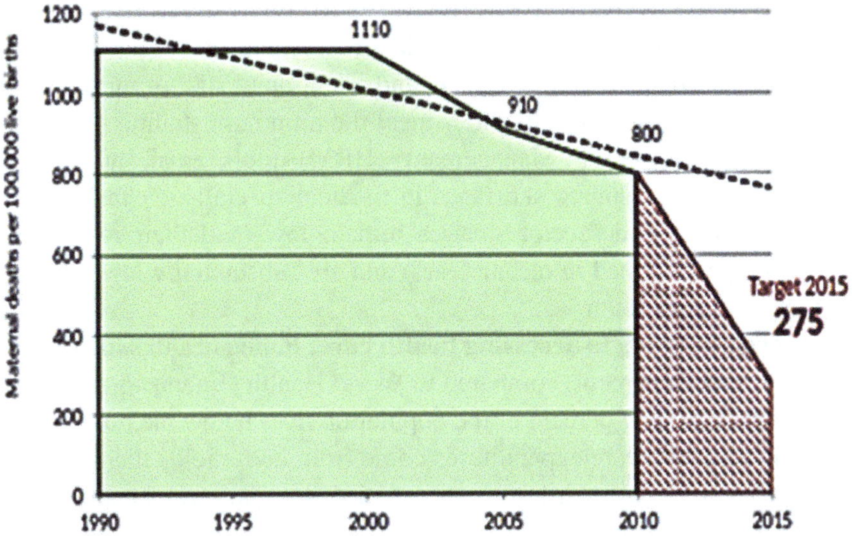

The rate of deaths of newborn babies and children below the age of 5 is still high. In 2011, the rate was 139 deaths per 1,000 live births (UNICEF, 2013). The major causes of death are pneumonia and diarrhoea which are mainly caused by malnutrition (58% of children under 5 years suffer from vitamin D deficiency), poor healthcare, and poor feeding practices.

Figure 2. Children (under 5 years) mortality rate: 1990–2015

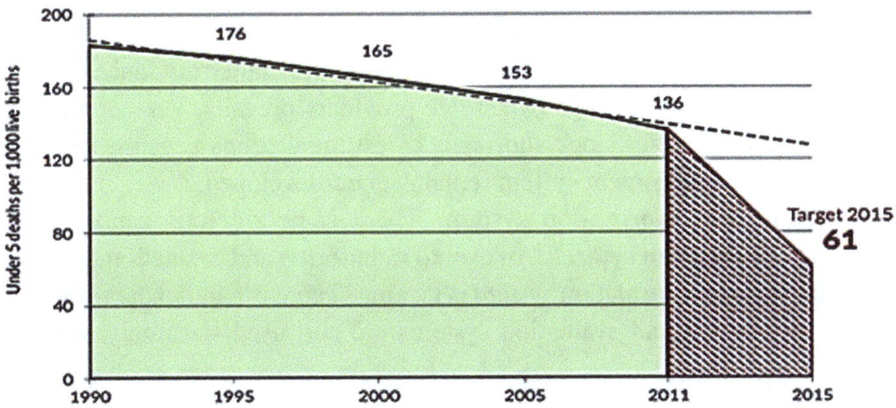

KEY CHALLENGES WITHIN THE BURUNDIAN HEALTH SECTOR

According to the Global health initiative strategy 2011-2015, the following are the key challenges that the country face:

- **Scarcity/low motivation of health professionals**: There are no clear strategies for distribution, coverage, and retention of staff in rural areas. Less than 50 percent of health facilities meet the minimum staffing requirements. No Human Resource Management (HRM) tools exist, and there are specific human resource shortages in medical specialists, pharmacists, and anaesthetists. Public sector salaries remain low (and their real value has significantly declined in recent years) and are substantially lower than those in neighbouring countries.
- **Financial barriers to accessing health care:** Public health expenditures are still low (seven percent) compared to World Health Organization's norms. In a country where 67 percent of the population lives below the poverty line, 40 percent of health care expenditures come from households themselves. Data show that about one-third of the population does not seek health care when it is needed, and among those who responded, 80 percent indicated that the prohibitive cost of health services was the main reason.
- **Poor quality of health services:** Utilization of health services remains low despite 80 percent of the population living within 5 km from a health centre, due to the perception of poor quality of public healthcare services. Systems for quality assurance are weak at all levels of the health system. Quality assurance policies, strategies, protocols, and guidelines are still lacking or not enforced, affecting diagnosis and treatment. The capacity of service providers is weak and needs strengthening.
    - **Poor access to essential medicines throughout the country:** There are insufficient resources to purchase essential drugs. There is an illicit network for essential drugs and the Government of Burundi is struggling to eradicate it. Due to limited knowledge and limited guidance, irrational prescription of drugs by service providers prevails. Very often, health facilities suffer stock shortages of essential drugs because the supply chain management system remains underdeveloped.
- **Weak health information system:** There is no rigorous national health information system in place. An overall monitoring and evaluation framework of the existing information system is lacking. There is parallel data collection; and monitoring and evaluation systems are still used separately, with each

health actor tracking its own indicators. There is a weak human resource and research capacity to generate and use information.

MHEALTH CAPABILITIES

The World Health Organisation defines mHealth as "medical and public health practice supported by mobile devices, such as mobile phones, patient monitoring devices, personal digital assistants, and other wireless devices. mHealth involves the use of and capitalisation on a mobile phone's core utility of voice and short messaging service (SMS) as well as more complex functionalities" (WHO, 2011:6). Wave (2009:9) points out that the key applications for mHealth in developing countries are:

Education and Awareness

The use of SMS is a cost-effective, efficient, and scalable way of providing outreach services for a wide range of health issues. Particularly, SMS messages can be used to inform mobile phone users about disease management, availability of health services and additional information such as testing and treatment methods (in the case of HIV and TB for instance). Wave (2009:10) further argues that "formal studies and anecdotal evidence demonstrate that SMS alerts have a measurable impact on and a greater ability to influence behaviour than radio and television campaigns". Short Message Service alerts are a convenient way to send confidential information (such as information on HIV/AIDS). In addition, SMS alerts are particularly effective in reaching populations from remote areas; providing health-related information to areas where there are no clinics, health care workers, and there is limited access to health-related information.

Short Message Service messages could be used for campaigns as "one-way alerts or interactive tools used for health-related education and communication" (Wave, 2009:10). "For example, a citizen may sign up to take a survey, delivered via SMS message, quizzing them on their knowledge about HIV/AIDS and the location of the nearest testing centre. Depending upon their responses, information regarding where and how to receive a free test will be transmitted. This interactive model has been deployed in several countries (e.g., India, South Africa, and Uganda) to promote AIDS education and testing, and provide information about other communicable diseases (such as TB), as well as to promote maternal health and educate youth about reproductive health" (Wave, 2009:10).

Remote Data Collection

There is a need for accurate data collection to assess the effectiveness of health-related interventions including existing health-related policies. Data collection is even more important in the developing world since a large portion of the population may not be able to visit hospitals even in case of an emergency. Thus, collecting data from the patients' homes is vital. Wave (2009:11) indicates that "information should ideally be updated and accessible on a real-time basis". He further argues that "the data collection process is more efficient and reliable if conducted via smartphones, PDAs, or mobile phones rather than paper-based surveys that must be submitted in person and manually entered into the central health database" (Wave, 2009:11). Thus, the use of mHealth to remotely collect data directly from the source, ensures the accuracy and reliability of the data.

Several data collection programs have been implemented in some developing countries. Wave (2009:11) contends that "these initiatives are closing the information gap that currently exists for patient's data in the developing world, enabling public officials to gauge the effectiveness of healthcare programs, allocate resources more efficiently, and adjust programs and policies accordingly".

Remote Monitoring

Developing countries are faced with several logistical problems that limit the number of patients that can be treated at hospitals and clinics. Thus, remote monitoring enables patients to be advised/treated out of the hospital. In this case, mobile technology in conjunction with other applications is a new way "to monitor health conditions, maintain caregiver appointments, or ensure medication regimen adherence" (Wave, 2009:12). Wave (2009:12) indicates that "monitoring patients at home for chronic conditions dramatically improves survival rates" as mobile technology may ensure strict adherence to medical (medicines) prescriptions. Remote monitoring using mobile technology may prove to be particularly beneficial in the case of patients with communicable and/or chronic diseases where strict adherence to a specific diet is essential.

Communication and Training of Healthcare Workers

Mobile technology is a tool that can be used to empower health workers/professionals with appropriate training by connecting them with sources of information. Thus, mobile technology does not only offer a platform to provide the needed support for health workers to perform their duties effectively, but also improves communication among health professionals/units for more efficient patient care. Mobile technology is an attractive platform for information seeking and sharing due to the shortage of landline phones and internet connectivity in developing countries. Thus, it is a platform that may sever the communication breakdown (which hampers effective care/treatment of patients in the developing world) between different health care units.

Disease and Epidemic Outbreak Tracking

The ability of mobile devices to instantaneously capture and transmit data on disease outbreaks is one of the ways that could be used to prevent and contain the spread of diseases. mHealth applications are used as an early warning system, allowing health professionals to monitor the spread of infectious diseases. Mobile networks are gradually replacing written, satellite, and radio communication emergency tracking systems. This migration contributes to the improvement of data quality and reduces costs.

Diagnostic and Treatment Support

mHealth applications can be designed to provide diagnosis and treatment advice to remote healthcare workers. This is done through access to medical information databases or medical personnel using wireless technology. mHealth-enabled diagnostics and treatment support enables patients to receive treatment from their homes or villages without being physically present at the hospital.

Given the mHealth benefits, it is anticipated that the adoption of scalable mHealth interventions will help alleviate some of the health-related challenges that Burundi currently faces.

Rapid SMS System: A Rwandan Successful mHealth Implementation Story

Rapid SMS is an open-source Information and Communications Technology (ICT) tool used for rapid configuration of SMS for data collection, analysis, transmission, and logistics coordination from a low entry mobile phone. Rapid SMS has had a positive in maternal and infants' treatment programs in countries such as Rwanda. In 2010, Rapid SMS was used by Community Health workers to monitor the health status of expectant mothers, newborn babies, and health risks and infants' nutrition. The system was a success as SMSs encouraged pregnant women to report to primary healthcare centres for checkups and treatments. The system also contributed to the reduction of home delivery; and the tracking system of newborn babies contributed to newborns receiving treatments from the first day. There was also a reduction in prenatal and maternal deaths. The real-time reporting feature of the system created a better link between expecting mothers and the healthcare system through the Commnunity-Based Healthcare Workers (CBHWs). In 2012, the system was rolled to the entire country.

Drawing from the Rapid SMS system experiences from Rwanda, Burundi in partnership with the United Nations Children's Fund (UNICEF) introduced the Kira-mama project, a Rapid SMS pilot project in two provinces Muyinga and Gitega towards the end of the year 2014. Figure 3 depicts how Rapid SMS was designed to work in the Ministry of Health's maternal and infants' health program to empower Community Health Workers (CHWs) for greater efficiency in reporting healthcare cases. A CHW would send a message reporting a health-related case. The message would be relayed to the Community Health Centre (CDS) and District Hospital (HD). Health promotion technicians who are CHWs' supervisors would monitor the messages and take adequate action. For instance, if an ambulance is required, the nearest health facility and district hospital would be notified and feedback is given to the CHW. The system also enables the Ministry of Health (MOH) to monitor the progress of reports by accessing the MOH's Rapid SMS central server. The Rapid SMS system would enable countrywide data collection on maternal and child's health. Thus, the central server would aggregate collected data in a format that makes it easier for decision making.
The main objectives of the Rapid SMS system are to:

1. Improve the monitoring of mothers-to-be till they give birth and at up to 42 days after giving birth.
2. To operationalize the auditing of maternal and neonatal deaths from Primary Healthcare centres and community levels.
3. To improve urgent obstetrical and neonatal care in healthcare facilities.
4. Improve the monitoring of children aged between 0 and 59 months. This includes monitoring of vaccination, immunization, and detection of malnutrition cases.

Text messages delivered through mobile phones have proved to bridge the communication gap in the health sector between health workers and patients, different managerial levels, and between the Ministry of Health and facilities in the peripheral areas (Hoffman et al., 2010; Pop-Eleches et al., 2011; Lester et al., 2010. Although the piloted system will primarily benefit mothers and infants, other stakeholders in public healthcare will benefit as well. These include the health departments in charge of the National Programme on Reproductive Health (PNSR), health departments in charge of the National Programme of Health Information Systems (SNIS), and the Ministry of Health in general. The system will collect key information that will help make informed decisions about future healthcare interventions.

Although there are no available data to evaluate the performance of the system, there are some lessons that Burundi can draw for its counterpart Rwanda regarding the implementation of mHealth interventions as they share similar historical and cultural backgrounds.

1. Only one major mobile service provider was involved in the project. The mobile service provider offered SMS services at 20% discounted rates which reduced the cost of the project (Burundi Ministry of Health, 2014). Thus, in the case of Burundi, there is a need for partnership (that brings benefits to both parties) between the Ministry of Health and mobile service providers to provide mHealth enabled interventions that are affordable to the consumers in the light of the country's socio-economic environment.
2. There was extensive consultation with CBHWs to ensure the success of the system (Burundi Ministry of Health, 2014). Such consultation brought forth an agreement about the system's requirements and how the system could be customized for ease of use. Involving users in the development process of telehealth initiatives is critical (Wootton et al., 2009). Gagnon et al. (2004) advocate that the diffusion of telehealth and its application depend on its acceptance among healthcare practitioners. Thus, the participatory design approach is particularly suitable for mHealth adoption. Particularly the involvement of users in interface design plays a role in the successful adoption and usability of mobile devices (Graves et al., 1998). In the case of Burundi, there is a need for such consultation as there is limited knowledge of mHealth capabilities, especially within the primary healthcare professionals. Such consultation will be an avenue for training stakeholders in the use of the system to ensure a high response rate to the project (Pop-Eleches et al., 2011).
3. Performance-based incentives were put in place to increase CBHWs adoption and ownership of the system (Burundi Ministry of Health, 2014). In this case, CBHWs were empowered for greater commitment to the mHealth based intervention. Lester et al. (2012) argue that providing adequate incentives is one of the factors that lead to a high response rate to mHealth projects. Hence in the case of Burundi, it is imperative to provide incentives to ensure adoption of the system especially because mHealth is a new concept within the country, hence healthcare professionals might not be enthusiastic about its adoption if they do not perceive any reward from using it.
4. Telecommunications infrastructure which provided the necessary support for communication, data flows, and links to the central database were also key in the success of the project (Burundi Ministry of Health, 2014). At the time of implementation, the country had 95% mobile network coverage. Hospitals had cell phone modems and CHBWs had cellphones. In Burundi, however, none of

the five mobile service operators (Smart, Africell, Onamob, Econet, and Leo) covers the entire country. Leo, the largest mobile service provider only covers 64% of the country's population. The mobile telecommunications' annual growth is 13% which gives hopes that in the future the country will experience full network coverage. Mobile cell phone penetration in the country is 31% which means that a large portion of the population still does not have access to mobile phones which impedes the scalability of mHealth interventions.

5. Additional logistics were put in place to support the outcomes of the mHealth based intervention (Burundi Ministry of Health, 2014). All hospitals were adequately equipped to deal with birth-related complications and serious newborn babies' illnesses. In Burundi, there is a need to assess whether there is enough logistics to deal with the increase of reported cases that will emanate from the system's implementation.

METHODOLOGY

Data was gathered from 212 primary healthcare workers systematically sampled from 48 primary healthcare institutions, through a survey questionnaire. Data collected from the primary healthcare workers captured their acceptance of eight mHealth capabilities. These capabilities are: SMS based awareness programs, collecting medical/health data using mobile devices, monitoring and treating patients using mobile devices, communicating with fellow health professionals using mobile devices, training health workers using mobile devices, tracking diseases and epidemic outbreaks using mobile devices, using mobile devices for diagnostic support, and using mobile devices for treatment support. The questionnaire further captured primary healthcare workers' perceptions of the following as potential impediments of mHealth adoption in Burundi: lack of skills, high cost of mobile devices, low rate of cellphone penetration, low rate of penetration of other mobile devices, unreliable network coverage, high cost of network connection, and high cost of mobile internet bundles. Principal components analysis was used to assign a score to each mHealth capability based on the percentage of the total variation within the data set. Pearson's correlation and multiple linear regression coefficients were generated based on the relationship between Mobile Health capabilities acceptance and impediments to mHealth adoption.

FINDINGS AND DISCUSSION

Mobile Health Capabilities Acceptance

In Table 1, the most highly ranked (thus accepted) mHealth capability is communication amongst fellow health professionals using mobile devices (% agree or strongly agree=94.2%) while the monitoring and treatment of patients using mobile devices received the least acceptance (51.2% agreed or strongly agreed).

Table 1. Mobile Health capabilities acceptance

M-Health Capabilities Acceptance	Frequencies							Main Principal Component	
	Strongly Disagree	**Disagree**	**Not Sure**	**Agree**	**Strongly Agree**	**Agree+ Strongly Agree**	**Rank**	**Loading**	**Reliability Statistics**
I would send SMS to make people aware of different methods of disease prevention	20	13	29	101	48	**70.6%**	**3**	0.645	Percentage of total variation =45.19% Cronbach's Alpha Statistic = 0.823
	9.5%	6.2%	13.7%	47.9%	22.7%				
I would collect medical/health data using mobile devices	10	10	15	119	58	**83.5%**	**2**	0.623	
	4.7%	4.7%	7.1%	56.1%	27.4%				
I would monitor and treat patients using mobile devices	40	25	35	78	27	**51.2%**	**8**	0.734	
	19.5%	12.2%	17.1%	38.0%	13.2%				
I would communicate with fellow health professionals using mobile devices	5	4	3	103	93	**94.2%**	**1**	0.376	
	2.4%	1.9%	1.4%	49.5%	44.7%				
I would train health workers using a mobile device	24	33	31	75	46	**57.9%**	**7**	0.659	
	11.5%	15.8%	14.8%	35.9%	22.0%				
I would track diseases and epidemic outbreaks using mobile devices	13	22	31	92	48	**68.0%**	**4**	0.700	
	6.3%	10.7%	15.0%	44.7%	23.3%				
I would use mobile devices for diagnostic support	14	25	29	93	45	**67.0%**	**5**	0.791	
	6.8%	12.1%	14.1%	45.1%	21.8%				
I would use mobile devices for treatment support	17	21	30	98	39	**66.8%**	**6**	0.762	
	8.3%	10.2%	14.6%	47.8%	19.0%				

The principal components analysis results (score) accounts for 45.19% of the total variation in the data set above. The Cronbach's Alpha coefficient is 0.823, which represents an internal consistency within the data set.

The use of mobile devices for diagnostic support has the highest Principal Component Analysis (PCA) score of 0.791, which means it has more influence (hence more importance) on the calculation of mHealth capabilities acceptance.

The overall measure of mHealth capabilities acceptance score per individual was obtained from the principal components analysis results. This overall score is a new variable derived from the original eight items. It is a weighted mean of the items under the mHealth capabilities construct. The mHealth capabilities score is computed as follows:

Mhealth capabilities acceptance index= 0.645×**Q12.1** +0.623×**Q12.2** + 0.734×**Q12.3**

+ 0.376×**Q12.4** + 0.659×**Q12.5** + 0.700×**Q12.6** + 0.791×**Q12.7** + 0.762×**Q12.8**

The overall PCA index in this section assists in the determination of correlation and regression coefficients to determine the relationship between the mHealth capabilities acceptance and factors that may hinder such acceptance.

Impediments to mHealth Acceptance

Table 2. Impediments of mHealth

Healthcare Impediments	Frequencies							Main Principal Component	
	Strongly Disagree	Disagree	Not Sure	Agree	Strongly Agree	Agree+ Strongly Agree	Rank	Loading	Reliability Statistics
Lack of skills to develop mHealth applications	5 2.4%	13 6.1%	17 8.0%	101 47.6%	76 35.8%	**83.5%**	**4**	0.628	Percentage of total variation =48.29% Cronbach's Alpha Statistic = 0.816
High cost of mobile devices	5 2.4%	11 5.2%	22 10.5%	94 44.8%	78 37.1%	**81.9%**	**6**	0.585	
Low rate of cell phone penetration	7 3.3%	17 8.0%	28 13.2%	96 45.3%	64 30.2%	**75.5%**	**2**	0.657	
Low rate of other mobile devices (excluding cell phones) penetration	3 1.4%	7 3.3%	22 10.5%	87 41.4%	91 43.3%	**84.8%**	**3**	0.702	
Unreliable network coverage in rural areas	4 1.9%	9 4.3%	16 7.6%	92 43.6%	90 42.7%	**86.3%**	**1**	0.761	
High cost of network connection	3 1.4%	8 3.8%	27 12.7%	91 42.9%	83 39.2%	**82.1%**	**5**	0.764	
High cost of mobile internet bundles	1 0.5%	10 4.7%	21 9.9%	69 32.5%	111 52.4%	**84.9%**	**2**	0.747	

Although above 75% of the respondents agreed that the factors listed in Table 2 are the impediments to mobile healthcare acceptance, the unreliability of network coverage in rural areas was the most agreed upon factor at 86.3% while the low rate of cell phone penetration is the least agreed upon (75.5%). The PCA was used to generate an individual score for each question within the data set. The PCA scores account for 48.29% of the total variation in the data set. The Cronbach's Alpha coefficient is 0.816.

Correlation Between Mobile Health Capabilities Acceptance and Impediments to mHealth Acceptance

Table 3. Correlation between Mobile Health capabilities acceptance and impediments of mHealth

	Pearson Correlations		mHealth Capabilities Acceptance
Impediments	Lack of skills	Correlation	0.238**
		p-value	0.001
		N	191
	High cost of mobile devices	Correlation	0.042
		p-value	0.569
		N	189
	Low rate of cell phone penetration	Correlation	0.177*
		p-value	0.014
		N	191
	Low rate of other mobile devices penetration	Correlation	0.124
		p-value	0.088
		N	190
	Unreliable network coverage	Correlation	0.202**
		p-value	0.005
		N	190
	High cost of network connection	Correlation	0.167*
		p-value	0.021
		N	191
	High cost of mobile internet bundles	Correlation	0.095
		p-value	0.191
		N	191

Table 3 indicates that lack of skills, low rate of cell phone penetration, unreliable network coverage, and high cost of network connection are significantly correlated with mHealth capabilities acceptance with a small effect size (correlation coefficient less than 0.30). This means that there is a weak association between these impediments and mHealth capabilities acceptance.

Stepwise Regression Between Mobile Health Capabilities Acceptance and Impediments of mHealth

A stepwise regression analysis was performed to identify impediments factors that fit into the regression model. The results indicate that lack of skills to develop mHealth applications is the only variable that significantly fits into the model (p=0.001) as depicted in Table 4. A regression equation was generated based on the following formulae: $Y = bX + constant\ value$ where Y is the dependent variable (mHealth capabilities), X the independent variable (lack of skills), and b is the regression coefficient value for the independent variable. Thus, $Y = 0.219X + 2.774$. The other variables as depicted in Table 5 were excluded from the regression model.

Table 4. Stepwise regression between mHealth capabilities acceptance and lack of skills

Coefficients [a]						
Model		Unstandardized Coefficients		Standardized Coefficients	T	Sig.
		B	Std. Error	Beta		
1	(Constant)	2.744	.264		10.389	.000
	15.1: Lack of skills to develop mHealth applications is an impediment towards mHealth adoption in Burundi	.219	.063	.249	3.496	.001

[a]Dependent Variable: mHealth Capabilities

Table 5. Stepwise regression mHealth capabilities and other factors (excluded factors)

Excluded Variables[a]						
Model		Beta In	T	Sig.	Partial Correlation	Collinearity Statistics
						Tolerance
	High cost of mobile devices is an impediment towards mHealth adoption in Burundi	-.055[b]	-.716	.475	-.053	.871
	Low rate of cell phone penetration in the country is an impediment towards mHealth adoption in Burundi	.115[b]	1.532	.127	.112	.890
	Low rate of other mobile devices (excluding cell phones) penetration in the country is an impediment towards mHealth adoption in Burundi	.052[b]	.693	.489	.051	.902
	Unreliable network coverage in rural areas is an impediment towards mHealth adoption in Burundi	.118[b]	1.540	.125	.113	.863
	High cost of network connection (airtime) is an impediment towards mHealth adoption in Burundi	.087[b]	1.153	.251	.085	.887
	High cost of mobile internet bundles is an impediment towards mHealth adoption in Burundi	.002[b]	.030	.976	.002	.919

a. Dependent Variable: mHealth Capabilities

b. Predictors in the Model: (Constant), 15.1: Lack of skills to develop mHealth applications is an impediment towards mHealth adoption in Burundi

CONCLUSION

Mobile health capabilities are generally accepted by primary health care professionals in Burundi. Although primary healthcare professionals recognise that some challenges that impede the adoption of mHealth need to be addressed; from a statistical point of view such impediments have a low effect on their acceptance of mHealth. However, from a practical implementation point of view, there are constraints that need to be addressed for mHealth interventions to have a countrywide impact in Burundi. Drawing from the Rwandan Rapid SMS case, the Burundian Ministry of Health needs to forge partnerships with mobile operators, foster user involvement in the mHealth system design, instil performance-based rewards for CBHWs greater commitment to the mHealth based interventions, advocate for wider mobile cellphone penetration in the country, and be equipped with enough logistics to deal with the increase of reported cases that will emanate from the mHealth system's implementation.

REFERENCES

Adedeji, A. A., Sanusi, B., Tella, A., Akinsanya, M., Ojo, O., Akinwunmi, M. O., Tikare, O. A., Ogunwande, I. A., Ogundahunsi, O. A., & Ayilara, O. O. (2011). Exposure to anti-malarial drugs and monitoring of adverse drug reactions using toll-free mobile phone calls in the private retail sector in Sagamu, Nigeria: Implications for pharmacovigilance. *Malaria Journal*, *10*, 230.

African Development Bank Group. (2011). *Burundi Country Strategy Paper 2012-2016*. Retrieved from http://www.afdb.org/fileadmin/uploads/afdb/Documents/Project-and-Operations/ Burundi%20-%20CSP%202012-16.pdf

Andreatta, P., Debpuur, D., Danquah, A., & Perosky, J. (2011). Using cell phones to collect postpartum haemorrhage outcome data in rural Ghana. *International Journal of Gynaecology and Obstetrics*, *113*(2), 148–151.

Bellina, L., & Missoni, E. (2009). Mobile cellphones (M-phones) in tele microscopy: Increasing connectivity of isolated laboratories. *Diagnostic Pathology*, *4*, 19.

Burundi Ministry of Health. (2014). *Kira-Mama project*. Available at https://unicefstories.files.wordpress.com/2014/05/burundi-final-english-300ppi.pdf

Colven, R., Shim, M. H., Brock, D., & Todd, G. (2011). Dermatological diagnostic acumen improves with the use of a simple telemedicine system for underserved areas of South Africa. *Telemedecine Journal- E Health*, *17*(5), 363–369.

Excelsior. (2014). *Less innovation, more scale. Realising the promise of health technology in Africa*. Available at excelsior-group.com/CMS/downloads/EXG_Whitepape.pdf

GHI. (2012). *Burundi Global Health Initiative strategy 2011-2015*. Available at www.ghi.gov/documents/organization/175128.pdf

Hoffman, J. A., Cunningham, J. R., Suleh, A. J., Sundsmo, A., Dekker, D., Vago, F., Munly, K., Igonya, E. K., & Hunt-Glassman, J. (2010). Mobile direct observation treatment for tuberculosis patients: A technical feasibility pilot using mobile phones in Nairobi, Kenya. *Pub Med, 39*(1), 78–80.

Imaja, I. M., Ndayizigamiye, P., & Maharaj, M. (2017). A design of a mobile health intervention for the prevention and treatment of Cholera in South Kivu in the Democratic Republic of Congo. In *2017 IEEE Global Humanitarian Technology Conference (GHTC)* (pp. 1-5). IEEE.

Kante, M., & Ndayizigamiye, P. (2020a). A systematic mapping of the adoption of Internet of Things to provide healthcare services in developing countries. In P. Ndayizigamiye, G. Barlow-Jones, R. Brink, S. Bvuma, R. Minty, & S. Mhlongo (Eds.), Perspectives on ICT4D and Socio-Economic Growth Opportunities in Developing Countries (pp. 99–126). IGI Global. https://doi.org/10.4018/978-1-7998-2983-6.ch004.

Kante, M., & Ndayizigamiye, P. (2020b). An analysis of the current status of Internet of Medical Things policies in developing countries. *NPG. Neurologie, Psychiatrie, Gériatrie, 20*(119), 259–265. https://doi.org/10.1016/j.npg.2020.03.002

Kante, M., & Ndayizigamiye, P. (2021). Internet of Medical Things, Policies and Geriatrics: An Analysis of the National Digital Health Strategy for South Africa 2019-2024 from the Policy Triangle Framework Perspective. *Scientific African*, e00759.

Lester, R., Ritvo, P., Mills, E., Kariri, A., Karanja, S., Chung, M. C., Jack, W., Habyarimana, J., Sadatsafavi, M., Najafzadeh, M., Marra, C. A., Estambale, B., Ngugi, E., Ball, T. B., Thabane, L., Gelmon, L. J., Kimani, J., Ackers, M., & Plummer, F. A. (2010). Effects of mobile phone short message service on antiretroviral treatment adherence in Kenya (WelTel Kenya1): A randomised trial. *Lancet, 376*, 1838–1845.

Matiyabu, I. I., & Ndayizigamiye, P. (2019). The potential use of Social Media for Healthcare Advocacy in the Democratic Republic of Congo. *Proceedings of 4th International Conference on the, 12*, 105-111.

Ndayizigamiye, P. (2016). *Potential adoption of mobile health technologies for public healthcare in Burundi* (Doctoral dissertation).

Ndayizigamiye, P., Hangulu, L., & Akintola, O. (2017). A design of a mobile health intervention to enhance home-carers' disposal of medical waste in South Africa. In *2017 IEEE Global Humanitarian Technology Conference (GHTC)* (pp. 1-6). IEEE.

Ndayizigamiye, P., Kante, M., & Shingwenyana, S. (2020). An adoption model of mHealth applications that promote physical activity. *Cogent Psychology*, *7*(1), 1764703.

Ndayizigamiye, P., & Maharaj, M. (2016a). Mobile health adoption in Burundi: A UTAUT perspective. In *2016 IEEE Global Humanitarian Technology Conference (GHTC)* (pp. 613-623). IEEE.

Ndayizigamiye, P., & Maharaj, M. (2016b). *Applying bridges framework to investigate challenges to the adoption of mHealth in Burundi. In 2016 IST-Africa Week Conference*. IEEE.

Ndayizigamiye, P., & Maharaj, M. (2017). Determinants of mobile health adoption in Burundi. *The African Journal of Information Systems*, *9*(3), 1–23.

Ndayizigamiye, P., & Maharaj, M. (2018). *A Systematic review of mHealth interventions for public healthcare in East Africa in AMCIS 2018 proceedings*. AIS.

Ndayizigamiye, P., Soni, T. C., & Jere, N. (2018). *Factors Motivating the Adoption of Self-Healthcare Monitoring Mobile Applications by the South African Youth. In 2018 IST-Africa Week Conference (IST-Africa)*. IEEE.

Pop-Eleches, C., Thirumurthy, H., Habyarimana, J. P., Zivin, J. G., Goldstein, M. P., de Walque, D., MacKeen, L., Haberer, J., Kimaiyo, S., & Sidle, J. (2011). Mobile phone technologies improve adherence to antiretroviral treatment in a resource-limited setting: A randomized controlled trial of text message reminders. *AIDS (London, England)*, *25*(6), 825–834.

Seidenberg, P., Nicholson, S., Schaefer, M., Semrau, K., Bweupe, M., Masese, N., Bonawitz, R., Chitembo, L., Goggin, C., & Thea, D. M. (2012). Early infant diagnosis of HIV infection in Zambia through mobile phone texting of blood test results. *Bulletin of the World Health Organization*, *90*(5), 348–356.

Soni, T. C., Ndayizigamiye, P., & Kante, M. (2019). Determinants of the Adoption of Self-healthcare Monitoring Mobile Applications. *Fortieth International Conference on Information Systems (ICIS)*, Munich, Germany.

UNICEF. (2013). *The State of the World's Children 2013*. Available at https://www.unicef.org/sowc2013/files/SWCR2013_ENG_Lo_res_24_Apr_2013.pdf

Wakadha, H., Chandir, S., Were, E. V., Rubin, A., Obor, D., Levine, O. S., Gibson, D. G., Odhiambo, F., Laserson, K. F., & Feikin, D. R. (2013). The feasibility of using mobile-phone based SMS reminders and conditional cash transfers to improve timely immunization in rural Kenya. *Vaccine*, *31*(6), 987–993.

Wave, V. (2009). *M-Health for Development: The Opportunity of Mobile Technology for Healthcare in the Developing World.* The United Nations Foundation and Vodafone Foundation Technology Partnership. Available: http://www.globalproblems-globalsolutionsfiles.org/unf_website/assets/publications/technology/mhealth/mHealth_for_Development_full.pdf

Chapter 9
Adoption of Blockchain to Support the National Health Insurance Implementation in South Africa:
An Integrative Review

Shaivar Girdhari
University of Johannesburg, South Africa

Patrick Ndayizigamiye
https://orcid.org/0000-0001-5721-6070
University of Johannesburg, South Africa

ABSTRACT

The National Department of Health aims to provide good quality healthcare to all citizens and especially those who cannot afford proper healthcare through the implementation of the National Health Insurance (NHI). This will be done by pooling funds to establish a social solidarity fund for all citizens in need of healthcare regardless of their socio-economic status. The South African healthcare sector currently makes use of skewed healthcare financing systems, which makes it difficult to have a convergent healthcare scheme such as the NHI. Therefore, it is proposed that for the implementation of the NHI in South Africa, a new healthcare financing system, is developed based on artificial intelligence (AI) and blockchain algorithms with embedded deep learning capabilities. It is anticipated that the proposed healthcare financing system will help build resilience in South Africa's healthcare financing system.

DOI: 10.4018/978-1-7998-8915-1.ch009

INTRODUCTION

South Africa's National Health Insurance (NHI) is a health insurance program that aims to provide good quality healthcare to all citizens, especially those who cannot afford. The South Africa's NHI is expected to be implemented by pooling funds together to establish a social solidarity fund for citizens in need of healthcare regardless of their socio-economic status (The Centre for Health Policy, 2019). However, South Africa's healthcare sector currently makes use of skewed healthcare financing systems which makes it difficult to have a convergent healthcare scheme such as the NHI. Skewed healthcare financing systems lead to inaccurate financial data being gathered, processed, and produced, which in turn directly inhibits the attainment of the NHI goals as it seeks to unify the healthcare sector.

The South African government plans to achieve the goals of the NHI by acquiring healthcare services from both the public and private sectors to enhance equity in the current distribution of health services. There are four primary goals/objectives of the NHI which are: a) to provide enhanced access to good quality healthcare for all South Africans regardless of social or employment status, b) to pool funds to establish an equitable social solidarity fund through the creation of a single national healthcare fund, c) to procure resources and services on behalf of the entire population and efficiently manage and control financial resources allocated to public healthcare, and d) aims to strengthen the strained and under-resourced public healthcare sector to improve health and healthcare systems performance (Department of Health, 2017).

In recent years, blockchain technology has been proposed as an alternative solution to deficiencies within financial information systems. The characteristics of blockchain are resilient by nature due to it being a decentralized peer-to-peer node network in the way it handles and processes transactions. In the healthcare financing context, the adoption of blockchain can result in a resilient - adaptive healthcare financing system, that would directly impact the health system as a whole. However, currently, there is a paucity of literature on the applications of blockchain within the context of healthcare financing. This chapter investigates the potential adoption of blockchain to support the NHI implementation in South Africa. Specifically, this chapter identifies the challenges faced by current South Africa's healthcare financing systems that may impede the implementation of the NHI. Then the chapter determines the role of blockchain in addressing the challenges. It finally provides a framework for the implementation of blockchain to support the NHI implementation in South Africa.

OVERVIEW OF THE SOUTH AFRICA'S HEALTHCARE FINANCING SYSTEM

Healthcare financing system is the basis upon which health insurance is provided with adequate management of financial resources. In South Africa, due to most of the healthcare funding coming from the private sector, many medical schemes offer health insurance that is mainly accessible to only the higher income group earners in the country. This leaves the lower-income group within South Africa exposed to poor quality of healthcare due to limited access to the necessary healthcare funding, which is normally provided by the medical schemes. This is because the lower-income group cannot afford health insurance premiums offered by current medical schemes. Therefore, South Africa's skewed healthcare financing systems need to be revised to allow lower-income families in the country access to proper health insurance, that provides a good standard of quality healthcare. Health insurances can be made accessible to lower-income families if the health financing systems are adjusted, so that resources are distributed more evenly throughout the country (Department of Health, 2017; Department of Planning, 2017).

Providing health insurance to all South Africans requires medical schemes in the private sector to become deprivatized to work towards a universal healthcare system for all. The two-tiered South Africa's healthcare system (private and public healthcare) will need to become cohesive to achieve the NHI implementation effectively; as well as more community healthcare workers need to be in place to serve the lower-income group of the population (Department of Health, 2019). According to Smith (2016), South Africa's private health insurance sector spends the most financial resources on healthcare in the world amounting to 44% of the total expenditure of health financing in the country. The public healthcare financing systems are of poor quality which could be caused by inefficient use and misdistribution of funds and resources within the sector (Manyazewal, 2017).

Lack of leadership and decision-making power are key impediments in the efficient and effective management of public healthcare financing systems which could be the cause of the ineffective use of funds and resources in South Africa's healthcare systems. These inefficiencies extend toward the whole public healthcare system, including primary healthcare services such as clinics and hospitals that provide secondary and tertiary services. Currently, there exists a colossal difference between the range and type of funding that is provided in the public and private healthcare sectors in South Africa. This provides a crucial insight into the reasons why the public healthcare sector has been underperforming (Manyazewal, 2017).

According to Passchier (2017), proper governance and accountability of how financial resources are spent is of vital importance and trumps the issue of sourcing funding streams for the NHI. There exist a lack of data and information resource monitoring mechanisms within the healthcare financing system, and this is mainly due to the lack of human resources to render those services. The NHI plans to purchase and acquire medical service technologies from the private sector even though there are high fees attached to the private healthcare sector which makes it hard to form strategic alliances. The partnerships between the public and private sectors will require a high level of transparency alongside experienced management so that they align with the national healthcare goals.

BLOCKCHAIN TECHNOLOGY

Blockchain is a distributed ledger technology that has a high computational ability to process records of transactions and facilitate data processing. According to Alketbi et al. (2018), blockchain can be equated to a database that groups records of transactions together to form a ledger. Records are stored in blocks, which are all linked together using cryptographic hash sequences to verify, authenticate, validate, and process the records - thus ensuring the integrity of transactions in all blocks in the chain. This is what is referred to as a consensus algorithm (Stone & Principal, 2017).

Blockchain allows all nodes (verified devices/users) within the network to access the ledger given that the nodes are first authenticated and validated by other nodes on the network. This allows blockchain to be interoperable without compromising the security of the network, therefore, protecting sensitive data.

According to McGhin et al. (2019) and Zhang et al. (2018), blockchain could make current health system models more patient-centric and interoperable. It can be used to eliminate the need for intermediaries to ensure trust in the authenticity of transactions, heavily reducing the costs associated with transactions (transfer of medical assets or services). Blockchain can also ensure a distributed and decentralised way of processing and securing patient's data. Smart contracts embedded with the blockchain can help validate all transactions over the network while ensuring that all data meets security standards to be shared laterally across the network. This eliminates varied data standards within the healthcare systems and aids in data sharing.

According to McGhin et al. (2019), blockchain could address varied data standards within the healthcare financing systems through its characteristic of shared data. This is true because data is shared across the blockchain network in a certain data format that remains consistent, which allows for newly inputted data to follow the same data structure. Various types of patient identifiers need to be correlated and synchronized so that stakeholders have secure, private access to patient records. Currently, the public healthcare sector has extremely restricted access to public data because the systems integration is not effective. Blockchain can address these data issues by its decentralized method of processing data while ensuring the integrity and availability of information in a timeous manner. Programmable smart contracts within blockchain allow for the automation of access to certain parties/organizations that are based on a set of rules. Once these rules have been validated, access to data is given only on what is validated and nothing more. This allows for proper management of patient's records and personal health records while preventing fraudulent behaviours (Agbo et al., 2019; Bell et al., 2018; Zhang et al., 2018).

The concept of immutability within blockchain means that present records in the blockchain network may not be altered, which means that the system does not depend on the trust of humans to secure data from unauthorised access (Chartier-Rueg & Zweifel, 2017; Katuwal et al., 2018). Public and private keys within the blockchain allow it to restrict access to different parties within the network so that there is some form of control of who has access to what data.

Blockchains security mechanisms (public and private key encryption) solve the current problem in the healthcare financing systems where networks are situated in multiple separate facilities. This allows a more trusted network to be established especially in terms of authenticating users of the network. Blockchain greatly reduces the cost per transaction due to it being a peer-to-peer based technology. This means that through real-time processing, systems become more efficient in processing data, which lowers transaction costs accordingly (Weiss et al., 2017).

PROBLEM STATEMENT

The purpose of South Africa's NHI scheme is to provide a healthcare financing scheme to all citizens of South Africa (NHI, 2020) regardless of race, gender, place of origin, class, or status among citizens. The core challenges of implementing the NHI scheme, are mainly due to skewed healthcare financing systems.

Blockchain has many characteristics that would directly support and benefit the entire South Africa's healthcare financing system model, including the NHI implementation specifically regarding the healthcare financing systems challenges that South Africa is facing. These characteristics are: immutability, transparency, high level of security using encryption algorithms (cryptographic hashes), and efficiency in handling data. Therefore, research is warranted to determine the potential adoption of blockchain in supporting the development of a new healthcare financing system model to directly address management and financing challenges in South Africa's healthcare sector. This new healthcare financing system will also support the NHI's implementation by satisfying the required data needs to promote a sustainable, reliable, and accurate healthcare financing system (Alketbi, Nasir and Talib, 2018).

The skewed healthcare financing systems in South Africa are key inhibitors of the implementation of South Africa's National Health Insurance Scheme (Department

of Health, 2019). Blockchain is an emerging technology that has various attributes such as transparency, security, and immutability that make it a viable solution to address the problems in healthcare financing systems (Alketbi, Nasir and Talib, 2018). Therefore, the purpose of this research is to identify how blockchain can aid in the design of a new healthcare financing system that will provide support to the implementation of the NHI.
This chapter is anchored on the following research objectives:

1. To identify the challenges faced in the current healthcare financing systems that may impede the implementation of the National Health Insurance in South Africa.
2. To determine the role that blockchain can play to address current healthcare financing systems challenges that may hamper the implementation of the National Health Insurance in South Africa.
3. To map a framework for the implementation of blockchain to address healthcare financing systems challenges.

METHODOLOGY

This study adopted the interpretivism philosophy coupled with the qualitative research approach. It further adopted the case study as the research strategy. Moreover, the study utilized the integrative literature review as the data collection method to identify the potential contribution of blockchain to enhance the implementation of the NHI scheme in South Africa. An integrative literature review makes use of secondary data to develop new frameworks and perspectives by synthesizing the data in an integrated way. In other words, it uses existing knowledge to create new knowledge (Russell, 2005). According to Torraco (2016), writing an integrative literature review can be broken down into 11 steps. These are:

1. The first step is to identify the need and purpose of the review.
2. Next is to examine the topic of the review to understand whether a new or existing topic will be examined in the literature review. It is important to specify the scope and boundaries of the review. This makes it easier to identify the literature that will be reviewed and which will not.
3. The authors' perspective on the review will need to be explained to the reader so that all assumptions by the author regarding the review are stated, i.e. whether the author takes a neutral or a specific point of view.
4. The review will need to be organized and structured effectively so that it follows a logical flow of ideas.

5. The discussion of research methods describing how the integrative literature review will be conducted should be sufficiently described.
6. A critical analysis will need to be done to analyse the existing literature on the topic being researched (critiquing). The critical analysis will need to identify the strengths and weaknesses of the literature, identifying whether there exists any omissions, inconsistencies or missing/incomplete information represented within the literature, and any graphical representations should be added that could enhance the readers understanding of the critical analysis of the literature.
7. The synthesis of the integrative literature review should provide a contribution that has value to the new knowledge about the topic.
8. The review should formulate questions for future research on the topic.
9. The logic and conceptual reasoning of the review should describe the logic that the author used to synthesize the framework from the review and how the author went about critiquing the literature.
10. The future of the topic or field should be discussed as well as factors that are shaping the future of the field, thus, assessing the direction of future events and trends of the topic.
11. The writing should be clear and concise.

Data was collected from the following databases: IEEE Xplore, EBSCOHOST, Google Scholar, Science Direct and Scopus. The literature selected for analysis was collected from peer-reviewed journals. The focus keywords/search strings used for finding relevant articles were centred on “blockchain”, “Healthcare”, and “financing systems”. Articles were selected based on their relevance to healthcare financing systems and blockchain applications to healthcare systems.

The first step in analyzing the data was to survey the identified literature based on the titles and their relevance to the research objectives of this chapter. Articles of which the full text could not be accessed, or duplicate articles were excluded. In addition, articles that were not written in English were not selected. Selected articles were interpreted based on their practical implications and relevance to the implementation of South Africa’s NHI.

RESULTS

Characteristics of Selected Papers

Table 1 describes the selected articles by showing the title of each selected article, the corresponding author(s), and the year of publication. The table shows that the selected papers were published between 2013 and 2020.

Table 1. List of selected papers

Article Title	Authors	Year of Publication
1. A Systematic Review of Equity in Healthcare Financing in Low- and Middle-Income Countries	(Rostampour & Nosratnejad)	2020
2. Do Healthcare Financing Systems Influence Hospital Efficiency? A Metafrontier Approach for the Case of Mexico	(Giménez et al.)	2019
3. Sustainability of Healthcare Systems: Aligning the Safety and Quality Debate with the Debate on the Financing Systems and Mechanisms	(Abbing)	2013
4. The private sector in national health financing systems: the role of health maintenance organizations and private healthcare providers in Nigeria	(Onoka)	2014
5. Health Financing Systems, Health Equity and Universal Health Coverage in Arab Countries.	(Alami)	2017
6. An Efficient Lightweight Cryptographic Technique for IoT based e-Healthcare System	(Chaudhary & Chatterjee)	2020
7. DITrust Chain: Towards Blockchain-Based Trust Models for Sustainable Healthcare IoT Systems	(Abou-Nassar et al.)	2020
8. Certificate-less Public Key Encryption for Secure e-Healthcare Systems	(Aditia et al.)	2019
9. ssHealth: Toward Secure, Blockchain-Enabled Healthcare Systems	(Abdellatif et al.)	2020
10. Convergence of Blockchain and Artificial Intelligence to Decentralize Healthcare Systems	(Lobo et al.)	2020
11. S2HS- A blockchain-based approach for smart healthcare system	(Tripathi et al.)	2020
12. Blockchain-based electronic healthcare record system for healthcare 4.0 applications	(Tanwar et al.)	2020
13. Using Healthcare Authority and Patient Blockchains to Develop a Tamper-Proof Record Tracking System	(Goel et al.)	2019
14. Towards a Blockchain-Based Healthcare Information System: Invited Paper	(Misic et al.)	2019
15. On the Design of a Blockchain-Based System to Facilitate Healthcare Data Sharing	(Theodouli et al.)	2018
16. Secure and Efficient Data Accessibility in Blockchain-Based Healthcare Systems	(Ramani et al.)	2018
17. Scaling Blockchains to Support Electronic Health Records for Hospital Systems	(Donawa et al.)	2019
18. The benefits and threats of blockchain technology in healthcare: A scoping review	(Abu-elezz et al.)	2020
19. Blockchain Utilization in Healthcare: Key Requirements and Challenges	(T. Kumar et al.)	2018

Continued on following page

Table 1. Continued

20. Artificial Neural Network Blockchain Techniques for Healthcare System: Focusing on the Personal Health Records	(Kim & Huh)	2020
21. Scalable and secure access control policy for healthcare system using blockchain and enhanced Bell-LaPadula model	(R. Kumar & Tripathi)	2020
22. Privacy-Preserving in Healthcare Blockchain Systems Based on Lightweight Message Sharing	(Fu et al.)	2020
23. Blockchain for e-Health-Care Systems: Easier Said Than Done	(Biswas et al.)	2020
24. Revocable Attribute-Based Signature for Blockchain-Based Healthcare System	(Su et al.)	2020
25. A Novel Smart Healthcare Design, Simulation, and Implementation Using Healthcare 4.0 Processes	(A. Kumar et al.)	2020
26. A Blockchain-Based Smart Contract System for Healthcare Management	(Khatoon)	2020
27. Blockchain Tree for eHealth	(Kushch et al.)	2019
28. Design of Blockchain-based Precision Health-Care using soft systems methodology	(Sharma et al.)	2020
29. Challenges Providing Ground Truth for Pervasive Healthcare Systems	(Yordanova et al.)	2019
30. Identifying Key Challenges Facing Healthcare Systems in Africa and Potential Solutions	(Oleribe et al.)	2019
31. Compiling a prioritized list of health data quality challenges in public healthcare systems	(Botha et al.)	2014
32. The three numbers you need to know about healthcare: the 60-30-10 Challenge	(Braithwaite et al.)	2020
33. Healthcare information systems: the cognitive challenge	(Lintern & Motavalli)	2018
34. Blockchain-enabled logistics finance execution platform for capital-constrained e-commerce retail	(Li et al.)	2020
35. A Systematic Review of Blockchain in Healthcare: Frameworks, Prototypes, and Implementations	(Chukwu & Garg)	2020
36. Design Choices and Trade-Offs in Health Care Blockchain Implementations: Systematic Review	(O'Donoghue et al.)	2019
37. Blockchain implementation in health care: Protocol for a systematic review	(Meinert et al.)	2019
38. Blockchain in healthcare: A systematic literature review, synthesizing framework and future research agenda	(Tandon et al.)	2020
39. Exploring Applications of Blockchain in Securing Electronic Medical Records	(Nguyen)	2017
40. A Comparative Analysis of Blockchain Architecture and its Applications: Problems and Recommendations	(Ali Syed et al.)	2019
41. Zero-trust hierarchical management in IoT	(Samaniego & Deters)	2018

As depicted in the word cloud in Figure 1 below, the major themes that emerged from the literature revolved around keywords about blockchain (mentioned 3,602 times), healthcare (mentioned 2,680 times), health (mentioned 3,147 times), and data (mentioned 3,240 times). Secondary themes that emerged were systems, information access, technology challenges, health insurance, and medical patient's records. Based on the word cloud, one may make a preliminary judgement that the themes that emerged from the analysis of the selected articles were aligned with the objectives of this study. The findings of the integrated literature review are presented and elaborated based on the study's guiding objectives.

Figure 1. Word cloud that shows themes covered by the selected papers

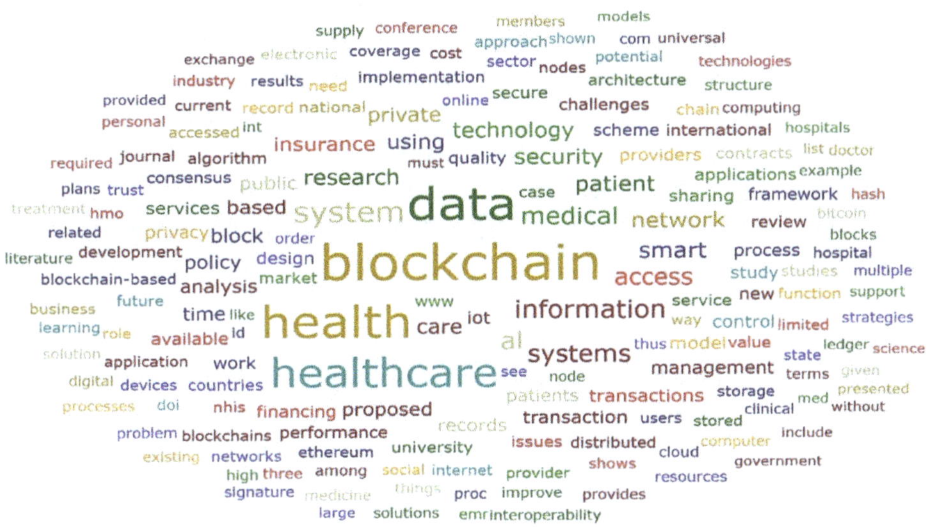

The first research objective of this study was to determine the current South African's healthcare financing systems challenges that may impede the implementation of the National Health Insurance.

According to the study by Rostampour and Nosratnejad (2020), most healthcare funding systems fail when customers use direct payment methods to transact for healthcare services. On the other hand, successful healthcare financing systems that provide quality healthcare are predominantly based on both social and individual insurance systems. Citizens within South Africa are mostly still using direct payment methods which becomes unfair to individuals who cannot afford the proper healthcare that they need. It is thus, evident that a crucial factor to consider when designing a new framework for the healthcare financing systems of the country is to create a financing system that is conducive to equitable healthcare financing. Such a financing system will allow the government alongside social institutions to implement health insurance for all individuals, especially for those who are poor. The financing system should also exempt low-income earners of the country from paying healthcare taxes so that quality healthcare services can be accessible to them (Dhai, 2011).

Healthcare financing systems require a cognitive and adaptive workforce to enforce healthcare systems strategies that are effective. It is inherent that current healthcare software infrastructure designs do not cater for the growing demand of knowledge and skills (cognition) required by healthcare practitioners to operate and run the healthcare financing systems at an optimum level. This results in the healthcare financing systems being unable to account for all processes, procedures, or workflows. Incorporating cognitive design into the healthcare financing system would allow the system to aid and improve work strategies for healthcare professionals. This would also allow for more accurate and relevant patient's data to be captured and stored on the system while surveying and eliminating redundant data. Therefore, for the healthcare financing system to be utilized to its full potential and capabilities, cognitive demands based on the types of work being done needs to be taken into account when designing and constructing the system, so that healthcare practitioners can develop more efficient work strategies that would aid the implementation of the NHI within South Africa (A. Kumar et al., 2020; Lintern & Motavalli, 2018).

According to Giménez et al. (2019), the efficiency of a healthcare funding system is determined by the capabilities of the technology used to assist the healthcare system. Due to the complex nature of healthcare systems and the related development and maintenance costs, healthcare financing systems based on high-technology infrastructures within healthcare facilities would be more useful if they were adequately funded.

The second objective of this study was to identify the role that blockchain can play to address the current healthcare financing systems challenges that may hamper the implementation of South Africa's NHI.

Blockchain can be used as a platform for secure data management and sharing within the context of healthcare financing systems. The Ethereum blockchain architectures have been developed and can cater for complex medical procedures, such as surgery which requires large amounts of medical data and information. This is done by developing and implementing a medical-specific smart contract health system for healthcare information management. This type of blockchain network framework could be used to develop a smart contract healthcare financing system that can handle the vast amount of healthcare-related data and render it in real-time. Cloud storage can be coupled with the smart contract system to make patient data easily accessible while still being secured on most devices and platforms through decentralized data storage and access (Abdellatif et al., 2020; Khatoon, 2020; T. Kumar et al., 2018; Misic et al., 2019).

Information system's features can be grouped into: application, data, technology, and business layers. An example of a technology feature would be the trade-off between firewalls and data availability. The NHI would require features and capabilities from all these categories and therefore, careful attention will need to be paid to choosing the best features from each layer to fulfil the purpose of the system more completely. These choices, if managed in an adaptable manner can be used to enhance the utilities of the blockchain platform.

Healthcare-related data is considered sensitive and should be secured and protected from unauthorized access. Therefore, data sharing privacy and security are key factors that will need to be emphasized when designing the healthcare financing system. Blockchains characteristic of immutability and transparency allow for a set of customized and personalized rules to be put in place so that when data is requested, only that specific data is provided once authorized and verified. Thus, creating a blockchain data-sharing model that is auditable on both public and private data sharing and access permissions will aid in preventing fraudulent or corrupt behaviours. Certificate-less public key encryption is a secure method by which to ensure data confidentiality, integrity, and availability on a Blockchain network (Aditia et al., 2019; Theodouli et al., 2018).

The third objective of this study was to determine the framework that could be used to adopt blockchain to support the implementation of the National Health Insurance. Artificial Intelligence (AI) blockchain algorithms can be incorporated into the Blockchain-enabled healthcare financing system to provide secure authentication and verification of patient healthcare records by encrypting and verifying the data to prevent data breaches. This will create a healthcare blockchain ecosystem in which the transmission of data between healthcare facilities will be securely verified, ensuring that accurate data is used across the spectrum for reliable, informed decision-making. Therefore, an AI information security system blockchain framework, encompassing deep learning capabilities could be used for the accurate extraction, authentication, and storage of healthcare data. This maximizes the confidentiality of all data within the blockchain network and allows for the AI blockchain algorithms to securely transmit and disseminate sensitive information, thus regulating access control mechanisms to suit South Africa's healthcare financing ecosystem. The Bell-LaPadula model, which is an access control framework, alongside sidechains allows for individual blockchains to be defined for specific individual tasks or use cases. It can be used to implement dynamic access control protocols and mechanisms within the healthcare blockchain system to address any scalability and bottleneck issues that may arise in the future. Smart contracts that will be created as part of the Blockchain financing system can also incorporate access control policies to provide enhanced data security within the network environment (Donawa et al., 2019; Kim & Huh, 2020; R. Kumar & Tripathi, 2021; Kushch et al., 2019; Tandon et al., 2020).

DISCUSSION

Regarding the first research objective of this study, a challenge that could potentially be encountered with the implementation of the NHI is the gathering, analyzing and storage of health-related records, and data and information. One of the problems faced by the current South Africa's healthcare financing system in this regard is that patient's records are incorrectly stored, making them inaccessible to healthcare providers if patients seek healthcare at other healthcare institutions within the country. This challenge contributes to the misalignment of the healthcare financing system of the country because patients may not get the healthcare that is needed as their records are not reliable, accurate, or available when needed (Yordanova et al., 2019).

Health and financial data quality within the country's healthcare financing system is a prominent factor that may hamper the implementation of the NHI. A key contributing element to this specifically regarding public healthcare facilities is that, SA has only recently begun the shift from paper-based records to electronic storage of patient's records and information. However, data quality issues may still arise with the electronic patient's records as storing the data in a reliable, accurate, and accessible manner while preserving data quality becomes a difficult task to achieve as it requires highly customized and personalized systems software (Botha et al., 2014).

The study by Oleribe et al. (2019), suggests that the lack of proper human resources, misallocation and misappropriation of funds in the healthcare sectors, and inadequate leadership and governance are the prominent elements that contribute to healthcare financing systems failures. Therefore, there is a need for an innovative approach that can provide a more streamlined, reliable healthcare financing system to support the NHI implementation within South Africa's healthcare financing context.

In South Africa, most of the healthcare financing systems development is being done by the private health insurance sector. Standardized health system policies must be put in place regarding the governance and funding of health insurance in the public and private healthcare sectors. This would allow for the creation of standardized pricing structures for healthcare insurance which directly supports the goal of the NHI towards achieving Universal Health Coverage (UHC) for South Africa. Moreover, it would also distribute the funding required from social institutions for health insurance so that it can be made available to the lower-income group of the country who cannot afford proper healthcare (Onoka, 2014).

The successful implementation of the NHI requires governments to look beyond the healthcare financing system and place emphasis on providing good quality healthcare that is distributable, accessible, and affordable for all citizens. The quality of healthcare that will be provided would be dependent on the type of financing system and model that will be used. Therefore, only increasing healthcare service offerings, budgets, or practitioners would not necessarily result in enhanced healthcare provision. The healthcare system needs to be equal, affordable, and be of good quality so that the right choice of healthcare financing systems is chosen which would contribute to providing UHC, thus aiding the NHI implementation (Abbing, 2013).

Current healthcare financing systems and insurance predominantly cater for the individuals that can afford proper healthcare, meaning that contributions are made from businesses and employees without regarding the percentage of the populace that are unemployed and therefore cannot afford healthcare. Current inequities within the healthcare financing systems highlight the gap between the needs of healthcare and the provision of healthcare services which has created a basis upon which access to healthcare is viewed on the ability of an individual to pay. Therefore, healthcare should be viewed as an investment and should be entitled to everyone, which requires a shift to an equity-based economy that emphasizes the political tolerance for corruption or misuse of healthcare financing systems resources (social injustice) (Alami, 2017).

Regarding the second research objective of this study, it is evident that the current healthcare financing system performance is of poor quality within the country. The study by Braithwaite et al. (2020), states that only 60% of healthcare follows the proper evidence-based guidelines and procedures; 30% of healthcare services incurs wastage of resources or generate low value, and 10% of healthcare procedures and processes cause harm to patients. Current healthcare financing systems are not cost-effective and are highly complex. Therefore, the implementation of the National Health Insurance cannot solely rely on standardization through technology or policies and structures, but also on creating a system that encompasses a dynamic AI and deep learning environment in which the national healthcare ecosystem will reside. This will allow for the healthcare financing system to gather the most relevant information and data (e.g. patient's records, lab data, payments, etc.) in real-time for prompt, and informed decision-making (based on empirical, evidenced-based guidelines and principles which will be available to all patients and healthcare professionals within the system). This will reduce the wastage of resources and the probability of harming patients (e.g. misdiagnosis). The design of the system would need a unique foundational infrastructure that utilizes AI features and capabilities (deep learning) alongside blockchain frameworks and algorithms that support private secure patient's data storage (zero-trust information security principle). This means that once a transaction is initiated, it cannot be changed after it is authenticated and verified (immutable) and is transparent (errors can be traced back to the relevant party if system resources are misused or if the unwanted activity is suspected). The design would aid in the provision of informed treatment and diagnosis. Such blockchain systems will enable a patient-centric approach to healthcare whereby patients will have more control over whom they can share data with, within the blockchain network. Thus, such a system would support the implementation of the mechanisms, principles, standards, and guidelines of the NHI by creating a healthcare digital environment that is conducive to solving challenges experienced in the current healthcare financing systems. This will imply moving away from a two-tiered system, towards a unified healthcare system in which health insurance is available to all citizens and is of the same quality for all regardless of the level of income (Abou-Nassar et al., 2020; Fu et al., 2020; A. Kumar et al., 2020; Lobo et al., 2020; Su et al., 2020; Tandon et al., 2020; Tanwar et al., 2020).

An electronic healthcare financing record management system can also be built using blockchain alongside the smart contract healthcare financing system, which would increase the interoperability of a patient-driven blockchain model and infrastructure (Ali Syed et al., 2019). This would also create a sustainable record management system that could be customized over the long term to refine and utilize healthcare predictive analytics. Moreover, it will significantly enhance the capturing, storage, and sharing of all healthcare data by using a soft systems methodology to generate innovative solutions. There are numerous advantages of blockchain solutions over traditional medical record keeping. The main benefit is that through the use of blockchain as a platform to create a decentralized electronic patient management system, the healthcare system will be able to manage, effectively disseminate, and communicate patient's information to wherever they may seek healthcare in the country, meaning that patients won't be restricted to certain healthcare facilities (where their medical records are held). This will help lessen the degree of data standard variation through the enhanced capability of blockchain to share data securely, accurately, and timeously. This will allow new forms and types of data that will be gathered by the NHI to be standardized and made accessible only to the relevant parties so that all data formats remain consistent and universally understandable. This would also require that patients be assigned unique identifying datasets or codes so that all records are synchronized and made available for secure access from the relevant stakeholders. Smart contracts would allow for the proposed system to reshape current payment systems and trust-building (A. Kumar et al., 2020; Meinert et al., 2019; Nguyen, 2018; Sharma et al., 2020; Tripathi et al., 2020).

With regard to the third research objective of this study, blockchains features of traceability and decentralization allow for a framework to be developed which provides personalized healthcare and patient's health status monitoring, while also enhancing information exchange and national health insurance management. This could allow for enhanced security behind peer-to-peer payment services through cryptographic keys and lightweight cryptographic techniques for constrained Internet of Things (IoT) devices. This will allow for the tracking of all healthcare financing system transactions while ensuring that only verified access is granted to relevant stakeholders in alignment with healthcare regulations and the NHI (Abu-elezz et al., 2020; Biswas et al., 2020; Chaudhary & Chatterjee, 2020; Goel et al., 2019).

An AI information security blockchain with deep learning capabilities shifts the electronic patient's records system power of authority from being centralized to decentralized. Blockchain frameworks for healthcare financing systems should incorporate the zero-trust information security principle, which states that all data entering the network should remain untrusted until verified and authenticated. This prevents threats from moving laterally across the network and causing damage to the healthcare financing system. Therefore, blockchain solves the problems of security, privacy, and trust experienced in traditional electronic patient's record keeping (Biswas et al., 2020; Chukwu & Garg, 2020; Samaniego & Deters, 2018).

The challenge of privacy can be addressed by the blockchain network due to the transparent nature of its infrastructure. This can be addressed using the zero-trust principle mentioned above. The other challenge is security within the blockchain framework which can also be addressed by the zero-trust principle alongside an attribute-based scheme as suggested by Su et al. (2020). The healthcare financing system should make use of e-commerce platforms to facilitate decentralized digitally regulated transactions to decrease the information and task load on the healthcare blockchain for processing smart contract requirements (Li et al., 2020; Samaniego & Deters, 2018).

Therefore, it is proposed that to successfully implement the NHI in South Africa, a new healthcare financing system be developed that combines AI and blockchain technology with embedded deep learning capabilities that can enable electronic health record systems to 'learn' from environmental factors and then optimize themselves. The proposed system will be able to combat the challenges identified that may hamper the NHI implementation and would satisfy the goals of the NHI by creating a unified healthcare system that enables Universal Health Care (UHC) for all. Figure 2 below shows how the identified challenges can be solved using the mentioned framework of AI blockchain algorithms and deep learning capabilities. Each of the challenges is linked to the solution proposed by the blockchain platform which could be used to address the identified issues in the healthcare financing systems.

The healthcare blockchain architecture mentioned by Sethi (2018), suggests a framework of blockchain that encompasses web 3.0 technologies such as data analytics, artificial intelligence and blockchain, that can specifically be used together to implement a customized blockchain framework, which could be used to support the NHI implementation. Therefore, for South Africa to adopt blockchain to aid the implementation of the NHI, the health systems policies will need to be revised so that the health policies align to universal and comprehensive coverage of healthcare for all citizens within the country. This will then allow for a decentralised national healthcare financing system to be implemented according to the characteristics whereby the government regulates the payments to healthcare providers and guarantees equal access to healthcare for the general population, while only owning some of the healthcare facilities (both private and public). This will provide the way for blockchain, which also uses a decentralised method of processing data and is not governed by a regulatory body, to be utilized to support the policy changes that will be instantiated by the NHI. In doing so, these policies will become the governing regulatory body (controlled by the government) for the healthcare blockchain to be implemented.

The proposed healthcare financing model will need to spread through innovative solutions within a local context so that the healthcare ecosystem being developed is adaptable and combats real-world problems while enhancing the quality of the overall healthcare system. The adoption of blockchain, AI, and other emerging technologies is still far from realization as public and private social institutions, which will be required to make contributions to the NHI are hesitant due to various reasons, such as socio-political and the legacy of the current healthcare systems issues (Sethi, 2018; Oleribe et al., 2019).

Figure 2. Proposed blockchain framework to aid the implementation of the NHI

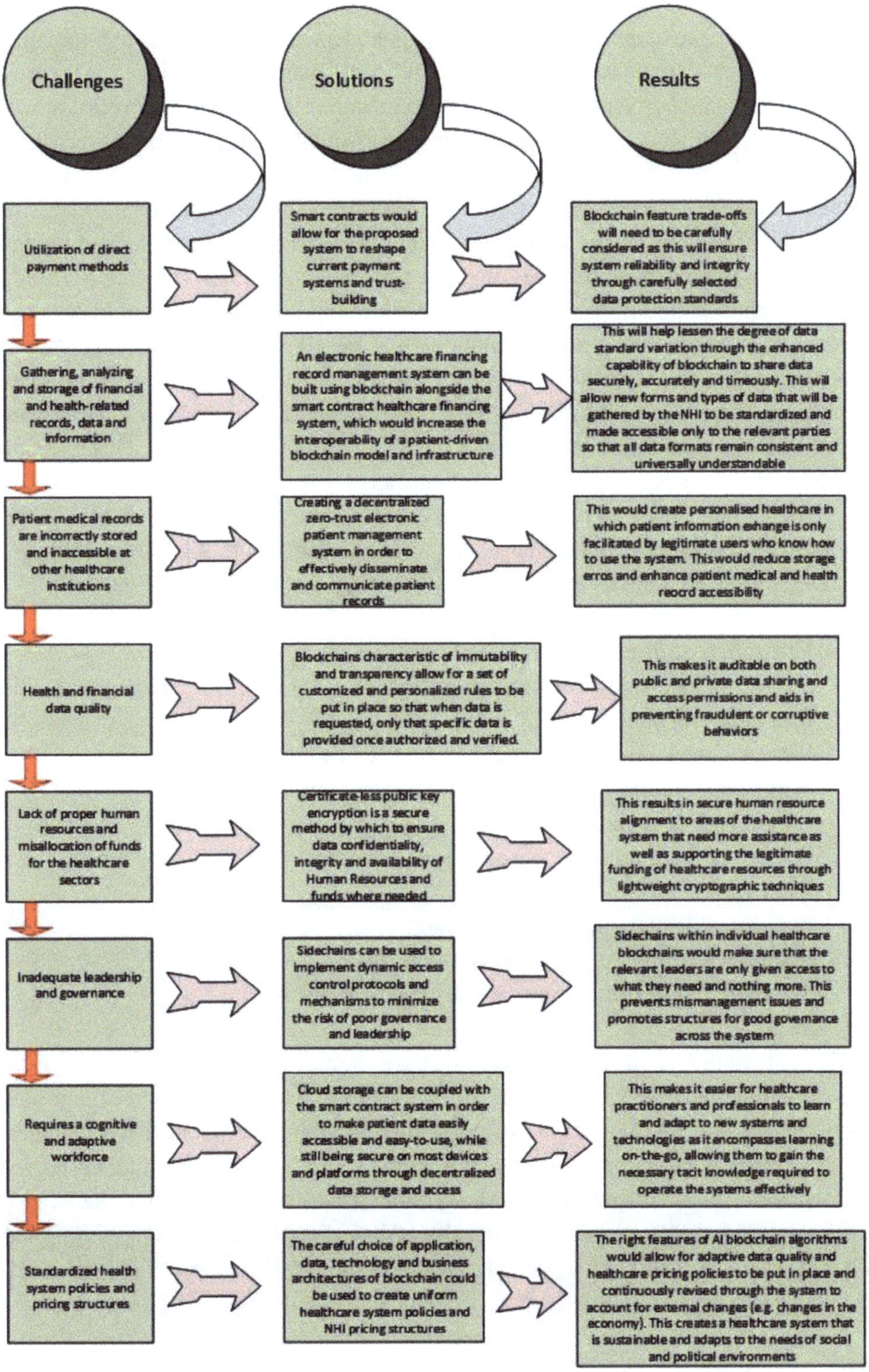

CONCLUSION

The main challenges experienced in the NHI implementation are caused predominantly by skewed healthcare financing systems. Healthcare financial mismanagement creates a lack of adequate human resources, leads to misallocation and misappropriation of funds in the healthcare sectors, and results in inadequate leadership and governance. These are the prominent elements that contribute to healthcare financing systems failures. There exists a lack of data and information resource monitoring mechanisms within the healthcare financing system, and this is mainly due to the lack of human resources to render those services.

Blockchain capabilities and features have many benefits that could be used in the development and implementation of a new healthcare financing system model which would directly support the NHI implementation. A newly developed healthcare financing system using blockchain technology could result in more effective and swifter implementation of the NHI within South Africa. This research aimed to investigate the role that blockchain can play to support South Africa's NHI implementation. The first research objective of this study was addressed through the identification of eight core challenges facing the current South African's healthcare systems. These challenges are:

1. Utilization of direct payment methods
2. Gathering, analysing and storage of financial and health-related records, and data and information
3. Patient's medical records are incorrectly stored and inaccessible at other healthcare institutions
4. Health and financial data quality
5. Lack of proper human resources and misallocation of funds for the healthcare sectors
6. Inadequate leadership and governance
7. Requires a cognitive and adaptive workforce
8. Standardized health system policies and pricing structures.

To address the second objective of this study, the eight challenges identified in the first research objective were then linked to the blockchain features and capabilities alongside the use of AI algorithms that could directly address the identified challenges.

The third research objective was addressed by stipulating the resultant effect of implementing the identified blockchain solutions to combat the identified challenges. This resulted in a framework being developed based on the identified solutions and their effect on the healthcare financing system challenges. The identified framework is based on an AI information security system blockchain model which encompasses deep learning capabilities and could be used to address the current challenges being faced with the healthcare financing systems and support the NHI implementation. The identified framework could also make the healthcare systems more reliable and stable by providing resilience in the facilitation of processing transactions and parsing data within the network. Once the system is implemented and has had sufficient time to operate and process transactions, it will be able to process certain transactions/data with greater resilience as those transactions may be automated through the use of smart contracts.

FUTURE RESEARCH DIRECTIONS

The research outlined a core set of features from multiple emerging technologies which can be incorporated into a blockchain framework and be utilized for the development of a new healthcare financing system to support the implementation of South Africa's National Health Insurance scheme. The research implications of this study are that blockchain could be used as the basis for the creation of new healthcare systems in future systems development practice. Below are recommendations for the healthcare blockchain suggested in this paper on how it could be practically implemented to enhance the implementation of the NHI:

- Current patient's data should be evaluated based on its value (i.e. the data or information deemed critical for either financial or medical processing/transacting reasons) before being put on the blockchain to reduce resource usage on implementation (i.e. only required financial and medical data and information should be put onto the system and the rest should be omitted or stored on sidechains within the network).
- Compatibility needs to be verified beforehand between the blockchain framework and social institutions' internal networks to ensure blockchain integration.

Future research should be conducted to determine the technical requirements for the development of each solution identified in this study. Furthermore, more research should be conducted to develop and assess the solutions artefact through computer simulations or ground testing.

REFERENCES

Abbing, H. R. (2013). Sustainability of healthcare systems: Aligning the safety and quality debate with the debate on the financing systems and mechanisms. European Journal of Health Law, 20(3), 253–259. doi:10.1163/15718093-12341271

Abdellatif, A. A., Al-Marridi, A. Z., Mohamed, A., Erbad, A., Chiasserini, C. F., & Refaey, A. (2020). SsHealth: Toward secure, blockchain-enabled healthcare systems. *IEEE Network*, *34*(4), 312–319. doi:10.1109/MNET.011.1900553

Abou-Nassar, E. M., Iliyasu, A. M., El-Kafrawy, P. M., Song, O. Y., Bashir, A. K., & El-Latif, A. A. A. (2020). DITrust Chain: Towards Blockchain-Based Trust Models for Sustainable Healthcare IoT Systems. *IEEE Access: Practical Innovations, Open Solutions*, *8*, 111223–111238. doi:10.1109/ACCESS.2020.2999468

Abu-elezz, I., Hassan, A., Nazeemudeen, A., Househ, M., & Abd-alrazaq, A. (2020). The benefits and threats of blockchain technology in healthcare: A scoping review. In *International Journal of Medical Informatics* (Vol. 142, p. 104246). Elsevier Ireland Ltd., doi:10.1016/j.ijmedinf.2020.104246

Aditia, M. K., Paida, S., Altaf, F., & Maity, S. (2019, December 1). Certificate-less public key encryption for secure e-Healthcare systems. *2019 IEEE Conference on Information and Communication Technology, CICT 2019*. 10.1109/CICT48419.2019.9066190

Agbo, C., Mahmoud, Q., & Eklund, J. (2019). Blockchain Technology in Healthcare: A Systematic Review. *Health Care*, *7*(2), 56. doi:10.3390/healthcare7020056 PMID:30987333

Alami, R. (2017). Health Financing Systems, Health Equity and Universal Health Coverage in Arab Countries. *Development and Change*, *48*(1), 146–179. doi:10.1111/dech.12290

Ali Syed, T., Alzahrani, A., Jan, S., Siddiqui, M. S., Nadeem, A., & Alghamdi, T. (2019). A Comparative Analysis of Blockchain Architecture and its Applications: Problems and Recommendations. *IEEE Access: Practical Innovations, Open Solutions*, *7*, 176838–176869. doi:10.1109/ACCESS.2019.2957660

Alketbi, A., Nasir, Q., & Talib, M. A. (2018). Blockchain for government services-Use cases, security benefits and challenges. *2018 15th Learning and Technology Conference, L and T 2018*, 112–119. 10.1109/LT.2018.8368494

Bell, L., Buchanan, W. J., Cameron, J., & Lo, O. (2018). Applications of Blockchain Within Healthcare. *Blockchain in Healthcare Today*, *1*(0). Advance online publication. doi:10.30953/bhty.v1.8

Biswas, S., Sharif, K., Li, F., & Mohanty, S. (2020). Blockchain for E-Health-Care Systems: Easier Said Than Done. *Computer*, *53*(7), 57–67. doi:10.1109/MC.2020.2989781

Botha, M., Botha, A., & Herselman, M. (2014). Compiling a prioritized list of health data quality challenges in public healthcare systems. *2014 IST-Africa Conference and Exhibition*, *2014*, 1–8. Advance online publication. doi:10.1109/ISTAFRICA.2014.6880649

Braithwaite, J., Glasziou, P., & Westbrook, J. (2020). The three numbers you need to know about healthcare: The 60-30-10 Challenge. In BMC Medicine (Vol. 18, Issue 1). BioMed Central Ltd. doi:10.118612916-020-01563-4

Chartier-Rueg, T. C., & Zweifel, T. D. (2017). Blockchain, leadership and management: Business as usual or radical disruption? *EUREKA: Social and Humanities*, *4*(4), 76–110. doi:10.21303/2504-5571.2017.00370

Chaudhary, R. R. K., & Chatterjee, K. (2020). An efficient lightweight cryptographic technique for iot based E-healthcare system. *2020 7th International Conference on Signal Processing and Integrated Networks, SPIN 2020*, 991–995. 10.1109/SPIN48934.2020.9071421

Chukwu, E., & Garg, L. (2020). A systematic review of blockchain in healthcare: Frameworks, prototypes, and implementations. *IEEE Access: Practical Innovations, Open Solutions*, *8*, 21196–21214. doi:10.1109/ACCESS.2020.2969881

Department of Health. (2017). White Paper for National Health Insurance for South Africa. *National Health Insurance Bill*, 1–80. www.gpwonline.co.za

Department of Health. (2019). *National Health Insurance (NHI) Pledge*. Author.

Department of Planning. (2017). *Socio-economic impact assessment system (SEIAS): Final impact assessment (Phase 2): White paper on national health insurance*. Author.

Dhai, A. (2011). Healthcare reform in South Africa : A step in the direction of social justice. *World Medical Journal*, *4*(2), 137–139. https://eds.a.ebscohost.com/eds/detail/detail?vid=0&sid=6a80e28a-7726-48c8-9186-ff52fac6166f%40sdc-v-sessmgr01&bdata=JkF1dGhUeXBlPXNzbyZzaXRlPWVkcy1saXZlJnNjb3BlPXNpdGU%3D#AN=edssas.ejc64551&db=edssas

Donawa, A., Orukari, I., & Baker, C. E. (2019). Scaling Blockchains to Support Electronic Health Records for Hospital Systems. *2019 IEEE 10th Annual Ubiquitous Computing, Electronics and Mobile Communication Conference, UEMCON 2019*, 550–556. 10.1109/UEMCON47517.2019.8993101

Fu, J., Wang, N., & Cai, Y. (2020). Privacy-preserving in healthcare blockchain systems based on lightweight message sharing. *Sensors (Switzerland)*, *20*(7), 1898. Advance online publication. doi:10.339020071898 PMID:32235389

Giménez, V., Keith, J. R., & Prior, D. (2019). Do healthcare financing systems influence hospital efficiency? A metafrontier approach for the case of Mexico. *Health Care Management Science*, *22*(3), 549–559. doi:10.100710729-019-9467-9 PMID:30659404

Goel, U., Ruhl, R., & Zavarsky, P. (2019). Using Healthcare Authority and Patient Blockchains to Develop a Tamper-Proof Record Tracking System. *2019 IEEE 5th Intl Conference on Big Data Security on Cloud (BigDataSecurity), IEEE Intl Conference on High Performance and Smart Computing, (HPSC) and IEEE Intl Conference on Intelligent Data and Security (IDS)*, 25–30. 10.1109/BigDataSecurity-HPSC-IDS.2019.00016

Katuwal, G. J., Pandey, S., Hennessey, M., & Lamichhane, B. (2018). *Applications of Blockchain in Healthcare: Current Landscape & Challenges*. https://arxiv.org/abs/1812.02776v1

Khatoon, A. (2020). A blockchain-based smart contract system for healthcare management. *Electronics (Switzerland)*, *9*(1), 94. Advance online publication. doi:10.3390/electronics9010094

Kim, S. K., & Huh, J. H. (2020). Artificial neural network blockchain techniques for healthcare system: Focusing on the personal health records. *Electronics (Switzerland)*, *9*(5), 763. Advance online publication. doi:10.3390/electronics9050763

Kumar, A., Krishnamurthi, R., Nayyar, A., Sharma, K., Grover, V., & Hossain, E. (2020). A Novel Smart Healthcare Design, Simulation, and Implementation Using Healthcare 4.0 Processes. *IEEE Access: Practical Innovations, Open Solutions*, *8*, 118433–118471. doi:10.1109/ACCESS.2020.3004790

Kumar, R., & Tripathi, R. (2021). Scalable and secure access control policy for healthcare system using blockchain and enhanced Bell–LaPadula model. *Journal of Ambient Intelligence and Humanized Computing*, *12*(2), 2321–2338. doi:10.100712652-020-02346-8

Kumar, T., Ramani, V., Ahmad, I., Braeken, A., Harjula, E., & Ylianttila, M. (2018, November 9). Blockchain utilization in healthcare: Key requirements and challenges. *2018 IEEE 20th International Conference on E-Health Networking, Applications and Services, Healthcom 2018*. 10.1109/HealthCom.2018.8531136

Kushch, S., Ranise, S., & Sciarretta, G. (2019, November 1). Blockchain Tree for eHealth. *2019 IEEE Global Conference on Internet of Things, GCIoT 2019*. 10.1109/GCIoT47977.2019.9058412

Li, M., Shao, S., Ye, Q., Xu, G., & Huang, G. Q. (2020). Blockchain-enabled logistics finance execution platform for capital-constrained E-commerce retail. *Robotics and Computer-integrated Manufacturing*, *65*, 101962. Advance online publication. doi:10.1016/j.rcim.2020.101962

Lintern, G., & Motavalli, A. (2018). Healthcare information systems: The cognitive challenge. In BMC Medical Informatics and Decision Making (Vol. 18, Issue 1). BioMed Central Ltd. doi:10.118612911-018-0584-z

Lobo, V. B., Analin, J., Laban, R. M., & More, S. S. (2020). Convergence of Blockchain and Artificial Intelligence to Decentralize Healthcare Systems. *Proceedings of the 4th International Conference on Computing Methodologies and Communication, ICCMC 2020*, 925–931. 10.1109/ICCMC48092.2020.ICCMC-000171

Manyazewal, T. (2017). Using the World Health Organization health system building blocks through survey of healthcare professionals to determine the performance of public healthcare facilities. *Archives of Public Health*, *75*(1), 50. Advance online publication. doi:10.118613690-017-0221-9 PMID:29075485

McGhin, T., Choo, K. K. R., Liu, C. Z., & He, D. (2019). Blockchain in healthcare applications: Research challenges and opportunities. In *Journal of Network and Computer Applications* (Vol. 135, pp. 62–75). Academic Press. doi:10.1016/j.jnca.2019.02.027

Meinert, E., Alturkistani, A., Foley, K. A., Osama, T., Car, J., Majeed, A., Van Velthoven, M., Wells, G., & Brindley, D. (2019). Blockchain implementation in health care: Protocol for a systematic review. *JMIR Research Protocols*, *8*(2), e10994. Advance online publication. doi:10.2196/10994 PMID:30735146

Misic, V. B., Misic, J., & Chang, X. (2019). Towards a blockchain-based healthcare information system: Invited paper. *2019 IEEE/CIC International Conference on Communications in China, ICCC 2019*, 13–18. 10.1109/ICCChina.2019.8855911

Nguyen, B. (2018). Exploring Applications of Blockchain in Securing Electronic Medical Records. *Maryland Journal of Contemporary Legal Issues*, *20*(1), 99. https://eds.b.ebscohost.com/eds/detail/detail?vid=0&sid=afc07135-ec43-4dd0-a9d1-21896f2fb4c9%40pdc-v-sessmgr01&bdata=JkF1dGhUeXBlPXNzbyZzaXRlPWVkcy1saXZlJnNjb3BlPXNpdGU%3D#AN=edshol.hein.journals.hclwpo20.8&db=edshol

O'Donoghue, O., Vazirani, A. A., Brindley, D., & Meinert, E. (2019). Design choices and trade-offs in health care blockchain implementations: Systematic review. In Journal of Medical Internet Research (Vol. 21, Issue 5). JMIR Publications Inc. doi:10.2196/12426

Oleribe, O. O., Momoh, J., Uzochukwu, B. S. C., Mbofana, F., Adebiyi, A., Barbera, T., Williams, R., & Taylor-Robinson, S. D. (2019). Identifying key challenges facing healthcare systems in Africa and potential solutions. *International Journal of General Medicine*, *12*, 395–403. doi:10.2147/IJGM.S223882 PMID:31819592

Onoka, C. (2014). The private sector in national health financing systems: the role of health maintenance organisations and private healthcare providers in Nigeria. *London School of Hygiene & Tropical Medicine*.

Passchier, R. V. (2017). Exploring the barriers to implementing national health insurance in South Africa: The people's perspective. *South African Medical Journal*, *107*(10), 836–838. doi:10.7196/SAMJ.2017.v107i10.12726 PMID:29022524

Ramani, V., Kumar, T., Bracken, A., Liyanage, M., & Ylianttila, M. (2018). Secure and Efficient Data Accessibility in Blockchain Based Healthcare Systems. *2018 IEEE Global Communications Conference, GLOBECOM 2018 - Proceedings*. 10.1109/GLOCOM.2018.8647221

Rostampour, M., & Nosratnejad, S. (2020). A Systematic Review of Equity in Healthcare Financing in Low- and Middle-Income Countries. *Value in Health Regional Issues*, *21*, 133–140. doi:10.1016/j.vhri.2019.10.001 PMID:31786404

Russell, C. L. (2005). An overview of the integrative research review. In Progress in Transplantation (Vol. 15, Issue 1, pp. 8–13). InnoVision Communications. doi:10.1177/152692480501500102

Samaniego, M., & Deters, R. (2018). Zero-trust hierarchical management in IoT. *Proceedings - 2018 IEEE International Congress on Internet of Things, ICIOT 2018 - Part of the 2018 IEEE World Congress on Services*, 88–95. 10.1109/ICIOT.2018.00019

Sethi, S. (2018). Healthcare Blockchain leads to Transform Healthcare Industry. *International Journal of Advance Research, Ideas and Innovations in Technology, 4*(1), 607–608. https://www.multichain.com/white-paper/

Sharma, R., Zhang, C., Wingreen, S. C., Kshetri, N., & Zahid, A. (2020). Design of Blockchain-based Precision Health-Care Using Soft Systems Methodology. *Industrial Management & Data Systems, 120*(3), 608–632. doi:10.1108/IMDS-07-2019-0401

Smith, A. M. (2016). Healthcare Reform Priorities for South Africa: Four Essays on the Financing, Delivery and User Acceptability of Healthcare. *Ph.D.*, (March), 1–244. doi:10.5588/ijtld.15.0312http

Stone, D., & Principal, D. (2017). *Blockchain: The challenges and opportunities in healthcare*. www.divurgent.com

Su, Q., Zhang, R., Xue, R., & Li, P. (2020). Revocable Attribute-Based Signature for Blockchain-Based Healthcare System. *IEEE Access: Practical Innovations, Open Solutions, 8*, 127884–127896. doi:10.1109/ACCESS.2020.3007691

Tandon, A., Dhir, A., Islam, N., & Mäntymäki, M. (2020). Blockchain in healthcare: A systematic literature review, synthesizing framework and future research agenda. *Computers in Industry, 122*, 103290. Advance online publication. doi:10.1016/j.compind.2020.103290

Tanwar, S., Parekh, K., & Evans, R. (2020a). Blockchain-based electronic healthcare record system for healthcare 4.0 applications. *Journal of Information Security and Applications, 50*, 102407. doi:10.1016/j.jisa.2019.102407

Tanwar, S., Parekh, K., & Evans, R. (2020b). Blockchain-based electronic healthcare record system for healthcare 4.0 applications. *Journal of Information Security and Applications, 50*, 102407. Advance online publication. doi:10.1016/j.jisa.2019.102407

The Centre for Health Policy. (2019). *Evaluation of the Phase 1 Implementation of the Interventions in the National Health Insurance Pilot Districts in South Africa*. Author.

Theodouli, A., Arakliotis, S., Moschou, K., Votis, K., & Tzovaras, D. (2018). On the Design of a Blockchain-Based System to Facilitate Healthcare Data Sharing. *Proceedings - 17th IEEE International Conference on Trust, Security and Privacy in Computing and Communications and 12th IEEE International Conference on Big Data Science and Engineering, Trustcom/BigDataSE 2018*, 1374–1379. 10.1109/TrustCom/BigDataSE.2018.00190

Torraco, R. J. (2016). Writing Integrative Literature Reviews: Using the Past and Present to Explore the Future. In Human Resource Development Review (Vol. 15, Issue 4, pp. 404–428). SAGE Publications Ltd. doi:10.1177/1534484316671606

Tripathi, G., Ahad, M. A., & Paiva, S. (2020). S2HS- A blockchain based approach for smart healthcare system. *Health Care*, *8*(1), 100391. Advance online publication. doi:10.1016/j.hjdsi.2019.100391 PMID:31753750

Weiss, M., Botha, A., Herselman, M., & Loots, G. (2017, November 8). Blockchain as an enabler for public mHealth solutions in South Africa. *2017 IST-Africa Week Conference*, *2017*, 1–8. Advance online publication. doi:10.23919/ISTAFRICA.2017.8102404

Yordanova, K., Favela, J., & Marcu, G. (2019). Challenges Providing Ground Truth for Pervasive Healthcare Systems. In IEEE Pervasive Computing (Vol. 18, Issue 2, pp. 100–104). Institute of Electrical and Electronics Engineers Inc. doi:10.1109/MPRV.2019.2912261

Zhang, P., Schmidt, D. C., White, J., & Lenz, G. (2018). Blockchain Technology Use Cases in Healthcare. In *Advances in Computers* (Vol. 111, pp. 1–41). Elsevier. doi:10.1016/bs.adcom.2018.03.006

KEY TERMS AND DEFINITIONS

Blockchain: Blockchain is a distributed ledger technology which promotes data transparency, validity, security, and accessibility by storing network information within individual nodes across the network.

Data Security: Data such as patient's medical records possess confidential information and thus requires protection in form of system security to ensure that only authorized personnel (such as doctors) may be granted access to such information.

Data Transparency: All transactions/processes need to be clearly visible within a healthcare system so that in the event of malpractice, all actions can be traced back to the source and held accountable thereof. Data transparency refers to having the ability to access all the transactions and/or processes that are conducted across the network to ensure proper management of the healthcare system.

Electronic Medical Record (EMR): EMRs can be described as patient's portfolios in which they describe a patient's medical history, prognosis, and diagnosis. These records are extremely confidential as they incorporate each individual patient's personal details which if stolen, can be used to facilitate fraud or impersonation.

Health Data: Patient's medical data such as diagnosis from the information make-up of a health system. Therefore, health data implies any and all information pertaining to an individual's medical history, records, and other personal information.

Healthcare: This refers to the healthcare industry as a whole, including all technical implications on a broad scale.

Healthcare Financing Systems: The basis upon which healthcare systems are operated is based on the healthcare financing systems that are utilized. An efficient, reliable healthcare financing system drives the facilitation of good healthcare service delivery and fundamentally eliminates or reduces many risks currently faced in the industry such as corruption.

National Health Insurance (NHI): The NHI serves as a basis for providing standardized equitable, affordable, accessible, and quality-based healthcare to all citizens of the country regardless of their socio-economic status by unifying the two-tiered healthcare system (public and private) within the country.

APPENDIX A: RAW DATA LOG TABLE

Table 2.

Article Title	Authors	Year of Publication	Main Objective(s) of Paper	Summary of Findings
1. A Systematic Review of Equity in Healthcare Financing in Low- and Middle-Income Countries	(Rostampour & Nosratnejad)	2020	Assessing the healthcare financing systems through specified indicators in low and middle-income countries. Focuses on the holistic perspective of the health system and suggests measures to implement successful healthcare systems	• The insurance system (organizations and individuals) provides the most equal healthcare financing to all • Direct payment is the most unfair healthcare financing mechanism • People tend to direct payments due to the lack of payment methods available
2. Do Healthcare Financing Systems Influence Hospital Efficiency? A Metafrontier Approach for the Case of Mexico	(Giménez et al.)	2019	Assessing the impact of healthcare financing systems on efficiency within Mexico	• The health system is divided into two tiers (1 private and 2 public) • Out-of-pocket funding systems incentivize more efficient behavior on average • For highly complex and high technology-based systems, public funding is the best option • An average price per person for healthcare is the best way to negotiate funding for the system
3. Sustainability of Healthcare Systems: Aligning the Safety and Quality Debate with the Debate on the Financing Systems and Mechanisms	(Abbing)	2013	Assessing the sustainability of healthcare systems with specific regard to the impacts of safety and quality on healthcare financing systems and mechanisms	• eHhealth is not yet close to being implemented and used; however, it is something to strive for accessible, affordable, and good quality services for all • Impact assessments need to be done before and after the introduction of healthcare technologies • It is essential to align quality of patient's care to financing options
4. The private sector in national health financing systems: the role of health maintenance organizations and private healthcare providers in Nigeria	(Onoka)	2014	Providing insights of policy processes for NHI proposals and considering the effectiveness of private healthcare financing in achieving Universal Health Coverage (UHC) in Nigeria	• Private funding for healthcare elongates the time taken to implement social health insurance plans • Healthcare providers respond to incentives created by business strategies
5. Health Financing Systems, Health Equity and Universal Health Coverage in Arab Countries.	(Alami)	2017	Providing an overview of healthcare financing structures within Arab countries to assess their readiness for UHC.	• Health protection insurance is usually most comprehensive for those who can afford it • Mainly catering for formally employed workers • Financing systems lack operational bases for resource pooling and risk sharing • Bad financing systems highlight the gap between healthcare needs and provision • Reducing health inequities will strengthen the healthcare financing systems
6. An Efficient Lightweight Cryptographic Technique for IoT based eHealthcare System	(Chaudhary & Chatterjee)	2020	Developing a new block cypher technique for secure transmission of data from IoT devices	• Secure transferring of health data is crucial for healthcare treatment and monitoring • Patient's data is stored on the cloud with access 24/7 • Lightweight cryptographic techniques can be used to encrypt health data on resource limited IoT devices

Continued on following page

Table 2. Continued

Article Title	Authors	Year of Publication	Main Objective(s) of Paper	Summary of Findings
7. DITrust Chain: Towards Blockchain-Based Trust Models for Sustainable Healthcare IoT Systems	(Abou-Nassar et al.)	2020	Developing a blockchain Decentralized Interoperable Trust (DIT) framework that works on IoT enabled devices.	• Trust inference systems help reduce semantic gaps • The combination of blockchain with IoT enabled devices helps to create sustainable integration between healthcare nodes • Lack of appropriate assets or resources hinder information exchange in regulated trust models
8. Certificate-less Public Key Encryption for Secure e-Healthcare Systems	(Aditia et al.)	2019	Developing a secure data sharing scheme that uses certificate-less public key encryption signatures for confidentiality and privacy for patient's health data to prevent unauthorized access	• eHealthcare systems store patient's confidential data and need to be secured • More users mean more security that is required • Certificate-less public key encryption provides more efficiency for data confidentiality
9. ssHealth: Toward Secure, Blockchain-Enabled Healthcare Systems	(Abdellatif et al.)	2020	Developing a healthcare system that leverages advances in edge computing and a blockchain based framework for remote monitoring, discover epidemics more earlier on, and to allow for faster emergency response through data sharing	• By acquiring, integrating, analyzing, and exchanging medical data at different levels, new practices can be introduced into the system • Blockchain is an essential mechanism in a successful healthcare system in the age of Fourth Industrial Revolution (4IR) emerging technologies
10. Convergence of Blockchain and Artificial Intelligence to Decentralize Healthcare Systems	(Lobo et al.)	2020	Developing a roadmap for blockchain-assisted bionetwork of healthcare data to initiate new drug discoveries and precautionary healthcare	• AI, deep learning, and blockchain can be harmoniously incorporated together to form a healthcare system that is adaptable and intuitive in providing and meeting healthcare requirements and challenges
11. S2HS- A blockchain based approach for smart healthcare system	(Tripathi et al.)	2020	Determining the technological and social barriers in adopting smart healthcare systems by analyzing user perceptions and proposes a blockchain based smart healthcare system for intrinsic system security and integrity	• Security and privacy are two of the key factors to consider for a successful smart healthcare system • Blockchain combats these two variables well • However, issues still exist with security, transparency, and privacy in smart healthcare systems
12. Blockchain-based electronic healthcare record system for healthcare 4.0 applications	(Tanwar et al.)	2020	Several options were explored for enhancing current limitation in healthcare systems using blockchain technology as well as evaluation measures for performance It proposes an access control policy algorithm for improving data accessibility among healthcare providers	• Blockchain can reform the interoperability of healthcare systems • Blockchain can increase secure access to patient's medical records • Blockchain can reform and manage prescription databases and hospital assets

Continued on following page

Table 2. Continued

Article Title	Authors	Year of Publication	Main Objective(s) of Paper	Summary of Findings
13. Using Healthcare Authority and Patient Blockchains to Develop a Tamper-Proof Record Tracking System	(Goel et al.)	2019	A dual blockchain model for the healthcare sector is proposed by combining healthcare authority and private patient blockchains to create a tamperproof tracking system	• The proposed system helps improve security and privacy of healthcare records • It also improves record and permission redundancy • Blockchain can be used to track healthcare transactions and ensure authorized access to patient's records
14. Towards a Blockchain-Based Healthcare Information System: Invited Paper	(Misic et al.)	2019	Proposing an architecture of blockchain-based healthcare information system in which block validation is performed through collective signatures	• Cryptocurrency blockchains are not completely suitable for use in healthcare systems • The proposed framework allows data owners to explicitly grant or revoke access permissions and authorizations of healthcare data
15. On the Design of a Blockchain-Based System to Facilitate Healthcare Data Sharing	(Theodouli et al.)	2018	Showing the potential of blockchain to facilitate private and auditable healthcare data sharing and healthcare data access permission handling through a blockchain-based system	• Sharing healthcare data for research purposes boosts research innovation • Healthcare data sharing raises many privacy and security concerns for patients who share their data
16. Secure and Efficient Data Accessibility in Blockchain Based Healthcare Systems	(Ramani et al.)	2018	Proposing a blockchain-based system for secure and efficient data accessibility for patients and professionals	• The proposed system will protect patient's privacy as well • The system has demonstrated its resistance to well-known cyberattacks
17. Scaling Blockchains to Support Electronic Health Records for Hospital Systems	(Donawa et al.)	2019	Quantifying scalability issues and bottlenecks related to blockchains and shows the limitations blockchains have when supporting healthcare systems	• Sidechains can be used to relieve blockchain bottlenecks • Blockchain is a promising solution for aiding electronic health records management
18. The benefits and threats of blockchain technology in healthcare: A scoping review	(Abu-elezz et al.)	2020	Exploring and categorizing the benefits and threats of blockchains in healthcare systems	• Eight benefits of blockchain were recording either within patient-related benefits or organizational-related benefits • There were eight threats identified of blockchain and were captured in either organizational threats, social threats or technological threats
19. Blockchain Utilization in Healthcare: Key Requirements and Challenges	(T. Kumar et al.)	2018	Exploring potential applications of blockchain in current healthcare systems and stating requirements needed to fulfill such healthcare systems	• Blockchain can be used as a powerful tool for many daily life applications • There are certain challenges that need to be resolved before blockchain can be implemented within the healthcare system
20. Artificial Neural Network Blockchain Techniques for Healthcare System: Focusing on the Personal Health Records	(Kim & Huh)	2020	Developing a framework of AI blockchain algorithms for safe verification of medical personal health records	• When using electronic health records, ensuring privacy will be easier • Data transmission and verification between hospitals will also become easier

Continued on following page

Table 2. Continued

Article Title	Authors	Year of Publication	Main Objective(s) of Paper	Summary of Findings
21. Scalable and secure access control policy for healthcare system using blockchain and enhanced Bell-LaPadula model	(R. Kumar & Tripathi)	2020	Proposing an enhanced Bell-LaPadula model to address scalability, privacy, and security issues	• Blockchain can address privacy and security within the network • The proposed model helps increase privacy and security to allow for more scalability without sacrificing on either one
22. Privacy-Preserving in Healthcare Blockchain Systems Based on Lightweight Message Sharing	(Fu et al.)	2020	They establish a lightweight privacy-preserving mechanism for a healthcare blockchain system	• Electronic Medical Record (EMR) systems are extremely important in healthcare systems • EMR's can be used with blockchain to facilitate cross-institution data sharing
23. Blockchain for E-Health-Care Systems: Easier Said Than Done	(Biswas et al.)	2020	Analyses the characteristics of e-health systems using blockchain frameworks and states the relevant challenges associated	• EMR's should be regulated • Healthcare system policies should be aligned with the requirements of privacy and security of data on the blockchain
24. Revocable Attribute-Based Signature for Blockchain-Based Healthcare System	(Su et al.)	2020	Proposed an attribute-based signature scheme to protect privacy of user identity in blockchain based healthcare system	• Attribute signature schemes do not rely on regulatory bodies or central authorities • The proposed scheme has been demonstrated to be unforgeable
25. A Novel Smart Healthcare Design, Simulation, and Implementation Using Healthcare 4.0 Processes	(A. Kumar et al.)	2020	Designing a smart healthcare system and it is found to be possible through integration and interoperability of Blockchain 3.0 and Healthcare 4.0 in consideration with healthcare ground-realities	• Healthcare 4.0 trends include industry 4.0 processes such as the Internet of Things (IoT), Industrial IoT (IIoT), cognitive computing, artificial intelligence, cloud computing, fog computing and' edge computing • Smart contracts and their designs are prepared for the proposed system to expedite the trust-building and payment systems
26. A Blockchain-Based Smart Contract System for Healthcare Management	(Khatoon)	2020	Reviews existing literature and applications available for the healthcare system using blockchain technology.	• Different medical workflows have been designed and implemented using the ethereum blockchain platform
27. Blockchain Tree for eHealth	(Kushch et al.)	2019	Introduces a novel approach based on the Blockchain technology for storing patient's medical data and creating an audit logging system able to protect health data from unauthorized modification and access.	• A balance between permissions and restrictions is needed for designing access control mechanisms • The proposed method has a tree structure • Main chain linked with what? • Patient's identity and one or several subchains used for storing additional critical data
28. Design of Blockchain-based Precision Health-Care using soft systems methodology	(Sharma et al.)	2020	The purpose of this paper is to describe the application of Soft Systems Methodology (SSM) to address the problematic situation of low opt-in rates for Precision Health-Care (PHC)	• The authors formulate design rules for the establishment of a trust-less platform for healthcare records • Blockchain and associated technologies present a cost-effective approach to low opt-in rates for health insurance coverage

Continued on following page

Table 2. Continued

Article Title	Authors	Year of Publication	Main Objective(s) of Paper	Summary of Findings
29. Challenges Providing Ground Truth for Pervasive Healthcare Systems	(Yordanova et al.)	2019	Training and validating pervasive successful healthcare systems and models	• Availability of high-quality ground truth data plays an essential role in creating healthcare systems that adapt to a person's needs and context
30. Identifying Key Challenges Facing Healthcare Systems in Africa and Potential Solutions	(Oleribe et al.)	2019	This study aimed to identify the principal challenges in the health sector in Africa and their solutions for evidence-based decisions, policy development, and program prioritization.	• The identified challenges identified were inadequate human resources (34.29%), inadequate budgetary allocation to health (30%) and poor leadership and management (8.45%). • The identified solutions were training and capacity building for health workers (29.69%), increase budgetary allocation to health (20.31%) and advocacy for political support and commitment (12.31%).
31. Compiling a prioritized list of health data quality challenges in public healthcare systems	(Botha et al.)	2014	The purpose of the paper is to identify Health Data Quality Challenges, by using a Literature Survey in public clinics in Gauteng	• 24 Broad data quality challenges have been identified from literature and will be used in further qualitative and quantitative studies to finally compile a prioritized list of Health Data Quality Challenges in Public Clinics
32. The three numbers you need to know about healthcare: the 60-30-10 Challenge	(Braithwaite et al.)	2020	Opinion paper: 60% of care on average is in line with evidence- or consensus-based guidelines, 30% is some form of waste or of low value, and 10% is harm. The 60-30-10 Challenge has persisted for three decades.	• Current top-down or chain-logic strategies to address this problem, based essentially on linear models of change and relying on policies, hierarchies, and standardization, have proven insufficient. • A deep learning health system is dynamic and shows great potential in alleviating the current challenges experienced with the current healthcare financing systems
33. Healthcare information systems: the cognitive challenge	(Lintern & Motavalli)	2018	By review and analysis of case studies, the review showed that healthcare systems developed without input from cognitive analysis and cognitive design fail to take account of important healthcare work processes and workflows	• Systems developed with a cognitively focused design strategy demonstrate how it is possible to introduce technology that supports and enhances the work strategies of those engaged in patient's care
34. Blockchain-enabled logistics finance execution platform for capital-constrained e-Commerce retail	(Li et al.)	2020	This paper proposed a blockchain-enabled logistics finance execution platform (BcLFEP) as an integrated solution to facilitate Logistics Finance (LF) for e-Commerce retail	• A hybrid finite state machine-based smart contract (HFSM-SC) is designed to associate and coordinate with all kinds of agents for LF operations throughout its lifecycle. • Blockchain is integrated with agent technology to construct a blockchain-enabled multi-agent system (BcMAS), providing a trusted runtime environment to more autonomously and efficiently executed smart contract

Continued on following page

Table 2. Continued

Article Title	Authors	Year of Publication	Main Objective(s) of Paper	Summary of Findings
35. A Systematic Review of Blockchain in Healthcare: Frameworks, Prototypes, and Implementations	(Chukwu & Garg)	2020	This study leveraged the Preferred Reporting Items for Systematic Reviews and Meta-Analyses (PRISMA) framework to systematically search and evaluate the different blockchain models proposed; prototyped and/ or implemented, to address centralizing power, failures, and attack-points	• Blockchain was found to solve the trust, security, and privacy constraints of traditional Electronic Health Records (centralizing power, failures, and attack-points) often at significant performance, storage, and cost trade-offs
36. Design Choices and Trade-Offs in Health Care Blockchain Implementations: Systematic Review	(O'Donoghue et al.)	2019	What are the trade-offs involved in different blockchain designs that are relevant to the creation of blockchain-based electronic medical records systems?	• Total of 17 trade-offs were identified impacting the design, development, and implementation of blockchain systems; these trade-offs are organized into themes, including business, application, data, and technology architecture.
37. Blockchain implementation in health care: Protocol for a systematic review	(Meinert et al.)	2019	In this work they present a Blockchain-based approach to sharing patient's data.	• This approach trades a single centralized source of trust in favor of network consensus, and predicates consensus on proof of structural and semantic interoperability.
38. Blockchain in healthcare: A systematic literature review, synthesizing framework and future research agenda	(Tandon et al.)	2020	This study presented a Systematic Literature Review (SLR) of research on blockchain applications in the healthcare domain	• The SLR findings indicate that blockchain is being used to develop novel and advanced interventions to improve the prevalent standards of handling, sharing, and processing of medical data and personal health records • Blockchain has added value through improved efficiency, access control, technological advancement, privacy protection, and security of data management processes
39. Exploring Applications of Blockchain in Securing Electronic Medical Records	(Nguyen)	2017	Understanding the elements of blockchain that can be used to secure Electronic Medical Record Systems	• Security and privacy remain a massive concern for the healthcare industry • Data breaches have only become more severe as technology has advanced, and with the current organization of security solutions, this trend seems unlikely to change in meaningful ways • Electronic medical records increase engagement between the public and private healthcare sector
40. A Comparative Analysis of Blockchain Architecture and its Applications: Problems and Recommendations	(Ali Syed et al.)	2019	This study presents a comparative analysis of core blockchain architectures, its fundamental concepts, and its applications in three major areas: The Internet-of-Things (IoT), healthcare, business and vehicular industry.	• Blockchain can be incorporated into IoT devices, creating an IoT chain • Decentralization and scalability remain the most prominent factors to address in healthcare systems

Continued on following page

Table 2. Continued

Article Title	Authors	Year of Publication	Main Objective(s) of Paper	Summary of Findings
41. Zero-trust hierarchical management in IoT	(Samaniego & Deters)	2018	This research introduces Amatista, a blockchain-based middleware for management in IoT	• Amatista presents a novel zero-trust hierarchical mining process that allows validating the infrastructure and transactions at different levels of trust. • Zero-trust can be applied to IoT blockchain enabled infrastructures

Chapter 10
Towards a Model for Self-Disclosure on Social Network Sites:
A Pilot Study

Mahamadou Kante
https://orcid.org/0000-0002-5544-8166
Université Virtuelle de Côte d'Ivoire, Côte d'Ivoire

Joel Christian Adepo
Université Virtuelle de Côte d'Ivoire, Côte d'Ivoire

Michel Babri
Université Félix Houphouët-Boigny, Côte d'Ivoire

ABSTRACT

One of the current discussions is the resilience of health systems in developing countries. Online platforms users including health system users (patients, doctors) are worried about their privacy being violated. While the users of social media enjoy the opportunity to learn, connect, and share, their privacy on those platforms is at risk. A possible cause of this is the information privacy paradox, which describes a disconnect between users' stated concerns and actual behaviour. In the pilot phase of this study, the authors have used the partial least squares structural equation modelling technique for the analysis of the relationships postulated to explain self-disclosure in social network sites. The survey instrument's content validity and adapted model's constructs validity and reliability were confirmed, and the preliminary findings revealed that the derived model explains 32.9% of the user's self-disclosure intention on social network sites.

DOI: 10.4018/978-1-7998-8915-1.ch010

INTRODUCTION

Resilience is an important concept in the context of healthcare systems implementation. Resilience has been defined as the ability of health systems to adapt in the face of crises such as Covid-19 and to plan for future shocks (Heeks, 2018). Resilience in health system relies on the constituents of health information systems ecosystem such as Information technology, people (nurses, medical doctors, policymakers, patients and others) and processes with people being at the centre of building resilient health systems. However, people who are part of healthcare ecosystems are affected by factors related to privacy and security when engaging with healthcare systems that need further investigation.

Hoy & Milne (2010) and Yao (2011) argue that online platforms including health systems' users (patients, doctors) are worried about their privacy being violated. Further, on Social Network Sites (SNS) like Twitter and Facebook, self-disclosure of personal information is a critical aspect for the users, in terms of security and privacy. This was also supported by Marwick & Hargittai (2019) who posited that some SNS users in addition to their concerns about security and privacy infringement perceive privacy violations as inevitable. Hence, people (users) disclosing their personal information (self-disclosure) has become an issue as it poses a risk to their privacy.

Recent privacy violation cases such as the Cambridge Analytica (CA) data harvest have shown that it is to the best of SNS users to protect themselves by controlling what information they disclose. The tech company, CA, reportedly harvested over 50 million Facebook profiles with the purpose to build software to influence and predict choices during the United States 2016 presidential election (Graham-Harrison & Cadwalladr, 2018). In fact, it has been reported by the CA whistleblower Wylie Christopher that the company used the data to predict and influence voters during President Donald Trump's campaign in the 2016 presidential election.

Issues associated with self-disclosure have been reported in many studies. For instance, Krasnova et al., 2010 and Min & Kim, 2015) investigated online users' information (personal) sharing enticement. Moreover, self-disclosure has been investigated considering traits such as culture (Krasnova et al., 2012b), and social context (Cui, 2015). While there is an agreement amongst scholars on online users behaviour and self-disclosure, debates continue regarding the factors that may affect that behaviour and the extent to which these factors affect online users. It was argued by Yao (2011) that self-disclosure of SNS user may be caused by his/her behaviour online. In the same vein, Krasnova et al. (2010) stated that behavior is determined by factors like platform enjoyment and the quest for maintaining existing relationship. Factors such as perceived similarity, keeping up with trends or social ties have also been mentioned as driving factors for online self-disclosure behaviors (Mahamadou Kante, 2022). Additionally, Zlatolas et al. (2015) reported privacy concerns as affecting the behaviour of SNS users to self-disclosure. Hence, the main objective of this study was to design and test a structural model for self-disclosure as a comprehensive pilot study phase. The specific objectives were:

1. To propose a conceptual model of SNSs' users self-disclosure
2. To establish the construct validity of the proposed conceptual model

FACTORS AFFECTING SELF-DISCLOSURE

An indispensable feature of any academic project is the literature review (Müller-Bloch & Kranz, 2015). We conducted an online literature search (Google scholar) in an attempt to single out factors that may affect SNSs' self-disclosure practices following the framework proposed by Levy & Ellis (Levy & Ellis, 2006). The proposed Framework (Figure 1) follows a systematic data processing approach which includes three main stages:

- Inputs: literature gathering and screening;
- Processing;
- Outputs: writing the literature.

The literature search was done exclusively digitally and details about the search strategy used are presented in Table 1.

Figure 1. The three stages of effective literature review process
Source (Levy & Ellis, 2006)

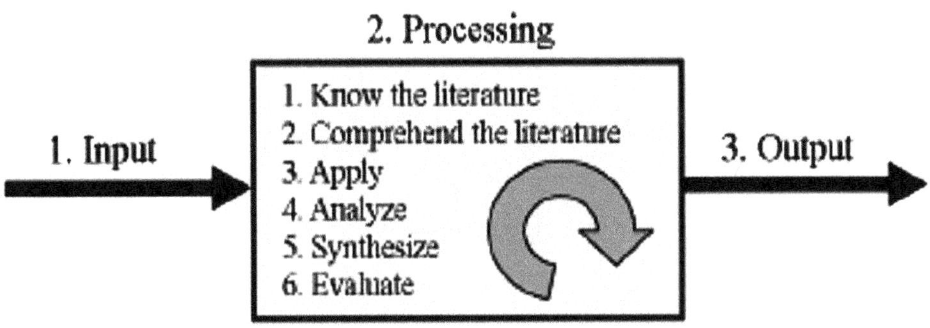

Table 1. Search strategy

Search Component	A	B	C
Search terms	Privacy Or Privacy protection Or Information privacy Or Information privacy protection	Social Network Services Or Social Media Or Online Social Networks	Facebook
Combinations of search terms	A + B + C Or A + B Or A + C		
Selection criteria	The content is focused on the search terms, or the combinations of the terms		

Source: format of this table was adapted from (Ismail & Zainab, 2013)

According to Roberts (2012) the formal research work that attempted to understand online consumer's concerns (but not behaviour) for information privacy using a theory is the work of Malhotra et al. (2004). Drawing on Social Contract (SC) theory (explanation), and the theory of reasoned action (TRA) (explanation), directed by the famous trust-risk framework; they proposed a causal model (see Figure 2) on how Internet Users' Information Privacy Concerns (IUIPC) influences user's decision to disclose or not personal information in a given situation.

Figure 2. Influence of Internet Users' Information Privacy Concerns (IUIPC) on user's decision to disclose personal information

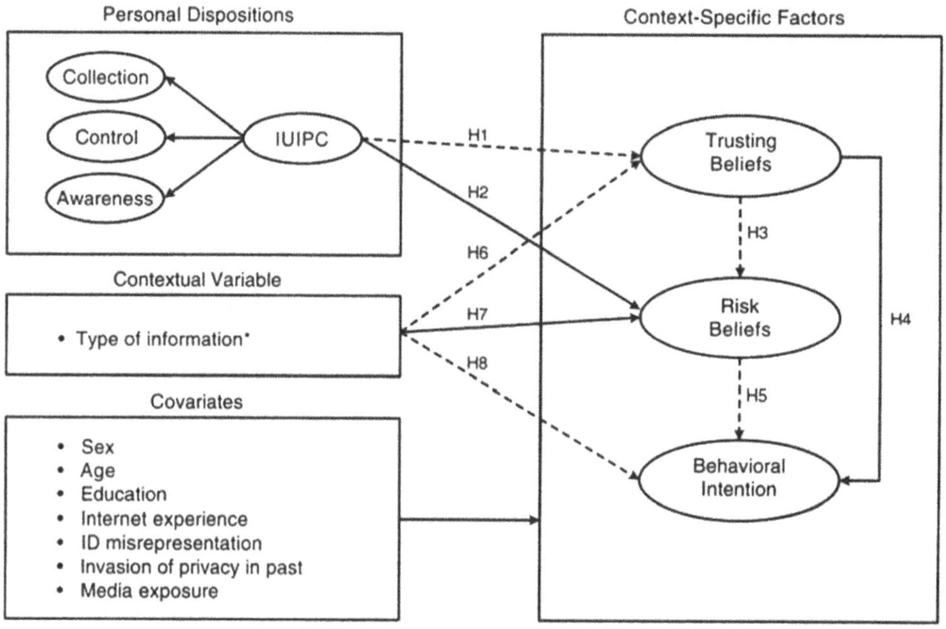

The IUIPC was originally developed to reflect recent changes at a time in an individual's views on fairness/justice because of the widespread use of the Internet. Their findings indicated that consumers' concerns caused by those unfair organizational practices can be succinctly summarized into the SC-based IUIPC concept. Furthermore, they also found that trusting beliefs and risk beliefs mediated the impact of IUIPC on behavioral intention. Their discoveries showed that people' worries brought by unfair practices of the firms can be briefly condensed into the SC-based IUIPC idea. Besides, their results suggest that risk beliefs and trusting beliefs mediated the effect of the model on behavioural expectation. Some limitations of IUIPC include but are not limited to: they investigated what factors informs one's level of concern and direct subsequent behaviour (Roberts, 2012). Though, according to the TRA a good indicator of behaviour starts with behavioural intention (Fishbein & Ajzen, 1975), but, considering the paradox, this might not always be the case.

Following that work, many studies have tried to understand privacy paradox in different settings using for example the theory of planned behaviour (TPB). The TPB is an extension of the TRA in which perceived behavioural control is incorporated as an antecedent to behavioural intentions (Ajzen & Fishbein, 1980; Madden et al., 1992). Indeed, Reynolds et al. (2011) attempted to find out users' attitude regarding day to day sharing against their actual behaviour on Facebook. They provided people a better comprehending of the notion of privacy paradox in the context of social media. Data were collected in the study using a multi-pronged approach. The majority of the respondents claimed to be Facebook users with an average of one to 2 years on the platform. Their findings suggest that users posting behaviour and their concern about privacy have little correlation. One key finding was in-line with previous research that gender and age have an influence on privacy attitudes.

Tufekci (2008) investigated student's online privacy concerns drawing on the social ecology framework of Altman (1975) which provides a conceptually rich multidimensional dynamic model for interpreting the interpersonal regulation of privacy. However, the model was developed before the widespread of social media phenomenon. In fact, privacy is more seen nowadays as boundary-control process by which an individual has control over whom and how one can access his (personal) information. In their study, Tufekci (2008) reported that concerns about privacy and information sharing had no relationship. They found that among the students, the majority use different privacy management configurations to decide who can see what they share with no regards to the type of information. Contrary to Tufekci (2008), Reynolds et al. (2011) found that the overall behaviour towards privacy was independent to posts that were accessible by a public audience.

Privacy behaviour is a highly contextual phenomenon. In fact, Kokolakis (2017) posited that people behave according to a given context. Actually, users are considered as the weakest link in security as reported by Sasse et al. (2001), in other terms, the platforms can have cutting edge technologies but the service users will always be the breach through which security flaws shall appear mostly. Therefore, considering the wideness and sharing concept behind social media platform, the issue increases exponentially.

Table 2. Evidence that supports the privacy paradox

Study	Methodology	Participants
(Barnes, 2006)	Survey	SNSs
(Malhotra et al., 2004)	One on one Interviews	Household respondent
(Tufekci, 2008)	Longitudinal survey	Facebook & Myspace users (students)
(Reynolds et al., 2011)	Survey	Facebook users
(Krasnova et al., 2010)	Focus group & survey	Users (students)
(Emad et al., 2018)	Survey	SNSs users
(Digital et al., 2011)	Survey	SNSs users
(Krasnova et al., 2012a)	Survey	Facebook users
(Roberts, 2012)	Experiment	SNSs users

Overall, the factors identified from the selected studies and their descriptions are reported below in Table 3. In this study, self-disclosure refers to "the extent of personal information an individual gives in the process of participation on a SNS" (Krasnova et al., 2010, p. 112).

Table 3. Identified Self-disclosure factors

Factor	Description
Relationships Maintenance	The reward users get from having the option to conveniently keep in contact with one another on SNSs (Krasnova et al., 2010)
New Relationship Building	The reward users get from having the option to develop new relationships with others on SNSs (Krasnova et al., 2010)
Enjoyment	The reward users get from having enjoyable encounters on SNSs (Krasnova et al., 2010)
Privacy concerns	A person's subjective perspective of fairness in a data privacy context (Campbell, 1997)
Information sensitivity	Data that contains high risk(in contrary to low risk) that causes the discloser to feel threatened in some way (Moon, 2000)
Trust in SNS provider	Convictions that the SNS provider has attributes that prevent it from taking part in opportunistic attitude (McKnight et al., 2002)
Trust in SNS members	Convictions that SNS members have attributes that prevent them from taking part in opportunistic attitude (McKnight et al., 2002)
Perceived control 1 Platform-Enabled 2 Legal Assurance	(1) *"Beliefs about one's ability to prevent undesired events on SNSs using privacy control options and privacy policies"* (analogue to Skinner, 1996) in (Krasnova et al., 2010, p. 112) (2) *"Beliefs that legal structures like regulations laws or other procedures adequately protect user privacy"* (Krasnova et al., 2010, p. 112)

THEORETICAL BACKGROUND

Scholars have used numerous disciplines to find a theory that can supplement the conceptualization of Information Privacy (disclosure). These include behavioural economics, social theory, psychology, and even quantum theory (Kokolakis, 2017; Wirth, 2018). The theory that stands out to be the most used theory in current research that is directed towards interpreting the gap between privacy behaviour and attitude is the privacy calculus theory.

Privacy Calculus and Self-Disclosure

The divulgation of personal information goes with a certain risk. Individuals, in their daily communications (online/offline) with others share personal information about themselves. This attitude has been explained in the literature and it shows the existence of privacy risks along with the disclosure of personal information but also that disclosure might provide significant benefits to the person disclosing (Warren, 2017). The notion of privacy calculus theory is the calculus that occurs between the potential benefits and privacy risks of data disclosure (Culnan & Armstrong, 1999). The theory was further elaborated on by Culnan & Bies (2003) with the intention of proposing other alternatives for implementing a fair information practices with particular attention to the internet. Considering the privacy calculus theory in social media contexts, it postulates that an online platform user will do a cost-benefit analysis when requested to disclose personal information to assess what they might deal with (or get) in exchange for their information.

The literature provides evidence of the use of the privacy calculus theory in studying factors that may influence self-disclosure. For instance, the privacy calculus theory was used in Felim et al. (2018) to identify the motivation of ASKfm (a social network on mobile devices and the Web that allows the user to ask questions to friends or others who also use the service) users to share their personal information and understand their willingness to disclose them based on their culture and gender. Many other studies (Hallam & Zanella, 2017; Koroleva et al., 2011; Krasnova et al., 2012b; Li et al., 2010; Marwick & Hargittai, 2019; Min & Kim, 2015; Warren, 2017; Wirth et al., 2019) have studied the nexus of self-disclosure and privacy in online settings using the privacy calculus theory. Therefore, in line with previous studies, this study uses the privacy calculus model (see Figure 3) to comprehend the concept of privacy paradox in the context of SNSs, especially Facebook. Specifically, this study will investigate factors that should be taken into consideration in the context of personal information disclosure.

Conceptual Framework and Hypotheses Development

In this section, we present our proposed model (see Figure 4), which is mainly based on the model of self-disclosure in SNSs proposed by (Krasnova et al., 2010) and theoretically relying on the privacy calculus theory described earlier. The self-disclosure factors identified within the literature which are used in our model were presented in Table 3.

Figure 3. The privacy calculus
Source: adapted from (Wirth et al., 2019)

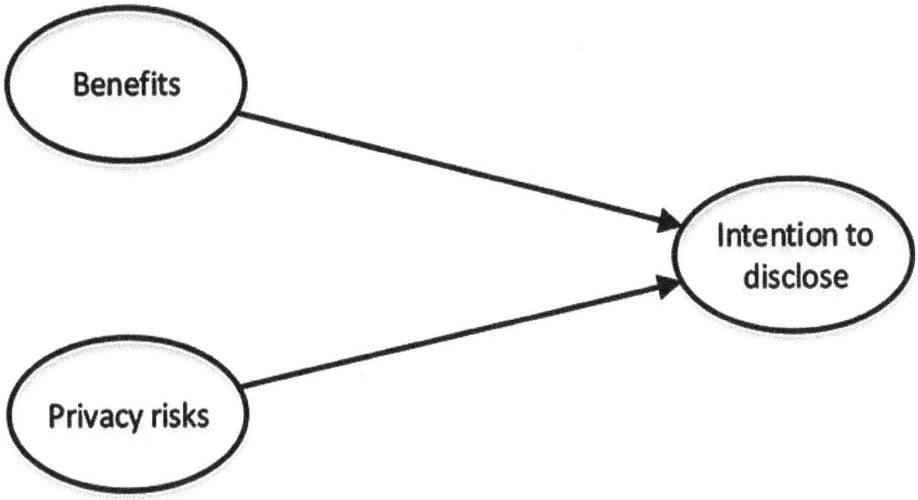

Benefits of Information Disclosure on SNSs

Relationships Maintenance

Krasnova et al. (2010) found that the most important benefit of using a SNS was the capability to maintain existing relationships in real-life. They indicated that SNS provide users with ways and tools to remain in contact with friends and maintain constant communication (Krasnova et al., 2010). With people generally being in distant locations in the pursuit of their career or educational purposes, maintaining their existing relationships is considered as an important factor. As argued by Qadheeb & Alsalloum (2018) SNS are convenient in keeping in touch with one another. Therefore, people disclose their personal information to make sure their family, friends, remain part of their lives. Therefore we hypothesized that:

H1a: User's beliefs regarding the ability to conveniently maintain existing relationships using SNS will affect in a positive manner their self-disclosure in SNS.

Building New Relationship

As SNSs allow users to manage existing connections between people, SNS also provide an environment where users can create new connections with people. Therefore, we hypothesized that:

H1b: Users' beliefs regarding new relationship-building opportunities on SNS will affect in a positive manner their self-disclosure in SNS.

Enjoyment

Enjoyment is essential in the use of any social media platform. For instance, many scholars have identified enjoyment as an important factor considered by users for the use of SNS (Krasnova et al., 2010, 2012b; Taddicken, 2014). Users may get various benefits by disclosing personal information on SNS, such as improved connectedness, self-esteem (Krasnova et al., 2012b). Some SNS give access to additional features to improve enjoyment. For example, Facebook uses gaming, online sharing, messaging and video sharing (Qadheeb & Alsalloum, 2018) to increase its user's enjoyment on their platform. Thus, we hypothesized that:

H1c: Users perceived enjoyment on SNS will affect in a positive manner their self-disclosure on SNS.

Concerns of Information Disclosure on SNS

Privacy Concerns

The use of SNS makes the users vulnerable to various threats to their privacy which could lead to them not disclosing personal information. For instance, studies have reported that while it remains true that the expectation of benefits motivates users to disclose their personal information, however, privacy concerns negatively affect users intention to disclose (Krasnova et al., 2012b; Taddicken, 2014; Warren, 2017; Wirth, 2018). In this study, we hypothesized that:

H2a: User' Information privacy concern will affect in a negative manner their self-disclosure on SNS.

Information Sensitivity

In the context of SNS, when sensitive information is accessed by an undesired or unauthorized person will result in negative consequences (Digital et al., 2011). We propose that:

H2b: Information sensitivity will affect in a negative manner their self-disclosure on SNS.

Trust

Trust plays a key role in information disclosure. SNS providers allow users to share various types of information. However, considering the limited control some SNS providers give their users over who can access and to what extent the disclosed information can be used members of a SNS must trust each other at a certain level for disclosure to happen (Qadheeb & Alsalloum, 2018). One will feel less concerned about privacy if she/he trusts other members. Moreover, trust in the service provider will as well lessen concerns about privacy. Thus, we hypothesized that:

H3a: Users' trust in other SNS members will reduce their privacy concerns on SNS.
H3b: Users' trust in the SNS Provider will reduce their privacy concerns on SNS.

Perceived Control

As argued by Krasnova et al. (2010) even if trust might be an important factor it does not allow users to control the behaviour of others. When users are given more control on the SNS platforms, the perceived privacy risk might decrease. More clear and effective policies could help increase the perceived control, which will positively impact on the trust beliefs of SNS providers as well as other members. Thus, we hypothesized that:

H4a: The perceived control of the users will reduce their privacy concerns on SNS.
H4b: The perceived control of the users will affect in a positive manner their trust in SNS service provider.
H4c: Users' perceived control will affect in a positive manner their trust in other SNS members.

Figure 4. Conceptual framework
(- - - = Negative effect, ____ = positive effect)

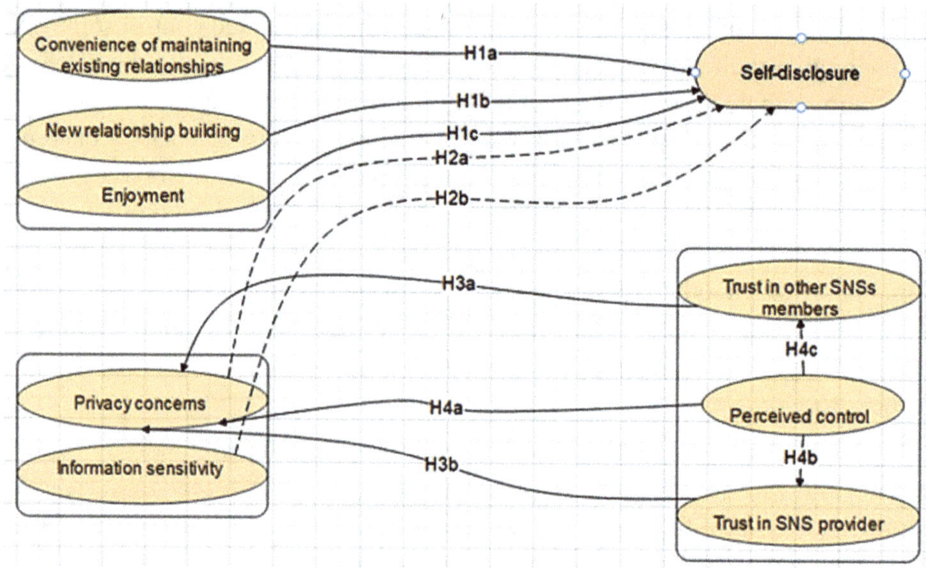

METHODS

Research Design

This study aimed to investigate online self-disclosure on SNSs, specifically Facebook. Moreover, this study is intended to serve as a pilot phase to test the proposed model. It adopted a quantitative approach. Quantitative research is explaining phenomena by collecting numerical data that are analyzed using mathematically based methods (in particular statistics) (Muijs, 2010).

Data Collection and Analysis

For data collection, a web-based survey questionnaire was developed and distributed through one SNS, namely Facebook. The sampling process will be executed randomly within. The research instrument was structured as follows: Section A presented the study's objectives, introduced the main researcher, and delineated how the respondents answers will be handled and furthers stated that participation in the study is voluntary. The primary aim of Section A was to get to know how the respondents use SNS and if they have been using Facebook specifically.

Section B collected respondents' basic data such as location; education, marital status and age. Finally, section C focused on the measurements of the study's variables.

We analyzed the data using SPSS v20 and SMART PLS 3.2.9. We used SPSS for cleaning the data and descriptive statistics such as mean calculations. We used SMART PLS 3 to conduct the Partial Least Square Structural Equation Modelling (PLS-SEM) analysis. SEM is mainly utilized for two purposes. Firstly, it is used to test theories or to develop one (covariance-based approach) (Krasnova et al., 2010). Secondly, SEM is solicited when dealing with predictive application (Partial Least Squares) (Krasnova et al., 2010). PLS-SEM has two models, the inner and outer model. In the inner model, the meaning of the constructs are determined by the outer model (G. David Garson, 2016). The inner model also called the structural model constitutes the causal model.

Measurements and Constructs

The following constructs will be evaluated: convenience of maintaining relationships, relationship building, enjoyment, privacy concern, information sensitivity, trust in SNS providers, trust in SNS members, perceived control and information disclosure. The resulting list of constructs measurement, and their sources are presented in Table 4.

Overall, 37 items were used to measure the study's constructs and they were mostly adapted from the existing literature (Chiu et al., 2006; Krasnova et al., 2010), (Nambisan & Baron, 2007), (Dinev & Hart, 2004; Wu & Zeng, 2012; Xu et al., 2012), (Digital et al., 2011), (Jarvenpaa et al., 1999; McKnight et al., 2002). A five-point Likert scale (1= strongly agree, 2 = agree, 3= neither agree nor disagree, 4= disagree, 5= strongly disagree) was used to measure all the constructs.

Table 4. Constructs and measures

Construct	Code	Item text
Convenience of maintaining existing relationship (Chiu et al., 2006; Krasnova et al., 2010)	CON1 CON2 CON3	1-Facebook is convenient for informing all my friends about my on-going activities of maintaining 2- Facebook allows me to save time when I want to share something new with my friends existing 3- I find Facebook effective in strengthen my relationship with my friends
New relationship building (Krasnova et al., 2010)	RB1 RB2 RB3	4- Through Facebook I get connected to new people who share my interests 5- Facebook helps me to expand my network 6- I get to know new people through Facebook
Enjoyment (Nambisan & Baron, 2007)	EN1 EN2 EN3	7- When I am bored I often login to Facebook. 8- I find Facebook entertaining 9- I spend enjoyable and relaxing time on Facebook
Privacy concern (Dinev & Hart, 2004; Wu & Zeng, 2012; Xu et al., 2012)	PC1 PC2 PC3 PC4 PC5	10- It bothers me when I have to put much personal information on Facebook 11- I am concerned that Facebook is collecting too much personal information about me 12- I am concerned that unauthorized people could access my personal information 13- I am concerned that Facebook use my personal information for purposes that I am not being notified of 14-I am concerned when I have to post personal information on Facebook
Information sensitivity Based on (Digital et al., 2011)	IS1 IS2 IS3 IS4 IS5 IS6 IS7	15- Basic information (sex, birthday, hometown, political and religious views) 16-Contact information (emails, home/school addresses and phone numbers, website URL) 17- Relationship information (status, interested in, looking for) 18- Personal information (activities, interests, about me, favourite movies, favourite Sports, TV shows, books, and quotes) 19- Educational information (university, class year, high school, primary) 20-Work information (employer, position, description, city/town) 21-Tagged photos
Trust in SNS provider (Jarvenpaa et al., 1999; McKnight et al., 2002)	TP1 TP2 TP3 TP4 TP5	Facebook 22- ...is open and receptive to the needs of its members 23- ...makes good-faith efforts to address most member concerns 24- ...is also interested in the well-being of its members, not just its own 25- ... is honest in its dealings with me 26- ... keeps its commitments to its members
Trust in other SNS Members (Chiu et al., 2006; McKnight et al., 2002)	TM1 TM2 TM3 TM4	Other members on Facebook 27- ...do care about the well-being of others 28- ... are open and receptive to the needs of each other 29- ... are honest in dealing with each other 30- ... are trustworthy

Continued on following page

Table 4. Continued

Construct	Code	Item text
Perceived Control (Krasnova et al., 2010)	PCo1 PCo2 PCo3	31- I feel in control over the information I provide on Facebook 32- Privacy settings allow me to have full control over the information I provide on the Facebook 33- I feel in control of who can view my information on Facebook
Self-Disclosure (Krasnova et al., 2010)	SD1 SD2 SD3 SD4	34- I have a comprehensive profile on Facebook 35- I find time to keep my profile up-to-date 36- I keep my friends updated about what is going on in my life through Facebook 37- When I have something to say, I like to share it on Facebook

RESULTS AND DISCUSSION

We report and discuss the results of this pilot study in this section.

Descriptive Statistics

Our final data set consisted of 86 valid responses. Respondents were from various continents namely Africa (75.9%), Asia (2.4%), Europe (17%), Australia (1.2%) and North America (3.5%). Most of the respondents were between 25 and 34 years of age, accounting for 57% of the respondents; 32.5% of the respondent were aged between the age of 18 and 24. This point to the fact that our respondents were young and below the age of 34, in fact only 10.5% were above 34 years of age. It is safe to say, based on these results that the youth tend to be more active on SNS than adults (above 35 years old). In terms of gender, we had 80.20% male respondents against 19.80 females.

Construct Validity

Convergent Validity

This section reports and discusses factors motivating (or discouraging) self-disclosure attitudes on SNS. These factors were determined by assessing the outer model (measurement model) of the proposed model (conceptual model). The establishment of the construct validity (convergent and discriminant validity) of the study's variables means that the variable passed the construct validity test are the (potential) determinants, i.e. the factors that (may) affect self-disclosure behaviours by SNS (Facebook) users.

Table 5. Construct reliability and validity

<table>
<tr><th></th><th>Indicators</th><th>Loadings</th><th>Indicator Reliability</th><th>Cronbach's Alpha</th><th>Composite Reliability</th><th>Average Variance Extracted (AVE)</th></tr>
<tr><td rowspan="3">Relationships Maintenance</td><td>CON1</td><td>0.845</td><td>0.714</td><td rowspan="3">0.755</td><td rowspan="3">0,856</td><td rowspan="3">0,664</td></tr>
<tr><td>CON2</td><td>0.798</td><td>0.636</td></tr>
<tr><td>CON3</td><td>0.801</td><td>0.641</td></tr>
<tr><td rowspan="3">Enjoyment</td><td>EN1</td><td>0.771</td><td>0.594</td><td rowspan="3">0.822</td><td rowspan="3">0.870</td><td rowspan="3">0.692</td></tr>
<tr><td>EN2</td><td>0.768</td><td>0.589</td></tr>
<tr><td>EN3</td><td>0.944</td><td>0.891</td></tr>
<tr><td rowspan="7">Information sensitivity</td><td>IS1</td><td>0.459</td><td>0.210</td><td rowspan="7">1.000</td><td rowspan="7">1.000</td><td rowspan="7">1.000</td></tr>
<tr><td>IS2</td><td>0.721</td><td>0.519</td></tr>
<tr><td>IS3</td><td>0.513</td><td>0.263</td></tr>
<tr><td>IS4</td><td>0.465</td><td>0.216</td></tr>
<tr><td>IS5</td><td>0.440</td><td>0.193</td></tr>
<tr><td>IS6</td><td>0.218</td><td>0.047</td></tr>
<tr><td>IS7</td><td>0.001</td><td>0</td></tr>
<tr><td rowspan="3">New relationship building</td><td>RB1</td><td>0.883</td><td>0.779</td><td rowspan="3">0.857</td><td rowspan="3">0.913</td><td rowspan="3">0.778</td></tr>
<tr><td>RB2</td><td>0.930</td><td>0.864</td></tr>
<tr><td>RB3</td><td>0.831</td><td>0.690</td></tr>
<tr><td rowspan="5">Privacy concerns</td><td>PC1</td><td>0.921</td><td>0.848</td><td rowspan="5">0.839</td><td rowspan="5">0.873</td><td rowspan="5">0.634</td></tr>
<tr><td>PC2</td><td>0.794</td><td>0.630</td></tr>
<tr><td>PC3</td><td>0.559</td><td>0.312</td></tr>
<tr><td>PC4</td><td>0.692</td><td>0.478</td></tr>
<tr><td>PC5</td><td>0.759</td><td>0.576</td></tr>
<tr><td rowspan="4">Self-disclosure</td><td>SD1</td><td>0.734</td><td>0.538</td><td rowspan="4">0.848</td><td rowspan="4">0.897</td><td rowspan="4">0.688</td></tr>
<tr><td>SD2</td><td>0.883</td><td>0.779</td></tr>
<tr><td>SD3</td><td>0.889</td><td>0.790</td></tr>
<tr><td>SD4</td><td>0.802</td><td>0.643</td></tr>
<tr><td rowspan="5">Trust in SNS provider</td><td>TP1</td><td>0.769</td><td>0.591</td><td rowspan="5">0.854</td><td rowspan="5">0.895</td><td rowspan="5">0.630</td></tr>
<tr><td>TP2</td><td>0.853</td><td>0.727</td></tr>
<tr><td>TP3</td><td>0.774</td><td>0.599</td></tr>
<tr><td>TP4</td><td>0.766</td><td>0.586</td></tr>
<tr><td>TP5</td><td>0.802</td><td>0.643</td></tr>
<tr><td rowspan="4">Trust in other SNSs members</td><td>TM1</td><td>0.856</td><td>0.732</td><td rowspan="4">0.897</td><td rowspan="4">0.928</td><td rowspan="4">0.764</td></tr>
<tr><td>TM2</td><td>0.929</td><td>0.863</td></tr>
<tr><td>TM3</td><td>0.869</td><td>0.755</td></tr>
<tr><td>TM4</td><td>0.840</td><td>0.705</td></tr>
</table>

Continued on following page

Table 5. Continued

	Indicators	Loadings	Indicator Reliability	Cronbach's Alpha	Composite Reliability	Average Variance Extracted (AVE)
Perceived control	PCo1	0.870	0.756	0.765	0.858	0.670
	PCo2	0.889	0.790			
	PCo3	0.681	0.463			

For construct validity to be established, firstly, the reliability of the indicators must be established to ensure that the items that comprise the indicators meet the appropriate requirements for operationalization of the constructs. The indicator reliability (the square of the loading) value of 0.6 (Macire Kante et al., 2018) or 0,7 (Wynne W. Chin, 1998) or greater is recommended for an item to pass the reliability test. However, in exploratory studies, values equal to 0.4 or greater is acceptable (Wynne W. Chin, 1998) in (Karuri et al., 2014). Items that have a value of 0.4 can only be removed if that would lead to an enhanced composite reliability value. In this study, we considered only loadings value above 0.4. As shown in table 5, we report the indicators loadings values and six indicators (IS1, IS3, IS4, IS5, IS7, PC3) had values lesser than 0.4. Hence, these indicators were dropped and did not feature in the next stages of the analysis.

In the second step of establishing construct validity, the Convergent Validity must be established through the Composite Reliability (value above 0.6) or the Average Variance Extracted (AVE) (value above 0.5) or the Cronbach's Alpha (value above 0.6) (G. David Garson, 2016; Macire Kante et al., 2018). As it can be seen in Table 3, we report the three criteria (Cronbach's Alpha, Composite Reliability and AVE) and they all point to a good convergent validity of our constructs (latent variables).

Divergent Validity

The discriminant or divergent validity assessment has the goal to ensure that a reflective construct has the strongest relationships with its own indicators (e.g., in comparison with than any other construct) in the PLS path model (Hair Jr et al., 2021). The divergent validity can be established through the Fornell-Larcker Criterion or the Heterotrait-Menotrait Ratio (HTMT) or the cross-loadings (G. David Garson, 2016; Macire Kante et al., 2018). This study used the Fornell-Larcker criterion to establish the divergent validity of the variables. When a latent variable has more variance with its indicators than any other latent variable, therefore the Fornell-Larcker criterion is satisfied. The results of the Fornell-Larcker criterion analysis are shown in Table 6 below. As this criterion was satisfied, we state that the divergent validity of the constructs was established. Summing up the convergent and divergent validity, we can conclude that the construct validity of each one of our conceptual model was established taking into account the 6 items eliminated during the convergent validity testing. Hence, the survey instrument was validated. Thus, based on the proposed Conceptual framework (Figure 4) pre-test, the factors that affect self-disclosure behaviours in SNSs (Facebook) are relationships maintenance, Enjoyment, New relationship Building, Information sensitivity, Privacy Concerns, Trust in other SNS members, Trust in SNS providers, perceived control and users self-disclosure intention.

Table 6. Fornell-Larcker discriminant validity criterion

	Convenience of Maintaining Existing Relationships	Enjoyment	Information Sensitivity	New Relationship Building	Privacy Concerns	Self-disclosure	Trust in SNS Provider	Trust in Other SNSs Members	Perceived Control
Relationships Maintenance	**0,815**								
Enjoyment	0,469	**0,832**							
Information sensitivity	0,282	0,165	**1,000**						
New relationship building	0,475	0,573	0,235	**0,882**					
Privacy concerns	0,033	0,076	0,234	-0,062	**0,796**				
Self-disclosure	0,372	0,381	0,119	0,495	-0,237	**0,829**			
Trust in SNS provider	0,452	0,479	0,241	0,539	-0,141	0,481	**0,794**		
Trust in other SNSs members	0,202	0,142	0,191	0,093	0,019	0,258	0,546	**0,874**	
perceived control	0,215	0,406	0,312	0,368	-0,140	0,528	0,603	0,337	**0,819**

Structural Model Fit

The final step of the PLS-SEM analysis is to assess the causal relationships between the constructs, and to eventually support or reject the study's conceptual model and the proposed hypotheses. Figure 3 represents the result of the PLS algorithm using SmartPLS 3 after the elimination of a few indicators (i.e. items) aforementioned as they did not meet the suggested reliability level during the convergent validity testing.

The variance explained (R2) or the coefficient of determination for the last level endogenous variable, namely Self-disclosure was 0.329 and that of Privacy concerns was 0.038. That means that the latent variables (LVs) Privacy concerns,

Enjoyment, Relationship maintenance, new relationship building explained 32.9% of the variance of SNS users' Self-disclosure while Trust in other SNS members, Perceived control and Trust in SNS provider explained only 3.8% of the variance of users' privacy concerns. Additionally, the exogenous variable Perceived control explained 36.4% of the variance in users' Trust in SNS provider and 11.3% of the variance in users' Trust in other SNS members.

Figure 5. PLS Results

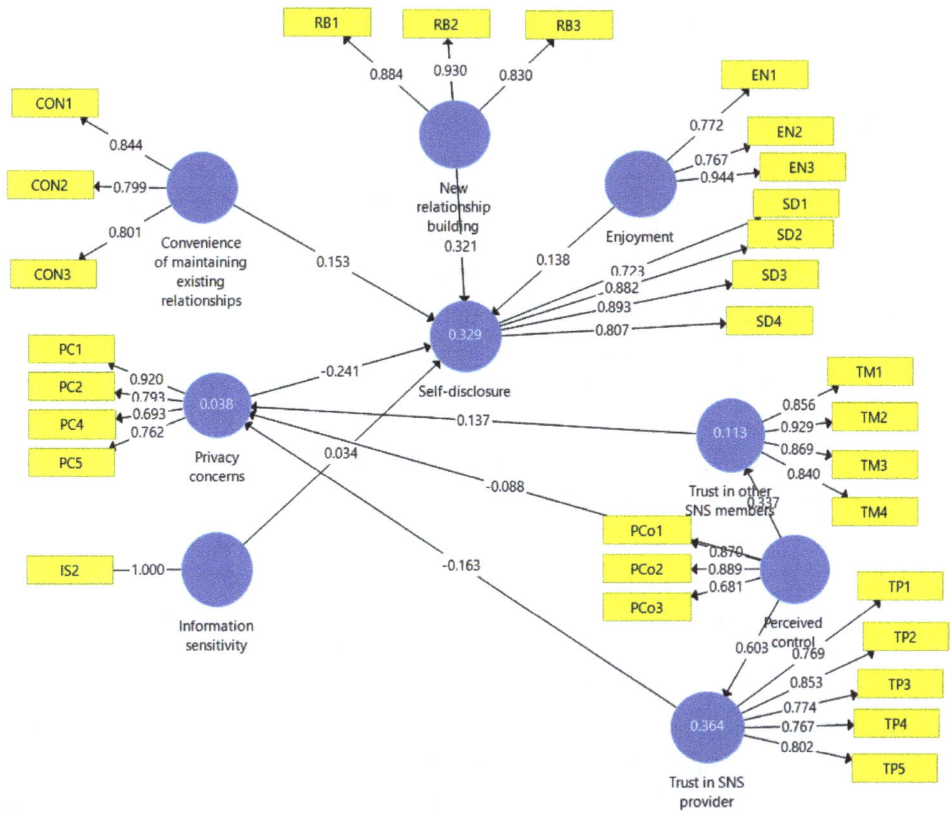

Concerning the inner model (see Figure 5), among the factors that positively motivate self-disclosure, Building New Relationships has the strongest effect (.321), followed by Convenience of maintaining existing relationships (.153) and Enjoyment (.138). On the other hand, as expected, Privacy concern (-0.241) has the strongest negative effect on self-disclosure behaviours on SNS followed by Information sensitivity with a weak but surprising positive effect (0.034).

The results show also that Trust (in SNS provider (-0.163) and other members (0.137)) and perceived control (-0.111) have surprising weak effects on users' privacy concerns either in increasing or lessening their concerns. As indicated in Figure 5, the significance of path coefficient is met when the path value is more than 0.1. Overall, that criterion was met in all the structural path relationship except for the relationship between Information sensitivity (independent variable) and the self-disclosure (dependent variable). This suggests that the construct Information sensitivity is to be dropped in our future research endeavours. In light of the small sample size (86), even though it is sufficient for a model test, could not allow us to carry out any further analysis to test the structural path relationships.

CONCLUSION

In this study, we aim to use the privacy calculus model to understand and identify determinant factors for self-disclosure behaviours in SNSs (Facebook). In this paper, we have discussed the comprehensive pilot phase of the study. The results revealed the suitability of the proposed research model, which is based on the privacy calculus theory, albeit the small sample size.

The Partial least square Structural Equation Modelling was used to ensure the reliability and validity of the items used to measure the proposed model constructs. We were then able to establish valid and reliable measures before embarking on the analysis of the structural model. Our preliminary findings suggest that the model explain 32.9% of variance in self-disclosure. More specifically, privacy concerns explained 3.8% of the variance in self-disclosure while Trust in SNS provider and Trust in other SNS members explained 36.4% and 11.3% of the variance in self-disclosure respectively. However, it is to be noted that the results might be biased considering that this is a pilot study. The study was conducted to serve as a basis to conduct a more reliable study using a larger and hence representative sample size.

The next stage of this study is to use the validated model to conduct a large-scale data collection targeting the right population based on the demographic data we got from this pilot study. Moreover, we might use other validated constructs/indicators identified by other researchers from new literature that would have emerged after the publication of this preliminary study's findings. Notwithstanding its limitations, this pilot study could serve as a starting point for other researchers to undertake studies about self-disclosure behaviours and not necessarily in the context of SNS, for example in health-care information systems.

CONFLICT OF INTERESTS

All authors declare no conflicts of interest in this paper.

ACKNOWLEDGMENT

This research received no specific grant from any funding agency in the public, commercial, or not-for-profit sectors. The authors would like to thank all the respondents who took their time to complete the survey. We would also like to thank all the participants who invest their time and efforts in the instrument translation process without which this study would not have been possible.

REFERENCES

Ajzen, I., & Fishbein, M. (1980). *Understanding attitudes and predicting social behaviour*. Academic Press.

Altman, I. (1975). The Environment and Social Behavior: Privacy, Personal Space, Territory, and Crowding. Academic Press.

Barnes, S. B. (2006). A privacy paradox: Social networking in the United States. *First Monday*, *11*(9). Advance online publication. doi:10.5210/fm.v11i9.1394

Campbell, A. J. (1997). Relationship marketing in consumer markets: A comparison of managerial and consumer attitudes about information privacy. *Journal of Direct Marketing*, *11*(3), 44–57. doi:10.1002/(SICI)1522-7138(199722)11:3<44::AID-DIR7>3.0.CO;2-X

Chin, W. W. (1998). The Partial Least Squares Approach to Structural Equation Modeling. In *Modern Methods for business Research*. Lawrence Erlbaum Associates.

Chiu, C.-M., Hsu, M.-H., & Wang, E. T. G. (2006). Understanding knowledge sharing in virtual communities: An integration of social capital and social cognitive theories. *Decision Support Systems*, *42*(3), 1872–1888. doi:10.1016/j.dss.2006.04.001

Cui, X. (2015). Self-Disclosure Relies on Social Context: Examining the Similarity and Differences of Chinese Students in the U.S. and China when Disclosing Information on WeChat. *ProQuest Dissertations and Theses*. https://dc.etsu.edu/etd/

Culnan, M. J., & Armstrong, P. K. (1999). Information privacy concerns, procedural fairness, and impersonal trust: An empirical investigation. *Organization Science, 10*(1), 104–115. doi:10.1287/orsc.10.1.104

Culnan, M. J., & Bies, R. J. (2003). Consumer privacy: Balancing economic and justice considerations. *The Journal of Social Issues, 59*(2), 323–342. doi:10.1111/1540-4560.00067

David Garson, G. (2016). *Partial least squares (PLS-SEM) 2016 edition*. www.statisticalassociates.com

Digital, M., Mcknight, D. H., Lankton, N. K., & Tripp, J. (2011). Social Networking Information Disclosure and Continuance Intention : A Disconnect. *44th Hawaii International Conference On System Sciences.*

Dinev, T., & Hart, P. (2004). Internet privacy concerns and their antecedents-measurement validity and a regression model. *Behaviour & Information Technology, 23*(6), 413–422. doi:10.1080/01449290410001715723

Emad, B., Arabia, S., Administratio, B., & Saud, K. (2018). Self-Disclosure in Social Networking Sites in Saudi Arabia. *International Journal of Business and Management, 13*(10), 96–115. doi:10.5539/ijbm.v13n10p96

Felim, P., Dimyati, D., & Shihab, M. (2018). ASKfm: Motives of Self-Disclosure to Anonymous Questions. *Jurnal Komunikasi, 13*(1), 93–108. doi:10.20885/komunikasi.vol13.iss1.art7

Fishbein, M., & Ajzen, I. (1975). *Belief, attitude, intention and behavior: An introduction to theory and research*. Academic Press.

Graham-Harrison, E., & Cadwalladr, C. (2018). Revealed: 50 million Facebook profiles harvested for Cambridge Analytica in major data breach. *The Guardian*, 1–5.

Hair, J. F. Jr, Hult, G. T. M., Ringle, C. M., & Sarstedt, M. (2021). *A primer on partial least squares structural equation modeling (PLS-SEM)*. Sage Publications. doi:10.1007/978-3-030-80519-7

Hallam, C., & Zanella, G. (2017). Online self-disclosure: The privacy paradox explained as a temporally discounted balance between concerns and rewards. *Computers in Human Behavior, 68*, 217–227. doi:10.1016/j.chb.2016.11.033

Heeks, R. (2018). *Information and Communication Technology for Development (ICT4D)*. doi:10.4324/9781315652603

Hoy, M. G., & Milne, G. (2010). Gender Differences in Privacy-Related Measures for Young Adult Facebook Users. *Journal of Interactive Advertising, 10*(2), 28–45. doi:10.1080/15252019.2010.10722168

Ismail, R., & Zainab, A. N. (2013). Assessing the status of library information systems security. *Journal of Librarianship and Information Science, 45*(3), 231–247. doi:10.1177/0961000613477676

Jarvenpaa, S. L., Tractinsky, N., & Saarinen, L. (1999). Consumer trust in an Internet store: A cross-cultural validation. *Journal of Computer-Mediated Communication, 5*(2), JCMC526.

Kante, M., Chepken, C., & Oboko, R. (2018). Partial Least Square Structural Equation Modelling' use in Information Systems: An Updated Guideline of Practices in Exploratory Settings. *Kabarak Journal of Research & Innovation, 6*(1), 49–67.

Kante, M. (2022). A mapping of the factors related to self-disclosure on social network sites. *International Journal of Big Data Management, 2*(1), 60–69. doi:10.1504/IJBDM.2022.119434

Karuri, J., Waiganjo, P., & Orwa, D. (2014). Determinants of Acceptance and Use of DHIS2: Survey Instrument Validation and Preliminary Findings using PLS-SEM. *Journal of Emerging Trends in Computing and Information Sciences, 5*(8), 647–660. doi:10.100710067-013-2361-9

Kokolakis, S. (2017). *Privacy attitudes and privacy behaviour: A review of current research on the privacy paradox phenomenon.* Academic Press.

Koroleva, K., Brecht, F., & Malinova, M. (2011). *'Generation Facebook'-A Cognitive Calculus Model of Teenage User Behavior on Social Network Sites. Enabling Batch Processing in Business Processes View project.* https://www.researchgate.net/publication/220890444

Krasnova, H., Spiekermann, S., Koroleva, K., & Hildebrand, T. (2010). Online social networks: Why we disclose. *Journal of Information Technology, 25*(2), 109–125. doi:10.1057/jit.2010.6

Krasnova, H., Veltri, N. F., & Günther, O. (2012a). Self-disclosure and privacy calculus on social networking sites: The role of culture. *Business & Information Systems Engineering, 4*(3), 127–135. doi:10.100712599-012-0216-6

Krasnova, H., Veltri, N. F., & Günther, O. (2012b). *Self-disclosure and Privacy Calculus on Social Networking Sites: The Role of Culture Intercultural Dynamics of Privacy Calculus.* doi:10.1007/s12599-012-0216-6

Levy, Y., & Ellis, T. J. (2006). A systems approach to conduct an effective literature review in support of information systems research. *Informing Science*, *9*, 181–211. doi:10.28945/479

Li, H., Sarathy, R., & Xu, H. (2010). Understanding situational online information disclosure as a privacy calculus Understanding situational online information disclosure as a privacy calculus. *Journal of Computer Information Systems*, *51*, 1–29. doi:10.1080/08874417.2010.11645450

Madden, T. J., Ellen, P. S., & Ajzen, I. (1992). A comparison of the theory of planned behavior and the theory of reasoned action. *Personality and Social Psychology Bulletin*, *18*(1), 3–9. doi:10.1177/0146167292181001

Malhotra, N. K., Kim, S. S., & Agarwal, J. (2004). Internet users' information privacy concerns (IUIPC): The construct, the scale, and a causal model. *Information Systems Research*, *15*(4), 336–355. doi:10.1287/isre.1040.0032

Marwick, A., & Hargittai, E. (2019). Nothing to hide, nothing to lose? Incentives and disincentives to sharing information with institutions online. *Information Communication and Society*, *22*(12), 1697–1713. doi:10.1080/1369118X.2018.1450432

McKnight, D. H., Choudhury, V., & Kacmar, C. (2002). Developing and validating trust measures for e-commerce: An integrative typology. *Information Systems Research*, *13*(3), 334–359. doi:10.1287/isre.13.3.334.81

Min, J., & Kim, B. (2015). How are people enticed to disclose personal information despite privacy concerns in social network sites? the calculus between benefit and cost. *Journal of the Association for Information Science and Technology*, *66*(4), 839–857. Advance online publication. doi:10.1002/asi.23206

Moon, Y. (2000). Intimate exchanges: Using computers to elicit self-disclosure from consumers. *The Journal of Consumer Research*, *26*(4), 323–339. doi:10.1086/209566

Muijs, D. (2010). Doing quantitative research in education with SPSS. *Sage (Atlanta, Ga.)*.

Müller-Bloch, C., & Kranz, J. (2015). A Framework for Rigorously Identifying Research Gaps in Qualitative Literature Reviews. *ICIS 2015 Proceedings*. https://aisel.aisnet.org/icis2015/proceedings/ResearchMethods/2

Nambisan, S., & Baron, R. A. (2007). Interactions in virtual customer environments: Implications for product support and customer relationship management. *Journal of Interactive Marketing*, *21*(2), 42–62. doi:10.1002/dir.20077

Qadheeb, B. E. A. L., & Alsalloum, O. I. (2018). Self-Dis closure in i Social Networking Sites in Saudi Arabia. *International Journal of Business and Management, 13*(10), 96–115. doi:10.5539/ijbm.v13n10p96

Reynolds, B., Venkatanathan, J., Gonçalves, J., & Kostakos, V. (2011). Sharing ephemeral information in online social networks: privacy perceptions and behaviours. *IFIP Conference on Human-Computer Interaction*, 204–215. 10.1007/978-3-642-23765-2_14

Roberts, T. H. (2012). A Cross-Disciplined Approach to Exploring the Privacy Paradox : Explaining Disclosure Behaviour Using the Theory of Planned Behaviour A Cross-Disciplined Approach to Exploring the Privacy Paradox : Explaining Disclosure Behaviour Using the Theory of Plann. *UK Academy for Information Systems Conference Proceedings, 7.*

Sasse, M. A., Brostoff, S., & Weirich, D. (2001). Transforming the 'weakest link'-a human/computer interaction approach to usable and effective security. *BT Technology Journal, 19*(3), 122–131. doi:10.1023/A:1011902718709

Skinner, E. A. (1996). A guide to constructs of control. *Journal of Personality and Social Psychology, 71*(3), 549–570. doi:10.1037/0022-3514.71.3.549 PMID:8831161

Taddicken, M. (2014). The "Privacy Paradox" in the Social Web: The Impact of Privacy Concerns, Individual Characteristics, and the Perceived Social Relevance on Different Forms of Self-Disclosure1. *Journal of Computer-Mediated Communication, 19*(2), 248–273. Advance online publication. doi:10.1111/jcc4.12052

Tufekci, Z. (2008). Can you see me now? Audience and disclosure regulation in online social network sites. *Bulletin of Science, Technology & Society, 28*(1), 20–36. doi:10.1177/0270467607311484

Warren, J. (2017). Communicating Personal Health Information in Virtual Health Communities. *An Integration of Privacy Calculus Model and Affective Commitment.*, *18*(1), 45–81.

Wirth, J. (2018). *Dependent Variables in the Privacy-Related Field: A Descriptive Literature Review*. Academic Press.

Wirth, J., Maier, C., & Laumer, S. (2019). *Subjective Norm and the Privacy Calculus: Explaining Self-Disclosure on Social Networking*. Academic Press.

Wu, A., & Zeng, Z. (2012). Dynamic behaviors of memristor-based recurrent neural networks with time-varying delays. *Neural Networks, 36*, 1–10. doi:10.1016/j.neunet.2012.08.009 PMID:23037770

Xu, H., Gupta, S., Rosson, M. B., & Carroll, J. M. (2012). *Measuring mobile users' concerns for information privacy*. Academic Press.

Yao, M. Z. (2011). Self-Protection of Online Privacy: A Behavioral Approach. In *Privacy Online* (pp. 111–125). Springer Berlin Heidelberg., doi:10.1007/978-3-642-21521-6_9

Zlatolas, L. N., Welzer, T., Heričko, M., & Hölbl, M. (2015). Privacy antecedents for SNS self-disclosure: The case of Facebook. *Computers in Human Behavior*, *45*, 158–167. Advance online publication. doi:10.1016/j.chb.2014.12.012

KEY TERMS AND DEFINITIONS

Enjoyment: The reward users get from having enjoyable encounters online.

Personal Information: Is any information related to an identifiable person.

Privacy Calculus Theory: States that individuals always rationally weigh the potential benefits and potential risks of data disclosure decisions.

Privacy Concerns: A person's subjective perspective of fairness in a data privacy context.

Self-Disclosure: The extent of personal information an individual gives in the process of participation on a Social Network Site.

Social Media: A computer-based technology that facilitates the sharing of ideas, thoughts, and information through the building of virtual networks and communities.

Social Network Services: Refers to social media sites.

Structural Model: Refers to the relationships among latent variables, and allows the researcher to determine their degree of correlation (calculated as path coefficients).

Compilation of References

Abbing, H. R. (2013). Sustainability of healthcare systems: Aligning the safety and quality debate with the debate on the financing systems and mechanisms. European Journal of Health Law, 20(3), 253–259. doi:10.1163/15718093-12341271

Abdellatif, A. A., Al-Marridi, A. Z., Mohamed, A., Erbad, A., Chiasserini, C. F., & Refaey, A. (2020). SsHealth: Toward secure, blockchain-enabled healthcare systems. *IEEE Network*, *34*(4), 312–319. doi:10.1109/MNET.011.1900553

Abone, C. (2003). Mass media: Effective instrument for promoting health programs in Africa. In I. E. Nwosu (Ed.), *Sustainable development in Nigeria*. Rhyce Kerex Publishers.

Abou-Nassar, E. M., Iliyasu, A. M., El-Kafrawy, P. M., Song, O. Y., Bashir, A. K., & El-Latif, A. A. A. (2020). DITrust Chain: Towards Blockchain-Based Trust Models for Sustainable Healthcare IoT Systems. *IEEE Access: Practical Innovations, Open Solutions*, *8*, 111223–111238. doi:10.1109/ACCESS.2020.2999468

Abu-elezz, I., Hassan, A., Nazeemudeen, A., Househ, M., & Abd-alrazaq, A. (2020). The benefits and threats of blockchain technology in healthcare: A scoping review. In *International Journal of Medical Informatics* (Vol. 142, p. 104246). Elsevier Ireland Ltd., doi:10.1016/j.ijmedinf.2020.104246

Ackland, P., Resnikoff, S., & Bourne, R. (2017). World blindness and visual impairment: Despite many successes, the problem is growing. *Community Eye Health*, *30*(100), 71. PMID:29483748

Adedeji, A. A., Sanusi, B., Tella, A., Akinsanya, M., Ojo, O., Akinwunmi, M. O., Tikare, O. A., Ogunwande, I. A., Ogundahunsi, O. A., & Ayilara, O. O. (2011). Exposure to anti-malarial drugs and monitoring of adverse drug reactions using toll-free mobile phone calls in the private retail sector in Sagamu, Nigeria: Implications for pharmacovigilance. *Malaria Journal*, *10*, 230.

Adepoju, P. (2020). Africa's COVID-19 health technologies' watershed moment. *The Lancet. Digital Health*, *2*(7), e346–e347. doi:10.1016/S2589-7500(20)30146-1

Aditia, M. K., Paida, S., Altaf, F., & Maity, S. (2019, December 1). Certificate-less public key encryption for secure e-Healthcare systems. *2019 IEEE Conference on Information and Communication Technology, CICT 2019*. 10.1109/CICT48419.2019.9066190

African Development Bank Group. (2011). *Burundi Country Strategy Paper 2012-2016*. Retrieved from http://www.afdb.org/fileadmin/uploads/afdb/Documents/Project-and-Operations/Burundi%20-%20CSP%202012-16.pdf

Agbo, C., Mahmoud, Q., & Eklund, J. (2019). Blockchain Technology in Healthcare: A Systematic Review. *Health Care*, *7*(2), 56. doi:10.3390/healthcare7020056 PMID:30987333

Aghadiuno, P. C., & Onyekweodiri, N. E. (2019). Social media for information dissemination in the digital era. In K.I. Igwe, S.A. Sadiku, & I.B. Edam-Agbor (Eds.), Themes and trends in information science (pp. 241-250). Ikorodu, Nigeria: Zeh.

Aghajani, J., Farnia, P., & Velayati, A. A. (2017). Impact of geographical information system on public health sciences. *Biomedical and Biotechnology Research Journal*, *1*(2), 94. doi:10.4103/bbrj.bbrj_34_17

Ahrq. (2019). *2019 National Healthcare Quality and Disparities Report*. https://www.ahrq.gov/research/findings/nhqrdr/nhqdr19/index.html

Ajzen, I., & Fishbein, M. (1980). *Understanding attitudes and predicting social behaviour*. Academic Press.

Akhtar, R. (1991). *Healthcare patterns and planning in developing countries*. Greenwood Press.

Akinyemi, O. O., Popoola, O. A., Fowotade, A., Adekanmbi, O., Cadmus, E. O., & Adebayo, A. (2021). A qualitative exploration of the health system response to COVID-19 pandemic applying the WHO health systems frame. A case: A case study of a Nigerian state. *Scientific African*, e00945-e00945.

Alami, R. (2017). Health Financing Systems, Health Equity and Universal Health Coverage in Arab Countries. *Development and Change*, *48*(1), 146–179. doi:10.1111/dech.12290

Ali Syed, T., Alzahrani, A., Jan, S., Siddiqui, M. S., Nadeem, A., & Alghamdi, T. (2019). A Comparative Analysis of Blockchain Architecture and its Applications: Problems and Recommendations. *IEEE Access: Practical Innovations, Open Solutions*, *7*, 176838–176869. doi:10.1109/ACCESS.2019.2957660

Alketbi, A., Nasir, Q., & Talib, M. A. (2018). Blockchain for government services-Use cases, security benefits and challenges. *2018 15th Learning and Technology Conference, L and T 2018*, 112–119. 10.1109/LT.2018.8368494

Al-Mamary, Y. H., Shamsuddin, A., & Aziati, N. (2014). The relationship between system quality, information quality, and organizational performance. *International Journal of Knowledge and Research in Management & E-Commerce, 4*, 7-10. https://www.researchgate.net/profile/Yaser-Hasan-Salem-Al-Mamary-d-yasr-hsn-almmry/publication/269463861_The_Relationship_between_System_Quality_Information_Quality_and_Organizational_Performance/links/5530f5380cf27acb0de8b002/The-Relationship-between-Sys

Al-Salman, S., & Ahmad, S. H. (2021). COVID-19 trending neologisms and word formation processes in English. *Russian Journal of Linguistics*, *25*(1), 24–42. doi:10.22363/2687-0088-2021-25-1-24-42

Altman, I. (1975). The Environment and Social Behavior: Privacy, Personal Space, Territory, and Crowding. Academic Press.

Alves, S. A. A., & Oliveira, M. L. B. (2018). Sociocultural aspects of health and disease and their pragmatic impact. *Journal of Human Growth and Development*, *28*(2), 183–188. doi:10.7322/jhgd.147236

Alzahrani, A. I., Mahmud, I., Ramayah, T., Alfarraj, O., & Alalwan, N. (2017). *Modelling digital library success using the DeLone and McLean information system success model*. doi:10.1177/0961000617726123

Ammenwerth, E., Gräber, S., Herrmann, G., Bürkle, T., & König, J. (2003). *Evaluation of health information systems — problems and challenges*. doi:10.1016/S1386-5056(03)00131-X

Anadolu Agency. (2020). *Health, Africa, latest on coronavirus outbreak*. Available at: www.aa.com.tr

Andreatta, P., Debpuur, D., Danquah, A., & Perosky, J. (2011). Using cell phones to collect postpartum haemorrhage outcome data in rural Ghana. *International Journal of Gynaecology and Obstetrics*, *113*(2), 148–151.

Aqil, A., Lippeveld, T., & Hozumi, D. (2009). PRISM framework: A paradigm shift for designing, strengthening and evaluating routine health information systems. *Health Policy and Planning*, *24*(3), 217–228. Advance online publication. doi:10.1093/heapol/czp010 PMID:19304786

Aranda-Jan, C., Mohutsiwa-Dibe, N., & Louakanova, S. (2014). Systematic review on what works, what does not work and why of implementation of mobile health (mHealth) projects in Africa. *BioMed Central Public Health*, *14*(1), 188–203. doi:10.1186/1471-2458-14-188 PMID:24555733

Armitage, R., & Nellums, L. B. (2020). Considering inequalities in the school closure response to COVID-19. *The Lancet. Global Health*, *8*(5), e644. doi:10.1016/S2214-109X(20)30116-9 PMID:32222161

Arviansyah, S. T., & Hillergersberg, J. V. (2015). Development and assessment of an instrument to measure equivocal situation and its causes in IS / IT project evaluation. *CES1*. doi:10.12821/ijispm030302

Asiimwe, C., Gelvin, D., Lee, E., Amor, Y. B., Quinto, E., Katureebe, C., Sundaram, L., Bell, D., & Berg, M. (2011). Use of an innovative, affordable, and open-source short message service-based tool to monitor malaria in remote areas of Uganda. *The American Journal of Tropical Medicine and Hygiene*, *85*(1), 26–33. doi:10.4269/ajtmh.2011.10-0528 PMID:21734120

Azim, M. D., Ahmed, H., & Khan, A. S. (2015). Operational performance and profitability: An empirical study on the Bangladeshi Ceramic companies. *Researchgate. Net, 3*(1), 63–73. https://www.researchgate.net/profile/Md-Azim-2/publication/323414631_OPERATIONAL_PERFORMANCE_AND_PROFITABILITY_AN_EMPIRICAL_STUDY_ON_THE_BANGLADESHI_CERAMIC_COMPANIES/links/5b910e20a6fdcce8a4ca27f7/OPERATIONAL-PERFORMANCE-AND-PROFITABILITY-AN-EMPIRICAL-STUDY-ON-THE-BANGLADESHI-CERAMIC-COMPANIES.pdf

Bakibinga-Gaswaga, E., Bakibinga, S., Bakibinga, D. B. M., & Bakibinga, P. (2020). Digital technologies in the COVID-19 responses in Sub-Saharan Africa: policies, problems and promises. *The Pan African Medical Journal, 35*(Suppl 2).

Banes, M. J., Culham, L. E., Crowston, J. G., Bunce, C., & Khaw, P. T. (2000). An optometrist's role of co-management in a hospital glaucoma clinic. *Ophthalmic & Physiological Optics, 20*(5), 351–359. doi:10.1046/j.1475-1313.2000.00527.x PMID:11045243

Barnes, S. B. (2006). A privacy paradox: Social networking in the United States. *First Monday, 11*(9). Advance online publication. doi:10.5210/fm.v11i9.1394

Barney, A., Buckelew, S., Mesheriakova, V., & Raymond-Flesch, M. (2020). The Covid-19 Pandemic and Rapid Implementation of Adolescent and Young Adult Telemedicine: Challenges and Opportunities for Innovation. *The Journal of Adolescent Health*, (2), 1–8. doi:10.1016/j.jadohealth.2020.05.006 PMID:32410810

Barrington, J., Wereko-Brobby, O., Ward, P., Mwafongo, W., & Kungulwe, S. (2010). SMS for Life: A pilot project to improve anti-malarial drug supply management in rural Tanzania using standard technology. *Malaria Journal, 9*(1), 1–9. doi:10.1186/1475-2875-9-298 PMID:20979633

Baumgart, D. C. (2020). Digital advantage in the COVID-19 response: Perspective from Canada's largest integrated digitized healthcare system. *NPJ Digital Medicine, 3*(1), 1–4. doi:10.103841746-020-00326-y PMID:32923691

Beaunoyer, E., Dupéré, S., & Guitton, M. J. (2020). COVID-19 and digital inequalities: Reciprocal impacts and mitigation strategies. *Computers in Human Behavior, 111*, 106424. doi:10.1016/j.chb.2020.106424 PMID:32398890

Bellina, L., & Missoni, E. (2009). Mobile cellphones (M-phones) in tele microscopy: Increasing connectivity of isolated laboratories. *Diagnostic Pathology, 4*, 19.

Bell, L., Buchanan, W. J., Cameron, J., & Lo, O. (2018). Applications of Blockchain Within Healthcare. *Blockchain in Healthcare Today, 1*(0). Advance online publication. doi:10.30953/bhty.v1.8

Ben, R. (2020). *Did coronavirus kickstart the economy? An innovation, a viral tweet, the story begins there. 34 seconds that potentially changed the fortunes of Innovative Nairobi Craftsman, Stephen Odhiambo.* African innovations liquid telecom. Available at: https://www.liquidtelecom.com/insights/innovation-blog/Did_Coronavirus_just_kick_start_the_digital_economy

Berg, A. O., Atkins, D., & Tierney, W. (1997). Clinical practice guidelines in practice and education. *Journal of General Internal Medicine, 12*(S2, Suppl 2), S25–S33. doi:10.1046/j.1525-1497.12.s2.4.x PMID:9127241

Betjeman, T. J., Soghoian, S. E., & Foran, M. P. (2013). mHealth in Sub-Saharan Africa. *International Journal of Telemedicine and Applications, 2013*, 1–7. Advance online publication. doi:10.1155/2013/482324 PMID:24369460

Bieling, T. (2009). Design Research and Disability. In *ICERI2009 Proceedings* (pp. 5761-5763). IATED.

Binyaruka, P., & Borghi, J. (2017). Improving quality of care through payment for performance: Examining effects on the availability and stock-out of essential medical commodities in Tanzania. *Tropical Medicine & International Health, 22*(1), 92–102. doi:10.1111/tmi.12809 PMID:27928874

Biswas, S., Sharif, K., Li, F., & Mohanty, S. (2020). Blockchain for E-Health-Care Systems: Easier Said Than Done. *Computer, 53*(7), 57–67. doi:10.1109/MC.2020.2989781

Bittner, A. K., Yoshinaga, P. D., Wykstra, S. L., & Li, T. (2020). Telerehabilitation for people with low vision. *Cochrane Database of Systematic Reviews*, 2. PMID:32102114

Blaya, J. A., Fraser, H. S. F., & Holt, B. (2010). E-health technologies show promise in developing countries. *Health Affairs, 29*(2), 244–251. Advance online publication. doi:10.1377/hlthaff.2009.0894 PMID:20348068

Bloom, G., Labrique, A., Hampshire, K., & Waldman, L. (2017). *Making mHealth Work for All.* doi:10.35648/20.500.12413/11781/ii286

Boland, A., Cherry, G., & Dickson, R. (2017). Doing a systematic review: A student's guide. *Sage (Atlanta, Ga.).*

Bonten, T. N., Rauwerdink, A., Wyatt, J. C., Kasteleyn, M. J., Witkamp, L., Riper, H., Gemert-Pijnen, L. J., van, Cresswell, K., Sheikh, A., Schijven, M. P., & Chavannes, N. H. (2020). Online Guide for Electronic Health Evaluation Approaches: Systematic Scoping Review and Concept Mapping Study. *Journal of Medical Internet Research, 22*(8), e17774. Advance online publication. doi:10.2196/17774 PMID:32784173

Boruchovitch, E., & Mednick, B. R. (2002, July/December). The meaning of health and illness: Some considerations for health psychology. *Psico-USF, 7*(2), 175–183. doi:10.1590/S1413-82712002000200006

Botha, M., Botha, A., & Herselman, M. (2014). Compiling a prioritized list of health data quality challenges in public healthcare systems. *2014 IST-Africa Conference and Exhibition, 2014*, 1–8. Advance online publication. doi:10.1109/ISTAFRICA.2014.6880649

Bourne, R. R., Adelson, J., Flaxman, S., Briant, P., Bottone, M., Vos, T., ... Taylor, H. R. (2020). Global Prevalence of Blindness and Distance and Near Vision Impairment in 2020: Progress towards the Vision 2020 targets and what the future holds. *Investigative Ophthalmology & Visual Science, 61*(7), 2317–2317.

Braithwaite, J., Glasziou, P., & Westbrook, J. (2020). The three numbers you need to know about healthcare: The 60-30-10 Challenge. In BMC Medicine (Vol. 18, Issue 1). BioMed Central Ltd. doi:10.118612916-020-01563-4

Bringhurst, R. (2004). Elements of typographical style. Roberts Point, WA: Hartley and Marks.

Brunner, M., & SÜβ, H.-M. (2005). Analyzing the reliability of multidimensional measures: An example from intelligence research. *Journals.Sagepub. Com*, *65*(2), 227–240. doi:10.1177/0013164404268669

Budd, J., Miller, B. S., Manning, E. M., Lampos, V., Zhuang, M., Edelstein, M., & McKendry, R. A. (2020). Digital technologies in the public-health response to COVID-19. *Nature Medicine*, *26*(8), 1183–1192. doi:10.103841591-020-1011-4 PMID:32770165

Burundi Ministry of Health. (2014). *Kira-Mama project.* Available at https://unicefstories.files.wordpress.com/2014/05/burundi-final-english-300ppi.pdf

Burundi Ministry of Health. (2014). *Kira-Mama project.* Retrieved June 09 2016 from https://unicefstories.files.wordpress.com/2014/05/burundi-final-english-300ppi.pdf

Buthelezi, B.E., Ndayizigamiye, P., & Twinomurinzi, H., & Dube. (2022). A Systematic Review of the Adoption of Blockchain for Supply Chain Processes. *Journal of Global Information Management.*

Campbell, A. J. (1997). Relationship marketing in consumer markets: A comparison of managerial and consumer attitudes about information privacy. *Journal of Direct Marketing*, *11*(3), 44–57. doi:10.1002/(SICI)1522-7138(199722)11:3<44::AID-DIR7>3.0.CO;2-X

Cassandra, W. (2020). *Employee Performance Evaluation: Definition, Benefits and How To Prepare.* https://www.indeed.com/career-advice/career-development/employee-performance-evaluation

Chang, J. C. J., & King, W. R. (2005). Measuring the performance of information systems: A functional scorecard. Journal of Management Information Systems. doi:10.1080/07421222.2003.11045833

Chang, A. Y., Littman-Quinn, R., Ketshogileng, D., Chandra, A., Rijken, T., Ghose, S., Kyer, A., Seymour, A. K., & Kovarik, C. L. (2012). Smartphone-based mobile learning with physician trainees in Botswana. *International Journal of Mobile and Blended Learning*, *4*(1), 1–14. doi:10.4018/jmbl.2012040101

Chaos. (2008). *Text to Change (TTC).* Retrieved February 23 2018 from http://images.aarogya.com/aids/pdf/unandzain.pdf

Chartier-Rueg, T. C., & Zweifel, T. D. (2017). Blockchain, leadership and management: Business as usual or radical disruption? *EUREKA: Social and Humanities*, *4*(4), 76–110. doi:10.21303/2504-5571.2017.00370

Chaudhary, R. R. K., & Chatterjee, K. (2020). An efficient lightweight cryptographic technique for iot based E-healthcare system. *2020 7th International Conference on Signal Processing and Integrated Networks, SPIN 2020*, 991–995. 10.1109/SPIN48934.2020.9071421

Chawinga, W. D., Chawinga, C., Kapondera, S. K., Chipeta, G. T., Majawa, F., & Nyasulu, C. (2020). Towards e-judicial services in Malawi: Implications for justice delivery. *The Electronic Journal on Information Systems in Developing Countries*, *86*(2), e12121. doi:10.1002/isd2.12121

Chawinga, W. D., & Zinn, S. (2016). Use of Web 2.0 by students in the Faculty of Information Science and Communications at Mzuzu University, Malawi. *South African Journal of Information Management*, *18*(1), 1–15. doi:10.4102ajim.v18i1.694

Chen, S., Osman, N. M., Nunes, J. M. B., & Peng, G. C. (2011). Information systems evaluation methodologies. *Proceedings of the IADIS International Workshop on Information Systems Research Trends, Approaches and Methodologies.*

Chen, Z., Fang, L., Chen, L., & Dai, H. (2008). Comparison of an SMS text messaging and phone reminder to improve attendance at a health promotion centres: A randomized controlled trial. *Journal of Zhejiang University. Science. B.*, *9*(1), 34–38. doi:10.1631/jzus.B071464 PMID:18196610

Chiang, M. F., Cole, R. G., Gupta, S., Kaiser, G. E., & Starren, J. B. (2005). Computer and world wide web accessibility by visually disabled patients: Problems and solutions. *Survey of Ophthalmology*, *50*(4), 394–405. doi:10.1016/j.survophthal.2005.04.004 PMID:15967193

Chib, A. (2010). The Aceh Besar midwives with mobile phones project: Design and evaluation perspectives using the information and communication technologies for healthcare development model. *Journal of Computer-Mediated Communication*, *15*(1), 500–525. doi:10.1111/j.1083-6101.2010.01515.x

Chin, W. W. (1998). The Partial Least Squares Approach to Structural Equation Modeling. In *Modern Methods for business Research*. Lawrence Erlbaum Associates.

Chitungo, I., Mhango, M., Mbunge, E., Dzobo, M., & Dzinamarira, T. (2021). Digital technologies and COVID-19: Reconsidering lockdown exit strategies for Africa. *The Pan African Medical Journal*, *39*, 39. doi:10.11604/pamj.2021.39.93.29773 PMID:34466195

Chiu, C.-M., Hsu, M.-H., & Wang, E. T. G. (2006). Understanding knowledge sharing in virtual communities: An integration of social capital and social cognitive theories. *Decision Support Systems*, *42*(3), 1872–1888. doi:10.1016/j.dss.2006.04.001

Chukwu, E., & Garg, L. (2020). A systematic review of blockchain in healthcare: Frameworks, prototypes, and implementations. *IEEE Access: Practical Innovations, Open Solutions*, *8*, 21196–21214. doi:10.1109/ACCESS.2020.2969881

Cohen, M. S., Smith, M. K., Muessig, K. E., Hallett, T. B., Powers, K. A., & Kashuba, A. D. (2013). Antiretroviral treatment of HIV-1 prevents transmission of HIV-1: Where do we go from here? *Lancet*, *382*(9903), 1515–1524. doi:10.1016/S0140-6736(13)61998-4 PMID:24152938

Colven, R., Shim, M. H., Brock, D., & Todd, G. (2011). Dermatological diagnostic acumen improves with the use of a simple telemedicine system for underserved areas of South Africa. *Telemedecine Journal- E Health, 17*(5), 363–369.

Communicating with Disaster Affected Communities (CDAC) Network. (2018). *Resources for those responding to COVID-19.* Available at www.cdacnetwork.org

Contreras, C. M., Metzger, G. A., Beane, J. D., Dedhia, P. H., Ejaz, A., & Pawlik, T. M. (2020). Telemedicine: Patient-Provider Clinical Engagement During the Covid-19 Pandemic and Beyond. *Journal of Gastrointestinal Surgery, 1*(7), 1692–1697. Advance online publication. doi:10.100711605-020-04623-5 PMID:32385614

Creswell, J. W. (2014). *Qualitative, Quantitative and Mixed Methods Approaches* (4th ed.). SAGE Publication.

Cronbach, L. J. (1951). Coefficient alpha and the internal structure of tests. *Psychometrika, 16*(3), 297–334. doi:10.1007/BF02310555

Cronin, P., Ryan, F., & Coughlan, M. (2008). Undertaking a literature review: A step-by-step approach. *British Journal of Nursing (Mark Allen Publishing), 17*(1), 38–43. doi:10.12968/bjon.2008.17.1.28059 PMID:18399395

CSEA AFRICA. (2020). *Africa's digital technology response strategy to COVID-19.* Centre for the Study of the Economies of Africa.

Cui, X. (2015). Self-Disclosure Relies on Social Context: Examining the Similarity and Differences of Chinese Students in the U.S. and China when Disclosing Information on WeChat. *ProQuest Dissertations and Theses.* https://dc.etsu.edu/etd/

Culnan, M. J., & Armstrong, P. K. (1999). Information privacy concerns, procedural fairness, and impersonal trust: An empirical investigation. *Organization Science, 10*(1), 104–115. doi:10.1287/orsc.10.1.104

Culnan, M. J., & Bies, R. J. (2003). Consumer privacy: Balancing economic and justice considerations. *The Journal of Social Issues, 59*(2), 323–342. doi:10.1111/1540-4560.00067

Das, A. V., & Christy, B. (2021). Commentary: Conquering insurmountable challenges: The importance of tele-rehabilitation. *Indian Journal of Ophthalmology, 69*(3), 729. doi:10.4103/ijo.IJO_280_21 PMID:33595511

David Garson, G. (2016). *Partial least squares (PLS-SEM) 2016 edition.* www.statisticalassociates.com

Dehbi, Z. E. O., Sedrati, H., Chaqsare, S., Azami, A. I., Merzouki, M., Raji, M., ... Ghazal, H. (2021). Moroccan digital health response to the COVID-19 crisis. *Frontiers in Public Health, 9.* PMID:34485221

DeLone, W. H., & McLean, E. R. (2003). The DeLone and McLean model of information systems success: A ten-year update. *Journal of Management Information Systems, 19*(4), 9–30. doi:10.1080/07421222.2003.11045748

DeLone, W. H., & McLean, E. R. (2016). Information Systems Success Measurement. *Foundations and Trends in Information Systems, 2*(1), 1–116. doi:10.1561/2900000005

Department of Health. (2017). White Paper for National Health Insurance for South Africa. *National Health Insurance Bill*, 1–80. www.gpwonline.co.za

Department of Health. (2019). *National Health Insurance (NHI) Pledge*. Author.

Department of Planning. (2017). *Socio-economic impact assessment system (SEIAS): Final impact assessment (Phase 2): White paper on national health insurance.* Author.

DeRenzi, B., Birnbaum, B., Findlater, L., Mangilima, J., Payne, J., Parikh, T., Borriello, G., & Lesh, N. (2012). Improving community health worker performance through automated SMS. *Proceedings for the Fifth International Conference on Information and Communication Technologies and Development (ICTD2012)*, 25-34. 10.1145/2160673.2160677

DeRenzi, B., Lesh, N., Parikh, T., Sims, C., Maokla, W., Chemba, M., Hamisi, Y., Mitchell, M., & Borriello, G. (2008). E-IMCI: Improving pediatric health care in low-income countries. In *Proceedings of the SIGCHI conference on human factors in computing systems* (pp. 753-762). New York: ACM. 10.1145/1357054.1357174

Dhai, A. (2011). Healthcare reform in South Africa : A step in the direction of social justice. *World Medical Journal, 4*(2), 137–139. https://eds.a.ebscohost.com/eds/detail/detail?vid=0&sid=6a80e28a-7726-48c8-9186-ff52fac6166f%40sdc-v-sessmgr01&bdata=JkF1dGhUeXBlPXNzbyZzaXRlPWVkcy1saXZlJnNjb3BlPXNpdGU%3D#AN=edssas.ejc64551&db=edssas

Digital, M., Mcknight, D. H., Lankton, N. K., & Tripp, J. (2011). Social Networking Information Disclosure and Continuance Intention : A Disconnect. *44th Hawaii International Conference On System Sciences.*

Dinev, T., & Hart, P. (2004). Internet privacy concerns and their antecedents-measurement validity and a regression model. *Behaviour & Information Technology, 23*(6), 413–422. doi:10.1080/01449290410001715723

Donawa, A., Orukari, I., & Baker, C. E. (2019). Scaling Blockchains to Support Electronic Health Records for Hospital Systems. *2019 IEEE 10th Annual Ubiquitous Computing, Electronics and Mobile Communication Conference, UEMCON 2019*, 550–556. 10.1109/UEMCON47517.2019.8993101

Donner, J., & Escobari, M. X. (2010). A review of evidence on mobile use by micro and small enterprises in developing countries. *Journal of International Development, 22*(5), 641–658. doi:10.1002/jid.1717

Dwivedi, Y. K., Hughes, D. L., Coombs, C., Constantiou, I., Duan, Y., Edwards, J. S., & Raman, R. (2020). Impact of COVID-19 pandemic on information management research and practice: Transforming education, work, and life. *International Journal of Information Management, 55*, 102211. doi:10.1016/j.ijinfomgt.2020.102211

Ebener, S., Roth, S., & Khetrapal, S. (2018). *Building Capacity for Geo-Enabling Health Information Systems: Supporting Equitable Health Services and Well-Being For ALL.* Academic Press.

EC. (2020). *Electoral Commission Statistics.* https://www.ec.or.ug/electoral-commission-statistics

Edwards, R. S., Davis, A. R., & Shilling, J. L. (1999). The role of orthoptists in biometry. *The British Orthoptic Journal*, (56), 19–21.

Eivazzadeh, S. (2019). *Evaluating Success Factors of Health Information Systems.* Academic Press.

Emad, B., Arabia, S., Administratio, B., & Saud, K. (2018). Self-Disclosure in Social Networking Sites in Saudi Arabia. *International Journal of Business and Management, 13*(10), 96–115. doi:10.5539/ijbm.v13n10p96

Erixon, C. (2012). *Information System Providers and Business Relationships: A Study on the Impact of Connections.* https://www.diva-portal.org/smash/record.jsf?pid=diva2:523537

Excelsior. (2014). *Less innovation, more scale. Realising the promise of health technology in Africa.* Available at excelsior-group.com/CMS/downloads/EXG_Whitepape.pdf

Felim, P., Dimyati, D., & Shihab, M. (2018). ASKfm: Motives of Self-Disclosure to Anonymous Questions. *Jurnal Komunikasi, 13*(1), 93–108. doi:10.20885/komunikasi.vol13.iss1.art7

Fincham, J. E. (2008). Response rates and responsiveness for surveys, standards, and the Journal. *American Journal of Pharmaceutical Education, 72*(2), 43. doi:10.5688/aj720243 PMID:18483608

Fishbein, M., & Ajzen, I. (1975). *Belief, attitude, intention and behavior: An introduction to theory and research.* Academic Press.

Fitzmaurice, K. (2000). A Method of Assessing Visual Performance Applicable to Multi-Handicapped Children: Response Mode. *Vision Rehabilitation*, 416.

Fitzmaurice, K. (1999). Low vision rehabilitation: An update. *Australian Orthoptic Journal, 34*, 9–14.

Flaxman, S. R., Bourne, R. R., Resnikoff, S., Ackland, P., Braithwaite, T., Cicinelli, M. V., Das, A., Jonas, J. B., Keeffe, J., Kempen, J. H., Leasher, J., Limburg, H., Naidoo, K., Pesudovs, K., Silvester, A., Stevens, G. A., Tahhan, N., Wong, T. Y., Taylor, H. R., ... Zheng, Y. (2017). Global causes of blindness and distance vision impairment 1990–2020: A systematic review and meta-analysis. *The Lancet. Global Health, 5*(12), e1221–e1234. doi:10.1016/S2214-109X(17)30393-5 PMID:29032195

Folorunso, G. I., Oyeyemi, A. I., Udoh, O. D., Ayodele, O. T., & Excellence-Oluye, N. O. (2020). Rethinking the role of traditional media on migration issues in Nigeria. In N. Okorie, B. R. Ojebuyi, & J. W. Macharia (Eds.), *Handbook of Research on the Global Impact of Media on Migration Issues* (pp. 85–95). IGI Global.

Fornell, C., & Larcker, D. F. (1981). Evaluating Structural Equation Models with Unobservable Variables and Measurement Error. *JMR, Journal of Marketing Research, 18*(1), 39–50. doi:10.1177/002224378101800104

Friderichs, G., Foh, K., & Gathinji, C. M. (2014). *mHealth Country Feasibility Report Malawi.* https://www.gsma.com/mobilefordevelopment/programme/mhealth/gsma-country-feasibility-report-malawi-2014

Fu, J., Wang, N., & Cai, Y. (2020). Privacy-preserving in healthcare blockchain systems based on lightweight message sharing. *Sensors (Switzerland), 20*(7), 1898. Advance online publication. doi:10.339020071898 PMID:32235389

Fujita, J., Aoki, S., & Shimizu, K. (2000). Orthoptist in Low Vision Clinic. *Japanese Orthoptic Journal, 28*, 239–243. doi:10.4263/jorthoptic.28.239

Gabbiadini, A., Baldissarri, C., Durante, F., Valtorta, R. R., De Rosa, M., & Gallucci, M. (2020). Together apart: The mitigating role of digital communication technologies on negative affect during the COVID-19 outbreak in Italy. *Frontiers in Psychology, 11*, 2763. doi:10.3389/fpsyg.2020.554678 PMID:33192807

Gates, B. (2020). Responding to COVID-19: A Once-in-a-Century Pandemic? *The New England Journal of Medicine, 382*(18), 1677–1679. doi:10.1056/NEJMp2003762 PMID:32109012

Geopoll. (2020a). *The financial impact of coronavirus in Sub-Saharan Africa.* Available at: https://f.hubspotusercontent30.net

Geopoll. (2020b). *Coronavirus in Sub-Sharan Africa: How Africans in 12 nations are responding to the COVID-19 outbreak.* Available at: https://cdn2.hubspot.net

Georgievski, Z., Koklanis, K., Fenton, A., & Koukouras, I. (2007). Victorian orthoptists' performance in the photo evaluation of diabetic retinopathy. *Clinical & Experimental Ophthalmology, 35*(8), 733–738. doi:10.1111/j.1442-9071.2007.01576.x PMID:17997777

GHI. (2012). *Burundi Global Health Initiative strategy 2011-2015.* Available at www.ghi.gov/documents/organization/175128.pdf

Giménez, V., Keith, J. R., & Prior, D. (2019). Do healthcare financing systems influence hospital efficiency? A metafrontier approach for the case of Mexico. *Health Care Management Science, 22*(3), 549–559. doi:10.100710729-019-9467-9 PMID:30659404

Girardi, F., De Gennaro, G., Colizzi, L., & Convertini, N. (2020). Improving the Healthcare Effectiveness: The Possible Role of EHR, IoMT and Blockchain. *Electronics (Basel), 9*(6), 884. doi:10.3390/electronics9060884

Githinji, S., Kigen, S., Memusi, D., Nyandigisi, A., Mbithi, A. M., Wamari, A., Muturi, A. N., Jagoe, G., Barrington, J., Snow, R. W., & Zurovac, D. (2013). Reducing stock-outs of life saving malaria commodities using mobile phone text-messaging: SMS for life study in Kenya. *PLoS One*, *8*(1), 1–8. doi:10.1371/journal.pone.0054066 PMID:23349786

Giudice, A., Barone, S., Muraca, D., Averta, F., Diodati, F., Antonelli, A., & Fortunato, L. (2020). Can teledentistry improve the monitoring of patients during the Covid-19 dissemination? A descriptive pilot study. *International Journal of Environmental Research and Public Health*, *17*(10), 1–9. doi:10.3390/ijerph17103399 PMID:32414126

Goel, U., Ruhl, R., & Zavarsky, P. (2019). Using Healthcare Authority and Patient Blockchains to Develop a Tamper-Proof Record Tracking System. *2019 IEEE 5th Intl Conference on Big Data Security on Cloud (BigDataSecurity), IEEE Intl Conference on High Performance and Smart Computing, (HPSC) and IEEE Intl Conference on Intelligent Data and Security (IDS)*, 25–30. 10.1109/BigDataSecurity-HPSC-IDS.2019.00016

Graham-Harrison, E., & Cadwalladr, C. (2018). Revealed: 50 million Facebook profiles harvested for Cambridge Analytica in major data breach. *The Guardian*, 1–5.

Greaves, C. J., Sheppard, K. E., Abraham, C., Hardeman, W., Roden, M., Evans, P. H., & Schwarz, P. (2011). Systematic review of reviews of intervention components associated with increased effectiveness in dietary and physical activity interventions. *BMC Public Health*, *11*(1), 1–12. doi:10.1186/1471-2458-11-119 PMID:21333011

GSMA. (2021). *Mobile Economy*. https://data.gsmaintelligence.com/api-web/v2/research-file-download?id=60621126&file=250621-Mobile-Economy-2021.pdf

Gustafsson, M., Norlinder, J., & Rehn, M. (2018). *Using an ICT System to Increase Efficiency and Effectiveness in Patient-Practitioner Communication*. www.it.uu.se

Hair, J. F. Jr, Hult, G. T. M., Ringle, C. M., & Sarstedt, M. (2021). *A primer on partial least squares structural equation modeling (PLS-SEM)*. Sage Publications. doi:10.1007/978-3-030-80519-7

Hallam, C., & Zanella, G. (2017). Online self-disclosure: The privacy paradox explained as a temporally discounted balance between concerns and rewards. *Computers in Human Behavior*, *68*, 217–227. doi:10.1016/j.chb.2016.11.033

Haman, M. (2020). The use of Twitter by state leaders and its impact on the public during the COVID-19 pandemic. *Heliyon*, *6*(11), 1–27. doi:10.1016/j.heliyon.2020.e05540 PMID:33294685

Hanson, W., & Heeks, R. (2020). Impact of ICTs-in-Agriculture on Rural Resilience in Developing Countries. In *Development Informatics* (No. 84; Working Paper Series, Issue July). doi:10.13140/RG.2.2.31885.90084

Heeks, R. (2018). *Information and Communication Technology for Development (ICT4D)*. doi:10.4324/9781315652603

Heeks, R., & Ospina, A. V. (2015). Analysing Urban Community Informatics from a Resilience Perspective. *The Journal of Community Informatics*, *11*(1), 1–18. doi:10.15353/joci.v11i1.2846

Helveston, E. M. (2005). Visual training: Current status in ophthalmology. *American Journal of Ophthalmology, 140*(5), 903–910. doi:10.1016/j.ajo.2005.06.003 PMID:16310470

Hernandez, L. M., & Blazer, D. G. (2006). *Genes, behavior, and the social environment: Moving beyond the nature/nurture debate*. National Academies Press.

Hindemark, F. (2013). *E-Health at Outpatient Clinics in Uganda*. https://www.diva-portal.org/smash/get/diva2:680178/FULLTEXT01.pdf

Hoffman, J. A., Cunningham, J. R., Suleh, A. J., Sundsmo, A., Dekker, D., Vago, F., Munly, K., Igonya, E. K., & Hunt-Glassman, J. (2010). Mobile direct observation treatment for tuberculosis patients: A technical feasibility pilot using mobile phones in Nairobi, Kenya. *Pub Med, 39*(1), 78–80.

Horwood, A. M. (2018). What do we expect new graduate orthoptists to do? *The British and Irish Orthoptic Journal, 14*(1), 11–19. doi:10.22599/bioj.108 PMID:32999959

Hoy, M. G., & Milne, G. (2010). Gender Differences in Privacy-Related Measures for Young Adult Facebook Users. *Journal of Interactive Advertising, 10*(2), 28–45. doi:10.1080/15252019.2010.10722168

Hynes, D., & Richardson, H. (2009). What use is domestication theory to information systems research? In *Handbook of research on contemporary theoretical models in information systems* (pp. 482–494). IGI Global. doi:10.4018/978-1-60566-659-4.ch027

Iacobucci, I. L. (1991). The role and growth of orthoptics in the ophthalmologist's private practice: The orthoptist's view. *The American Orthoptic Journal, 41*(1), 15–18. doi:10.1080/0065955X.1991.11981846

ICTworks. (2020). *10 Educational Technology Solutions for COVID-19 Out-of-School Children.* Wayan Vota. Available at: www.ictworks.org

IGI-Global. (2021). *What is Financial Factors*. https://www.igi-global.com/dictionary/financial-factors/39752

Imaja, I. M., Ndayizigamiye, P., & Maharaj, M. (2017). A design of a mobile health intervention for the prevention and treatment of Cholera in South Kivu in the Democratic Republic of Congo. In *2017 IEEE Global Humanitarian Technology Conference (GHTC)* (pp. 1-5). IEEE. 10.1109/GHTC.2017.8239251

International Labour Organization (ILO). (2020). *ILO Monitor: COVID-19 and the world of work* (4th ed.). International Labour Organization. Available at: http://www.ilo.org/global/topics/coronavirus/impacts-and-responds/WCMS_745963/lang--en/index.thm

Ismail, R., & Zainab, A. N. (2013). Assessing the status of library information systems security. *Journal of Librarianship and Information Science, 45*(3), 231–247. doi:10.1177/0961000613477676

ISO. (2011). *Product Quality Model*. ISO/IEC 25010:2011. https://www.iso.org/standard/35733.html

ITU. (2014). *ICT Facts and Figures*. Retrieved May 16, 2016 from https://www.itu.int/en/ITU-D/Statistics/Documents/facts/ICTFactsFigures2014-e.pdf

Jamison, J., Karlan, D., & Raffler, P. (2013). Mixed Method Evaluation of a Passive mHealth Sexual Information Texting Service in Uganda. *Information Technologies and International Development*, *9*(3), 1–19.

Jarvenpaa, S. L., Tractinsky, N., & Saarinen, L. (1999). Consumer trust in an Internet store: A cross-cultural validation. *Journal of Computer-Mediated Communication, 5*(2), JCMC526.

Jarvis, S. N., Tamhne, R. C., Thompson, L., Francis, P. M., Anderson, J., & Colver, A. F. (1991). Preschool vision screening. *Archives of Disease in Childhood, 66*(3), 288–294. doi:10.1136/adc.66.3.288 PMID:2025002

Jethwa, T., Ton, A., Paredes Molina, C. S., Speicher, L., Walsh, K., Knight, D., Davlantes, T., & Francis, D. (2020). Establishing Mayo Clinic's Coronavirus Disease 2019 Virtual Clinic: A Preliminary Communication. *Telemedicine Journal and E-Health : The Official Journal of the American Telemedicine Association*. . doi:10.1089/tmj.2020.0145

Jewitt, C. (2005). Multimodality, "reading," and "writing" for the 21st Century. *Discourse (Abingdon), 26*(3), 315–331. doi:10.1080/01596300500200011

Jewitt, C., Kress, G., Ogborn, J., & Tsatsarelis, C. (2001). Exploring learning through visual, actional and linguistic communication: The multimodal environment of a science classroom. *Educational Review*, *53*(1), 5–18. doi:10.1080/00131910123753

Kaium, M. A., Bao, Y., Alam, M. Z., Hasan, N., & Hoque, M. R. (2019). Understanding the insight of factors affecting mHealth adoption: A systematic review. *International Journal of Research in Business and Social Science, 8*(6), 181-200.

Kalantaryan, S., & McMahon, S. (2020). *COVID-19 and Remittances in Africa*. EUR 30262 EN, Publications Office of the European Union. Available at https://ec.europa.eu/jrc

Källander, K., Tibenderana, J. K., Akpogheneta, O. J., Strachan, D. L., Hill, Z., ten Asbroek, A. H. A., Conteh, L., Kirkwood, B. R., & Meek, S. R. (2013). Mobile health (mHealth) approaches and lessons for increased performance and retention of community health workers in low-and middle-income countries: A review. *Journal of Medical Internet Research*, *15*(1), e17. doi:10.2196/jmir.2130 PMID:23353680

Kamanga, A., Moono, P., Stresman, G., Mharakurwa, S., & Shiff, C. (2010). Rural health centres, communities and malaria case detection in Zambia using mobile telephones: A means to detect potential reservoirs of infection in unstable transmission conditions. *Malaria Journal*, *9*(1), 1–7. doi:10.1186/1475-2875-9-96 PMID:20398318

Kanaan, A. G., & Hassan, S. B., & Shahzad, A. (2016). A Conceptual Model for E-Government Success Factors in Developing Countries. *International Journal of Scientific and Research Publications*, *6*(12), 39–44.

Kante, M., & Ndayizigamiye, P. (2020a). A systematic mapping of the adoption of Internet of Things to provide healthcare services in developing countries. In P. Ndayizigamiye, G. Barlow-Jones, R. Brink, S. Bvuma, R. Minty, & S. Mhlongo (Eds.), Perspectives on ICT4D and Socio-Economic Growth Opportunities in Developing Countries (pp. 99–126). IGI Global. https://doi.org/10.4018/978-1-7998-2983-6.ch004.

Kante, M., & Ndayizigamiye, P. (2021). Internet of Medical Things, Policies and Geriatrics: An Analysis of the National Digital Health Strategy for South Africa 2019-2024 from the Policy Triangle Framework Perspective. *Scientific African*, e00759.

Kante, M., Chepken, C., & Oboko, R. (2018). Partial Least Square Structural Equation Modelling' use in Information Systems: An Updated Guideline of Practices in Exploratory Settings. *Kabarak Journal of Research & Innovation, 6*(1), 49–67. http://eserver.kabarak.ac.ke/ojs/

Kante, M. (2022). A mapping of the factors related to self-disclosure on social network sites. *International Journal of Big Data Management*, *2*(1), 60–69. doi:10.1504/IJBDM.2022.119434

Kante, M., Chepken, C., & Oboko, R. (2018). Partial Least Square Structural Equation Modelling' use in Information Systems: An Updated Guideline of Practices in Exploratory Settings. *Kabarak Journal of Research & Innovation*, *6*(1), 49–67.

Kante, M., & Ndayizigamiye, P. (2020a). A systematic mapping of the adoption of Internet of Things to provide healthcare services in developing countries. In P. Ndayizigamiye, G. Barlow-Jones, R. Brink, S. Bvuma, R. Minty, & S. Mhlongo (Eds.), *Perspectives on ICT4D and Socio-Economic Growth Opportunities in Developing Countries* (pp. 99–126). IGI Global. doi:10.4018/978-1-7998-2983-6.ch004

Kante, M., & Ndayizigamiye, P. (2020b). An analysis of the current status of Internet of Medical Things policies in developing countries. *NPG. Neurologie, Psychiatrie, Gériatrie*, *20*(119), 259–265. doi:10.1016/j.npg.2020.03.002

Karmarkar, U. R., & Dan, Y. (2006). Experience-dependent plasticity in adult visual cortex. *Neuron*, *52*(4), 577–585. doi:10.1016/j.neuron.2006.11.001 PMID:17114043

Karuri, J., Waiganjo, P., & Orwa, D. (2014). Determinants of Acceptance and Use of DHIS2: Survey Instrument Validation and Preliminary Findings using PLS-SEM. *Journal of Emerging Trends in Computing and Information Sciences*, *5*(8), 647–660. doi:10.100710067-013-2361-9

Kasusse, M., Rosette, M., Burke, E., Mwangi, C., Batamwita, R., Tumwesigye, N., & Aisu, S. (2014). Understanding ICT behaviors among health workers in sub-Saharan Africa: A cross-sectional study for laboratory persons in Uganda. *IJSSH, 8*(2), 258-261. https://citeseerx.ist.psu.edu/viewdoc/download?doi=10.1.1.975.6541&rep=rep1&type=pdf

Katuwal, G. J., Pandey, S., Hennessey, M., & Lamichhane, B. (2018). *Applications of Blockchain in Healthcare: Current Landscape & Challenges*. https://arxiv.org/abs/1812.02776v1

Katz, R.L., Callorda, F.M. & Jung, J. (2020, May 14). Can Digitization Mitigate COVID-19 Damages? Evidence from Developing Countries. *Evidence from Developing Countries.*

Khabsa, M., & Giles, C. L. (2014). The number of scholarly documents on the public web. *PLoS One*, *9*(5), e93949. doi:10.1371/journal.pone.0093949 PMID:24817403

Khalifehsoltani, S. N., & Gerami, M. R. (2010). E-health challenges, opportunities and experiences of developing countries. *International Conference on E-Education, e-Business, e-Management and e-Learning*, 264-268. 10.1109/IC4E.2010.119

Khatoon, A. (2020). A blockchain-based smart contract system for healthcare management. *Electronics (Switzerland)*, *9*(1), 94. Advance online publication. doi:10.3390/electronics9010094

Khordoc, C. (2001). The comic book's soundtrack: Visual sound effects in Asterix. In R. Varnum & C. T. Gibbons (Eds.), *The language of comics: Word and image* (pp. 156–173). University Press of Mississippi.

Khubone, T., Tlou, B., & Mashamba-Thompson, T. P. (2020). Electronic Health Information Systems to Improve Disease Diagnosis and Management at Point-of-Care in Low and Middle Income Countries: A Narrative Review. *Diagnostics (Basel)*, *10*(5), 327. Advance online publication. doi:10.3390/diagnostics10050327 PMID:32443856

Kiberu, V. M., Mars, M., & Scott, R. E. (2017). Barriers and opportunities to implementation of sustainable e-Health programmes in Uganda: A literature review. African Journal of Primary Health Care and Family Medicine. doi:10.4102/phcfm.v9i1.1277

Kiberu, V. M., Matovu, J. K., Makumbi, F., Kyozira, C., Mukooyo, E., & Wanyenze, R. K. (2014). Strengthening district-based health reporting through the district health management information software system: The Ugandan experience. *BMC Medical Informatics and Decision Making*, *14*(1), 40. doi:10.1186/1472-6947-14-40 PMID:24886567

Kim, S. K., & Huh, J. H. (2020). Artificial neural network blockchain techniques for healthcare system: Focusing on the personal health records. *Electronics (Switzerland)*, *9*(5), 763. Advance online publication. doi:10.3390/electronics9050763

Knight, D., & Holt, A. (2010). Internet and mobile technologies in healthcare service delivery: A case study exploring elements within their use and potential use in midwifery service delivery. Proceedings of Postgraduate Day 2010, 53-54.

Knopke, V. (2013). Gender and Technology Education-theory and background. *Journal of Industrial Technology Design Teachers Association of Queensland*, *54*, 7–11.

Kokolakis, S. (2017). *Privacy attitudes and privacy behaviour: A review of current research on the privacy paradox phenomenon.* Academic Press.

Koroleva, K., Brecht, F., & Malinova, M. (2011). *'Generation Facebook'-A Cognitive Calculus Model of Teenage User Behavior on Social Network Sites. Enabling Batch Processing in Business Processes View project.* https://www.researchgate.net/publication/220890444

Kothari, C. R. (2004). *Research Methodology: Methods and Techniques (3rd ed.).* New Age International Publishers.

Krasnova, H., Spiekermann, S., Koroleva, K., & Hildebrand, T. (2010). Online social networks: Why we disclose. *Journal of Information Technology*, *25*(2), 109–125. doi:10.1057/jit.2010.6

Krasnova, H., Veltri, N. F., & Günther, O. (2012a). Self-disclosure and privacy calculus on social networking sites: The role of culture. *Business & Information Systems Engineering*, *4*(3), 127–135. doi:10.100712599-012-0216-6

Kress, G. (2010). *Multimodality: A social semiotic approach to contemporary communication.* Routledge.

Kress, G. R., & van Leeuwen, T. (1996). *Reading images: The grammar of visual design.* Routledge.

Kress, G. R., & van Leeuwen, T. (2001). *Multimodal discourse: The modes and media of contemporary communication.* Arnold.

Kruse, C., Betancourt, J., Ortiz, S., Luna, S. M. V., Bamrah, I. K., & Segovia, N. (2019). Barriers to the use of mobile health in improving health outcomes in developing countries: Systematic review. *Journal of Medical Internet Research*, *21*(10), e13263. doi:10.2196/13263 PMID:31593543

Kuca, K. (2020). *The 2019 Novel Coronavirus (COVID-19) Outbreak in China and the world: A new lesson for public health system letters in drug design and discovery.* Academic Press.

Kumar, T., Ramani, V., Ahmad, I., Braeken, A., Harjula, E., & Ylianttila, M. (2018, November 9). Blockchain utilization in healthcare: Key requirements and challenges. *2018 IEEE 20th International Conference on E-Health Networking, Applications and Services, Healthcom 2018.* 10.1109/HealthCom.2018.8531136

Kumar, A., Krishnamurthi, R., Nayyar, A., Sharma, K., Grover, V., & Hossain, E. (2020). A Novel Smart Healthcare Design, Simulation, and Implementation Using Healthcare 4.0 Processes. *IEEE Access: Practical Innovations, Open Solutions*, *8*, 118433–118471. doi:10.1109/ACCESS.2020.3004790

Kumar, R., & Tripathi, R. (2021). Scalable and secure access control policy for healthcare system using blockchain and enhanced Bell–LaPadula model. *Journal of Ambient Intelligence and Humanized Computing*, *12*(2), 2321–2338. doi:10.100712652-020-02346-8

Kushch, S., Ranise, S., & Sciarretta, G. (2019, November 1). Blockchain Tree for eHealth. *2019 IEEE Global Conference on Internet of Things, GCIoT 2019.* 10.1109/GCIoT47977.2019.9058412

L'Engle, K., Plourde, K. F., & Zan, T. (2017). *Evidence-based adaptation and scale-up of a mobile phone health information service.* Retrieved November 25, 2018, from https://mhealth.amegroups.com/article/view/14104/14325

Lau, F., & Kuziemsky, C. (2016). *Handbook of eHealth Evaluation: An Evidence-based Approach.* http://venus.library.uvic.ca/handle/1828/7814

Lau, F., Hagens, S., & Muttitt, S. (2007). *A proposed benefits evaluation framework for health information systems in Canada.* Healthcare Quarterly.

Lester, R. T., Ritvo, P., Mills, E. J., Kariri, A., Karanja, S., Chung, M. H., Jack, W., Habyarimana, J., Sadatsafavi, M., Najafzadeh, M., Marra, C. A., Estambale, B., Ngugi, E., Ball, T. B., Thabane, L., Gelmon, L. J., Kimani, J., Ackers, M., & Plummer, F. A. (2010). Effects of a mobile phone short message service on antiretroviral treatment adherence in Kenya (WelTel Kenya1): A randomised trial. *Lancet*, *376*(9755), 1838–1845. doi:10.1016/S0140-6736(10)61997-6 PMID:21071074

Lester, R., Ritvo, P., Mills, E., Kariri, A., Karanja, S., Chung, M. C., Jack, W., Habyarimana, J., Sadatsafavi, M., Najafzadeh, M., Marra, C. A., Estambale, B., Ngugi, E., Ball, T. B., Thabane, L., Gelmon, L. J., Kimani, J., Ackers, M., & Plummer, F. A. (2010). Effects of mobile phone short message service on antiretroviral treatment adherence in Kenya (WelTel Kenya1): A randomised trial. *Lancet*, *376*, 1838–1845.

Levy, Y., & Ellis, T. J. (2006). A systems approach to conduct an effective literature review in support of information systems research. *Informing Science*, *9*, 181–211. doi:10.28945/479

Liang, T., Huang, C., Yeh, Y., & Lin, B. (2007). Adoption of mobile technology in business: A fit-viability model. *Industrial Management & Data Systems*, *107*(8), 1154–1169. doi:10.1108/02635570710822796

Li, H., Sarathy, R., & Xu, H. (2010). Understanding situational online information disclosure as a privacy calculus Understanding situational online information disclosure as a privacy calculus. *Journal of Computer Information Systems*, *51*, 1–29. doi:10.1080/08874417.2010.11645450

Li, M., Shao, S., Ye, Q., Xu, G., & Huang, G. Q. (2020). Blockchain-enabled logistics finance execution platform for capital-constrained E-commerce retail. *Robotics and Computer-integrated Manufacturing*, *65*, 101962. Advance online publication. doi:10.1016/j.rcim.2020.101962

Lintern, G., & Motavalli, A. (2018). Healthcare information systems: The cognitive challenge. In BMC Medical Informatics and Decision Making (Vol. 18, Issue 1). BioMed Central Ltd. doi:10.118612911-018-0584-z

Lissouba, P., Taljaard, D., Rech, D., Doyle, S., Shabangu, D., Nhlapo, C., Otchere-Darko, J., Mashigo, T., Matson, C., Lewis, D., Billy, S., & Auvert, B. (2010). A Model for the Roll-Out of Comprehensive Adult Male Circumcision Services in African Low-Income Settings of High HIV Incidence: The ANRS 12126 Bophelo Pele Project. *PLoS Medicine*, *7*(7), e1000309. doi:10.1371/journal.pmed.1000309 PMID:20652013

Lobo, V. B., Analin, J., Laban, R. M., & More, S. S. (2020). Convergence of Blockchain and Artificial Intelligence to Decentralize Healthcare Systems. *Proceedings of the 4th International Conference on Computing Methodologies and Communication, ICCMC 2020*, 925–931. 10.1109/ICCMC48092.2020.ICCMC-000171

Lund, S., Nielsen, B. B., Hemed, M., Boas, I. M., Said, A., Said, K., Makungu, M. H., & Rasch, V. (2014). Mobile phones improve antenatal care attendance in Zanzibar: A cluster randomized controlled trial. *BMC Pregnancy and Childbirth*, *14*(29), 1–10. doi:10.1186/1471-2393-14-29 PMID:24438517

Lwoga, E. T., & Sangeda, R. Z. (2019). ICTs and development in developing countries: A systematic review of reviews. *The Electronic Journal on Information Systems in Developing Countries*, *85*(1), e12060. doi:10.1002/isd2.12060

Madden, T. J., Ellen, P. S., & Ajzen, I. (1992). A comparison of the theory of planned behavior and the theory of reasoned action. *Personality and Social Psychology Bulletin*, *18*(1), 3–9. doi:10.1177/0146167292181001

Malanga, D. F. (2017). Implementation of Mobile Health Initiatives in Malawi: Current Status, Issues, and Challenges. Health Information Systems and Advancement of Medical Practice in Developing Countries, 115-128. doi:10.4018/978-1-5225-2262-1.ch007

Malanga, D. F. (2017b). *Assessing information literacy skills: A survey of undergraduate education students at the University of Livingstonia in Malawi*. https://digitalcommons.unl.edu/libphilprac/1806/

Malanga, D. F. (2020). *Tackling Gender-Based Cyber Violence against Women and Girls in Malawi amidst the Covid-19 Pandemic*. African Declarations on Internet Rights and Freedoms & APC, 1-12. https://africaninternetrights.org/sites/default/files/Donald_Flywell-1.pdf

Malanga, D. F. (2022). The Prevalence of Online Violence Against Female Students at a Private University in Malawi. In Handbook of Research on Digital Violence and Discrimination Studies (pp. 451-465). doi:10.4018/978-1-7998-9187-1.ch019

Malanga, D. F., & Banda, M. (2021). *ICT Use and Livelihoods of Women Microenterprises in Malawi*. arXiv preprint arXiv:2108.09807.

Malanga, D. F., & Banda, M. J. (2021b). *The use of mobile phones by women microenterprises in Malawi: a sustainable livelihoods perspective*. Global Knowledge, Memory and Communication. doi:10.1108/GKMC-09-2020-0143

Malanga, D. F., & Chigona, W. (2018). Mobile Health Initiatives in Malawi: Understanding Impact, Funding Model and Challenges. *International Journal of Privacy and Health Information Management*, *6*(1), 49–60. doi:10.4018/IJPHIM.2018010104

Malawi Communications Regulatory Authority. (2015). *National Survey on Access and Usage of ICT Services in Malawi*. http://www.macra.org.mw/wp-content/uploads/2016/01/MACRA-Survey-Report-National-Household-and-Individual-access-to-and-usage-of-ICT.pdf

Malawi National Health Policy. (2017). https://npc.mw/wp-content/uploads/2020/07/national-health-policy.pdf

Malhotra, N. K., Kim, S. S., & Agarwal, J. (2004). Internet users' information privacy concerns (IUIPC): The construct, the scale, and a causal model. *Information Systems Research*, *15*(4), 336–355. doi:10.1287/isre.1040.0032

Manyazewal, T. (2017). Using the World Health Organization health system building blocks through survey of healthcare professionals to determine the performance of public healthcare facilities. *Archives of Public Health*, *75*(1), 50. Advance online publication. doi:10.118613690-017-0221-9 PMID:29075485

Marinoni, G., Van't Land, H., & Jensen, T. (2020). *The impact of COVID-19 on higher education around the world.* IAU Global Survey Report. Available at www.iau.aiu.net

Marks, S. (2020). Ethiopian diaspora champions digital apps in the fight against COVID. *Voice of America News.*

Marra, D. E., Hamlet, K. M., Bauer, R. M., & Bowers, D. (2020). Validity of teleneuropsychology for older adults in response to Covid-19: A systematic and critical review. *The Clinical Neuropsychologist*, *0*(0), 1–42. doi:10.1080/13854046.2020.1769192 PMID:32519594

Martinez, M. S., Robinson, M. R., & Arora, V. M. (2020). Rethinking Hospital-Associated Disability for Patients With COVID-19. *Journal of Hospital Medicine*, *15*(12), 757–759. doi:10.12788/jhm.3504 PMID:33231543

Marwick, A., & Hargittai, E. (2019). Nothing to hide, nothing to lose? Incentives and disincentives to sharing information with institutions online. *Information Communication and Society*, *22*(12), 1697–1713. doi:10.1080/1369118X.2018.1450432

Mateus, M. D., Santos, J. Q., & Mari, J. J. (2005). Popular conceptions of schizophrenia in Cape Verde, Africa. *Revista Brasileira de Psiquiatria (Sao Paulo, Brazil)*, *27*(2), 101–107. doi:10.1590/S1516-44462005000200006 PMID:15962133

Matiyabu, I. I., & Ndayizigamiye, P. (2019). The potential use of Social Media for Healthcare Advocacy in the Democratic Republic of Congo. In *Proceedings of 4th International Conference on the* (*Vol. 12*, pp. 105-111). Academic Press.

Matiyabu, I. I., & Ndayizigamiye, P. (2019). The potential use of Social Media for Healthcare Advocacy in the Democratic Republic of Congo. *Proceedings of 4th International Conference on the, 12*, 105-111.

Matiyabu, I. I., & Ndayizigamiye, P. (2019). The potential use of Social Media for Healthcare Advocacy in the Democratic Republic of Congo. *Proceedings of 4th International Conference, 12*, 105-111.

McCarry, B. (1999). Orthoptists' current shared care role in ophthalmology. *The British Orthoptic Journal*, (56), 11–18.

McGhin, T., Choo, K. K. R., Liu, C. Z., & He, D. (2019). Blockchain in healthcare applications: Research challenges and opportunities. In *Journal of Network and Computer Applications* (Vol. 135, pp. 62–75). Academic Press. doi:10.1016/j.jnca.2019.02.027

McGowan, H. E. (2020). *How the coronavirus pandemic is accelerating the future of work.* Available at: https://www.forbes.com/sites/heathermcgowan/2020/03/23/ the-coronavirus-pandemic-accelerates-the-future-of-work-and-provides-opportunity/?sh=43fe449b317f

McHaney, R. W., Reychev, I., Azuri, J., McHaney, M. E., & Moshonov, R. (2019). *Impacts of Information Technology on Patient Care and Empowerment*. IGI Global. https://books.google.com/books?hl=en&lr=&id=kmqtDwAAQBAJ&oi=fnd&pg=PR1&dq=Roger+W.+McHaney+(Kansas+State+University,+USA),+Iris+Reychev+(Ariel+University,+Israel),+Joseph+Azuri+(Maccabi+Healthcare+Services,+Israel),+Mark+E.+McHaney+(U.S.+Air+Force,+USA)+a

McKnight, D. H., Choudhury, V., & Kacmar, C. (2002). Developing and validating trust measures for e-commerce: An integrative typology. *Information Systems Research, 13*(3), 334–359. doi:10.1287/isre.13.3.334.81

Meinert, E., Alturkistani, A., Foley, K. A., Osama, T., Car, J., Majeed, A., Van Velthoven, M., Wells, G., & Brindley, D. (2019). Blockchain implementation in health care: Protocol for a systematic review. *JMIR Research Protocols, 8*(2), e10994. Advance online publication. doi:10.2196/10994 PMID:30735146

Mhlanga, D., & Moloi, T. (2020). COVID-19 and the digital transformation of education: What are we learning on 4IR in South Africa? *Education Sciences, 10*(7), 180. doi:10.3390/educsci10070180

Mieseigha, E. G., & Ogbodo, U. K. (2013). An empirical analysis of the benefits of a cashless economy on Nigeria's economic development. *Research Journal of Finance and Accounting, 4*(17), 11–16.

Min, J., & Kim, B. (2015). How are people enticed to disclose personal information despite privacy concerns in social network sites? the calculus between benefit and cost. *Journal of the Association for Information Science and Technology, 66*(4), 839–857. Advance online publication. doi:10.1002/asi.23206

Mishra, S., & Singh, I. (2008). *mHealth: A Developing Country Perspective*. Retrieved June, 14, 2016 from http://www.ehealth-connection.org/files/conf-materials/mHealth_%20A%20Developing%20Country%20Perspective_0.pdf

Misic, V. B., Misic, J., & Chang, X. (2019). Towards a blockchain-based healthcare information system: Invited paper. *2019 IEEE/CIC International Conference on Communications in China, ICCC 2019*, 13–18. 10.1109/ICCChina.2019.8855911

Molefi, M. (2010). *An Assessment of eHealth Projects and Initiatives in Africa*. https://scholar.google.com/scholar?hl=en&as_sdt=0%2C5&q=10.%09Molefi+M.+An+Assessment+of+eHealth+Projects+and+Initiatives+in+Africa.+World+Heal+Organ+Geneva%2C+Switz.+2010.&btnG=

Moon, Y. (2000). Intimate exchanges: Using computers to elicit self-disclosure from consumers. *The Journal of Consumer Research, 26*(4), 323–339. doi:10.1086/209566

Moucheraud, C., Schwitters, A., Boudreaux, C., Giles, D., Kilmarx, P. H., Ntolo, N., Bangani, Z., St Louis, M. E., & Bossert, T. J. (2017). Sustainability of health information systems: A three-country qualitative study in southern Africa. *BMC Health Services Research, 17*(1). Advance online publication. doi:10.118612913-016-1971-8 PMID:28073361

Mpungose, C. B., & Khoza, S. B. (2020). *Digitalized curriculum to the rescue of a higher education institution*. African Identities.

Mueller, B., & Urbach, N. (2013). The why, what, and how of theories in is research. In *Thirty Fourth International Conference on Information Systems* (*Vol. 192*, Issue 111, pp. 181–192). AISel.

Muhammad, F., Abdulkareem, J. H., & Chowdhury, A. A. (2017). Major public health problems in Nigeria: A review. *South East Asia Journal of Public Health*, *7*(1), 6–11. doi:10.3329eajph.v7i1.34672

Muijs, D. (2010). Doing quantitative research in education with SPSS. *Sage (Atlanta, Ga.)*.

Müller-Bloch, C., & Kranz, J. (2015). A Framework for Rigorously Identifying Research Gaps in Qualitative Literature Reviews. *ICIS 2015 Proceedings*. https://aisel.aisnet.org/icis2015/proceedings/ResearchMethods/2

Mullet, D. R. (2018). A general critical discourse analysis framework for educational research. *Journal of Advanced Academics*, *29*(2), 116–142. doi:10.1177/1932202X18758260

Munyua, S., Rotich, G., & Kimwele, M. (2015). Factors affecting the adoption of mhealth in maternal health care in nakuru provincial general hospital. *Int J Sci Technol Res*, *2015*, 4.

Muranaka, Y., Furuta, N., Aoki, S., & Gohke, K. (1985). Use of the simplified color video magnifier by young children with severely impaired vision. *Journal of Visual Impairment & Blindness*, *79*(9), 391–395. doi:10.1177/0145482X8507900902

Murphy, E., Kuber, R., McAllister, G., Strain, P., & Yu, W. (2008). An empirical investigation into the difficulties experienced by visually impaired Internet users. *Universal Access in the Information Society*, *7*(1), 79–91. doi:10.100710209-007-0098-4

Mustapha, L. (2008). Mass media and optimization of health policy, the participating option. In R. A. Akinfeleye (Ed.), *Mass media and society: A multiperspective approach*. Department of Mass Communication University of Lagos.

Nabukenya, J., & Ashaba, J. (2019). *Evaluation of eHealth Implementations in Uganda: Investigating Practices, Challenges and Insights*. https://europepmc.org/article/ppr/ppr147961

Nambisan, S., & Baron, R. A. (2007). Interactions in virtual customer environments: Implications for product support and customer relationship management. *Journal of Interactive Marketing*, *21*(2), 42–62. doi:10.1002/dir.20077

National Cancer Institute and the Centers for Disease Control and Prevention. (2010). *Making health communication programs work*. National Cancer Institute and the Centers for Disease Control and Prevention.

National Statistics Office. (2015). *Survey on Access and Usage of ICT services in Malawi*. https://www.yumpu.com/en/document/view/55017822/national-survey-on-access-to-andusage-of-ict-services-in-malawi-2015

NationalICT Policy. (2013). https://www.itu.int/en/ITU-D/Cybersecurity/Documents/National_Strategies_Repository/Malawi_2013_Malawi_ICT_Policy.pdf

Ndayizigamiye, P. (2016). *Potential adoption of mobile health technologies for public healthcare in Burundi* (Doctoral dissertation).

Ndayizigamiye, P., Hangulu, L., & Akintola, O. (2017). A design of a mobile health intervention to enhance home-carers' disposal of medical waste in South Africa. In *2017 IEEE Global Humanitarian Technology Conference (GHTC)* (pp. 1-6). IEEE. 10.1109/GHTC.2017.8239241

Ndayizigamiye, P., Kante, M., & Shingwenyana, S. (2020). An adoption model of mHealth applications that promote physical activity. *Cogent Psychology*, *7*(1), 1764703. doi:10.1080/23311908.2020.1764703

Ndayizigamiye, P., & Maharaj, M. (2016a). Mobile health adoption in Burundi: A UTAUT perspective. In *2016 IEEE Global Humanitarian Technology Conference (GHTC)* (pp. 613-623). IEEE. 10.1109/GHTC.2016.7857342

Ndayizigamiye, P., & Maharaj, M. (2016b). *Applying bridges framework to investigate challenges to the adoption of mHealth in Burundi. In 2016 IST-Africa Week Conference*. IEEE.

Ndayizigamiye, P., & Maharaj, M. (2017). Determinants of mobile health adoption in Burundi. *The African Journal of Information Systems*, *9*(3), 1–23.

Ndayizigamiye, P., & Maharaj, M. (2018). *A Systematic review of mHealth interventions for public healthcare in East Africa in AMCIS 2018 proceedings*. AIS.

Ndayizigamiye, P., Soni, T. C., & Jere, N. (2018). *Factors Motivating the Adoption of Self-Healthcare Monitoring Mobile Applications by the South African Youth. In 2018 IST-Africa Week Conference (IST-Africa)*. IEEE.

Netemeyer, R. G., Bearden, W. O., & Sharma, S. (2003). *Scaling procedures: Issues and applications*. Sage Publications. doi:10.4135/9781412985772

Neubeck, L., Hansen, T., Jaarsma, T., Klompstra, L., & Gallagher, R. (2020). Delivering healthcare remotely to cardiovascular patients during Covid-19: A rapid review of the evidence. *European Journal of Cardiovascular Nursing*, *0*(0), 1–9. doi:10.1177/1474515120924530 PMID:32380858

Nguyen, B. (2018). Exploring Applications of Blockchain in Securing Electronic Medical Records. *Maryland Journal of Contemporary Legal Issues*, *20*(1), 99. https://eds.b.ebscohost.com/eds/detail/detail?vid=0&sid=afc07135-ec43-4dd0-a9d1-21896f2fb4c9%40pdc-v-sessmgr01&bdata=JkF1dGhUeXBlPXNzbyZzaXRlPWVkcy1saXZlJnNjb3BlPXNpdGU%3D#AN=edshol.hein.journals.hclwpo20.8&db=edshol

Nguyen, T. D., Nguyen, T. M., & Cao, T. H. (2015). Information systems success: a literature review. In *International Conference on Future Data and Security Engineering* (pp. 242-256). Springer. 10.1007/978-3-319-26135-5_18

Nilsson, U. L., Frennesson, C., & Nilsson, S. E. G. (2003). Patients with AMD and a large absolute central scotoma can be trained successfully to use eccentric viewing, as demonstrated in a scanning laser ophthalmoscope. *Vision Research, 43*(16), 1777–1787. doi:10.1016/S0042-6989(03)00219-0 PMID:12818347

Njidda, A. M., Oyebanji, O., Obasanya, J., Ojo, O., Adedeji, A., Mba, N., Oladejo, J., & Ihekweazu, C. (2018). The Nigeria Centre for Disease Control. *BMJ Global Health, 3*(2), e000712. doi:10.1136/bmjgh-2018-000712 PMID:29707246

Njoroge, M., Zurovac, D., Ogara, E. A. A., Chuma, J., & Kirigia, D. (2017). Assessing the feasibility of eHealth and mHealth: A systematic review and analysis of initiatives implemented in Kenya. *BMC Research Notes, 10*(1), 90. doi:10.118613104-017-2416-0 PMID:28183341

Norris, F. H., Stevens, S. P., Pfefferbaum, B., Wyche, K. F., & Pfefferbaum, R. L. (2008). Community resilience as a metaphor, theory, set of capacities, and strategy for disaster readiness. *American Journal of Community Psychology, 41*(1), 127–150. doi:10.100710464-007-9156-6 PMID:18157631

Novis, C. (2020). Orthoptists. *South African Ophthalmology Journal, 15*(2), 44–46.

Nunnally, J. C. (1988). *Psychometric Theory*. McGraw-Hill Book Company. http://www.sciepub.com/reference/131748

Nwosu, I. A. (2013). Indigenous communication as an enabling factor for rural development in Nigeria. *International Journal of Development and Management Review, 8*(1).

Nyaga, G. N. (2021). *mHealth Impact on Demand-Capacity Mismatch in Accessing Health Services in Africa*. https://research.wpcarey.asu.edu/carisca/wp-content/uploads/2021/07/Session-1-Gilbert-Nyaga-mHealth.pdf

Nyemba-Mudenda, M., & Chigona, W. (2018). mHealth outcomes for pregnant mothers in Malawi: A capability perspective. *Information Technology for Development, 24*(2), 245–278. doi:10.1080/02681102.2017.1397594

O'Donoghue, O., Vazirani, A. A., Brindley, D., & Meinert, E. (2019). Design choices and trade-offs in health care blockchain implementations: Systematic review. In Journal of Medical Internet Research (Vol. 21, Issue 5). JMIR Publications Inc. doi:10.2196/12426

O'Halloran, K. L., Tan, S., Smith, B. A., & Podlasov, A. (2010). Challenges in designing digital interfaces for the study of multimodal phenomena. *Information Design Journal, 18*(1), 2–21. doi:10.1075/idj.18.1.02hal

Odeny, T. A., Bailey, R. C., Bukusi, E. A., Simoni, J. M., Tapia, K. A., Yuhas, K., Holmes, K. K., & McClelland, R. S. (2012). Text messaging to improve attendance at post-operative clinic visits after adult male circumcision for HIV prevention: A randomized controlled trial. *PLoS One, 7*(9), e43832. doi:10.1371/journal.pone.0043832 PMID:22957034

Oh, H., Rizo, C., Enkin, M., & Jadad, A. (2005). What Is eHealth (3): A Systematic Review of Published Definitions. J Med Internet Res, 7(1). doi:10.2196/jmir.7.1.e1

Oleribe, O. O., Momoh, J., Uzochukwu, B. S. C., Mbofana, F., Adebiyi, A., Barbera, T., Williams, R., & Taylor-Robinson, S. D. (2019). Identifying key challenges facing healthcare systems in Africa and potential solutions. *International Journal of General Medicine*, *12*, 395–403. doi:10.2147/IJGM.S223882 PMID:31819592

Olu, O., Muneene, D., Bataringaya, J. E., Nahimana, M. R., Ba, H., Turgeon, Y., & Dovlo, D. (2019). How can digital health technologies contribute to the sustainable attainment of universal health coverage in Africa? A perspective. *Frontiers in Public Health*, *7*, 341. doi:10.3389/fpubh.2019.00341 PMID:31803706

Oluwole, V. (2021). *Top richest countries in Africa.* Business Insider Africa. Available at: https://africa.businessinsider.com/local/markets/top-20-richest-countries-in-africa/ndhb6cx

Omaswa, C. (2016). *Ministry of Health: Uganda National eHealth policy.* Academic Press.

Onoka, C. (2014). The private sector in national health financing systems: the role of health maintenance organisations and private healthcare providers in Nigeria. *London School of Hygiene & Tropical Medicine.*

Oryila, S. S., & Aghadiuno, P. C. (2021). Multimodal communication practice in Nigeria's digital space. In P. Ndayizigamiye, G. Barlow-Jones, R. Brink, S. Bvuma, R. Minty, & S. Mhlongo (Eds.), *Perspectives on ICT4D and socio-economic growth opportunities in developing countries* (pp. 31–61). IGI Publications. doi:10.4018/978-1-7998-2983-6.ch002

Osah, O., & Kyobe, M. (2017). Predicting user continuance intention towards M-pesa in Kenya. *African Journal of Economic and Management Studies*, *8*(1), 36–50. doi:10.1108/AJEMS-03-2017-148

Oxman, A. D., & Guyatt, G. H. (1991). Validation of an index of the quality of review articles. *Journal of Clinical Epidemiology*, *44*(11), 1271–1278. doi:10.1016/0895-4356(91)90160-B PMID:1834807

Oyewole, O. S., Gambo, J., Abba, M., & Onuh, M. E. (2013). Electronic payment system and economic growth: A review of transition to a cashless economy in Nigeria. *International Journal of Scientific Engineering and Technology*, *2*(9), 913–918.

Ozili, P. K. (2020). COVID-19 in Africa: Socio-economic impact, policy response, and opportunities. *The International Journal of Sociology and Social Policy*. Advance online publication. doi:10.1108/IJSSP-05-2020-0171

Pagliari, C., Sloan, D., Gregor, P., Sullivan, F., Detmer, D., Kahan, J. P., Oortwijn, W., & MacGillivray, S. (2005). What Is eHealth (4): A Scoping Exercise to Map the Field. J Med Internet Res, 7(1). doi:10.2196/jmir.7.1.e9

Panesi, S. Caruso, G.P., Ferlino, L., & Dini, S. (2018). Choosing apps for rehabilitation, learning and leisure activities involving visually-impairedvisually impaired children. *Edulearn 2018.*

Panesi, S., Caruso, G., Earp, J., Ferlino, L., & Dini, S. (2020). Visually-impaired children and apps: sharing informal and formal information to guide choice. INNODOCT 2019.

Pankomera, R., & van Greunen, D. (2018). A model for implementing sustainable mHealth applications in a resource-constrained setting: A case of Malawi. *The Electronic Journal on Information Systems in Developing Countries*, *84*(2), e12019. doi:10.1002/isd2.12019

Papadopoulos, T., Baltas, K. N., & Balta, M. E. (2020). The use of digital technologies by small and medium enterprises during COVID-19: Implications for theory and practice. *International Journal of Information Management*, *55*, 102192. doi:10.1016/j.ijinfomgt.2020.102192 PMID:32836646

Parant, A., Schiano-Lomoriello, S., & Marchan, F. (2017). How would I live with a disability? Expectations of bio-psychosocial consequences and assistive technology use. *Disability and Rehabilitation. Assistive Technology*, *12*(7), 681–685. doi:10.1080/17483107.2016.1218555 PMID:27677931

Passchier, R. V. (2017). Exploring the barriers to implementing national health insurance in South Africa: The people's perspective. *South African Medical Journal*, *107*(10), 836–838. doi:10.7196/SAMJ.2017.v107i10.12726 PMID:29022524

Pattillo, S. T., Heller, K. W., & Smith, M. (2004). The impact of a modified repeated-reading strategy paired with optical character recognition on the reading rates of students with visual impairments. *Journal of Visual Impairment & Blindness*, *98*(1), 28–46. doi:10.1177/0145482X0409800104

Perasso, G., Bagino, C., Capris, E., Cocchi, E., Dini, S., Facchini, V., Panizzi, A., & Salvagno, S. (2021). Visual telerehabilitation in the Covid-19 era: tradition meets innovation. *INNODOCT*: Congress at University of Valencia, Spain, 27 October - 1 November 2021

Petersen, K., Vakkalanka, S., & Kuzniarz, L. (2015). Guidelines for conducting systematic mapping studies in software engineering: An update. *Information and Software Technology*, *64*, 1–18. doi:10.1016/j.infsof.2015.03.007

Peterson, R. A., & Kim, Y. (2013). On the relationship between coefficient alpha and composite reliability. *The Journal of Applied Psychology*, *98*(1), 194–198. doi:10.1037/a0030767 PMID:23127213

Pettifor, A., MacPhail, C., Corneli, A., Sibeko, J., Kamanga, G., Rosenberg, N., Miller, W. C., Hoffman, I., Rees, H., & Cohen, M. S. (2011). Continued high risk sexual behavior following diagnosis with acute HIV infection in South Africa and Malawi: Implications for prevention. *AIDS and Behavior*, *15*(6), 1243–1250. doi:10.100710461-010-9839-0 PMID:20978833

Pilz, K. S., Braun, C., Altpeter, E., MacKeben, M., & Trauzettel-Klosinski, S. (2006). Modulation of visual stimulus discrimination by sustained focal attention: An MEG study. *Investigative Ophthalmology & Visual Science*, *47*(3), 1225–1229. doi:10.1167/iovs.04-1338 PMID:16505062

Pop-Eleches, C., Thirumurthy, H., Habyarimana, J. P., Zivin, J. G., Goldstein, M. P., de Walque, D., MacKeen, L., Haberer, J., Kimaiyo, S., & Sidle, J. (2011). Mobile phone technologies improve adherence to antiretroviral treatment in a resource-limited setting: A randomized controlled trial of text message reminders. *AIDS (London, England)*, *25*(6), 825–834.

Powers, K. A., Ghani, A. C., Miller, W. C., Hoffman, I. F., Pettifor, A. E., Kamanga, G., Martinson, F. E., & Cohen, M. S. (2011). The role of acute and early HIV infection in the spread of HIV and implications for transmission prevention strategies in Lilongwe, Malawi: A modelling study. *Lancet, 378*(9787), 256–268. doi:10.1016/S0140-6736(11)60842-8 PMID:21684591

Punia, V., Nasr, G., Zagorski, V., Lawrence, G., Fesler, J., Nair, D., & Najm, I. (2020). Evidence of a Rapid Shift in Outpatient Practice During the Covid-19 Pandemic Using Telemedicine. *Telemedicine Journal and e-Health, 00*(00), 1–3. doi:10.1089/tmj.2020.0150 PMID:32429769

Rabuñal, R., Suarez-Gil, R., Golpe, R., Martínez-García, M., Gómez-Méndez, R., Romay-Lema, E., Pérez-López, A., Rodríguez-Álvarez, A., & Bal-Alvaredo, M. (2020). Usefulness of a Telemedicine Tool TELEA in the Management of the Covid-19 Pandemic. *Telemedicine Journal and e-Health, 00*(00), 1–4. doi:10.1089/tmj.2020.0144 PMID:32501747

Ramani, V., Kumar, T., Bracken, A., Liyanage, M., & Ylianttila, M. (2018). Secure and Efficient Data Accessibility in Blockchain Based Healthcare Systems. *2018 IEEE Global Communications Conference, GLOBECOM 2018 - Proceedings*. 10.1109/GLOCOM.2018.8647221

Rapid S. M. S. (2013). Retrieved February 09 2018 from https://www.rapidsms.org/

Ren, X., Zhai, Y., Song, X., Wang, Z., Dou, D., & Li, Y. (2020). The Application of Mobile Telehealth System to Facilitate Patient Information Presentation and Case Discussion. *Telemedicine Journal and e-Health, 26*(6), 725–733. doi:10.1089/tmj.2020.0084 PMID:32298208

ResearchICTAfrica. (2020). *How Covid-19 exposes the defects in South Africa's digital economy*. Available at: https://researchictafrica.net/2020/03/26/how-covid-19-exposes-the-defects-in-south-africas-digital-economy/

Reynolds, B., Venkatanathan, J., Gonçalves, J., & Kostakos, V. (2011). Sharing ephemeral information in online social networks: privacy perceptions and behaviours. *IFIP Conference on Human-Computer Interaction*, 204–215. 10.1007/978-3-642-23765-2_14

Rizzo, J. R., Beheshti, M., Fang, Y., Flanagan, S., & Giudice, N. A. (2021). COVID-19 and Visual Disability: Can't Look and Now Don't Touch. *PM & R, 13*(4), 415–421. doi:10.1002/pmrj.12541 PMID:33354903

Roberts, T. H. (2012). A Cross-Disciplined Approach to Exploring the Privacy Paradox : Explaining Disclosure Behaviour Using the Theory of Planned Behaviour A Cross-Disciplined Approach to Exploring the Privacy Paradox : Explaining Disclosure Behaviour Using the Theory of Plann. *UK Academy for Information Systems Conference Proceedings, 7*.

Rostampour, M., & Nosratnejad, S. (2020). A Systematic Review of Equity in Healthcare Financing in Low- and Middle-Income Countries. *Value in Health Regional Issues, 21*, 133–140. doi:10.1016/j.vhri.2019.10.001 PMID:31786404

Rothman, C., & Maltser, S. (2021). Exercise while living with breast and gynecological cancers. In A. Cristian (Ed.), Breast cancer and gynecologic cancer rehabilitation (pp. 19-38). Elsevier.

Royce, T. D. (2007). *Intersemiotic complementarity: A framework for multimodal discourse analysis. In New directions in the analysis of multimodal discourse*. Routledge.

Russell, C. L. (2005). An overview of the integrative research review. In Progress in Transplantation (Vol. 15, Issue 1, pp. 8–13). InnoVision Communications. doi:10.1177/152692480501500102

Said, B., Hajar, E., & Amine, S. (2020). The COVID-19 outbreak: A catalyst for digitization in African countries. *The Journal of the Egyptian Public Health Association*, *95*(1).

Salgueiro, C., Urrùtia, G., & Cabanas-Valdés, R. (2021). Available apps for stroke telerehabilitation during corona virus disease 2019 confinement in Spain. *Disability and Rehabilitation. Assistive Technology*, 1–11. doi:10.1080/17483107.2021.1883751 PMID:33576299

Saltes, N. (2018). Navigating disabling spaces: Challenging ontological norms and the spatialization of difference through 'Embodied Practices of Mobility'. *Mobilities*, *13*(1), 81–95. doi:10.1080/17450101.2017.1333279

Samaniego, M., & Deters, R. (2018). Zero-trust hierarchical management in IoT. *Proceedings - 2018 IEEE International Congress on Internet of Things, ICIOT 2018 - Part of the 2018 IEEE World Congress on Services*, 88–95. 10.1109/ICIOT.2018.00019

Sasse, M. A., Brostoff, S., & Weirich, D. (2001). Transforming the 'weakest link'-a human/computer interaction approach to usable and effective security. *BT Technology Journal*, *19*(3), 122–131. doi:10.1023/A:1011902718709

Saunders, C. S., & Jones, J. W. (2015). Measuring Performance of the Information Systems Function. *Journal of Management Information Systems*. Advance online publication. doi:10.1080/07421222.1992.11517939

Saunders, M., Lewis, P., & Thornhill, A. (2016). *Research Methods for Business Students* (7th ed.). Apprentice Hall.

SC4CCM. (2018). *Emerging Lessons of Cstock*. http://sc4ccm.jsi.com/emerging-lessons/cstock/

Scheetz, J., Koklanis, K., McGuinness, M., Long, M., & Morris, M. E. (2019). A Randomized Trial to Increase the Assessment Accuracy of Glaucoma and Optic Disc Characteristics by Orthoptists. *The Journal of Continuing Education in the Health Professions*, *39*(3), 161–167. doi:10.1097/CEH.0000000000000258 PMID:31318721

Schopf, T. R., Nedrebø, B., Hufthammer, K. O., Daphu, I. K., & Lærum, H. (2019). How well is the electronic health record supporting the clinical tasks of hospital physicians? A survey of physicians at three Norwegian hospitals. *BMC Health Services Research*, *19*(1), 934. doi:10.118612913-019-4763-0 PMID:31801518

Schweitzer, J., & Synowiec, C. (2012). The economics of eHealth and mHealth. *Journal of Health Communication*, *17*(1), 73–81. doi:10.1080/10810730.2011.649158 PMID:22548602

Scott, B. K., Miller, G. T., Fonda, S. J., Yeaw, R. E., Gaudaen, J. C., Pavliscsak, H. H., Quinn, M. T., & Pamplin, J. C. (2020). Advanced Digital Health Technologies for Covid-19 and Future Emergencies. *Telemedicine Journal and e-Health*, *00*(00), 1–8. doi:10.1089/tmj.2020.0140 PMID:32456560

Scott-Emuakpor, A. (2010). The evolution of healthcare systems in Nigeria: Which way forward in the twenty-first century. *Nigerian Medical Journal*, *51*, 53–65.

Seidenberg, P., Nicholson, S., Schaefer, M., Semrau, K., Bweupe, M., Masese, N., Bonawitz, R., Chitembo, L., Goggin, C., & Thea, D. M. (2012). Early infant diagnosis of HIV infection in Zambia through mobile phone texting of blood test results. *Bulletin of the World Health Organization*, *90*(5), 348–356.

Senjam, S. S., Manna, S., Vashist, P., Gupta, V., Varughese, S., & Tandon, R. (2021). Tele-rehabilitation for visually challenged students during COVID-19 pandemic: Lesson learned. *Indian Journal of Ophthalmology*, *69*(3), 722. doi:10.4103/ijo.IJO_2527_20 PMID:33595510

Serafini, F., & Clausen, J. (2012). Typography as semiotic resource. *Journal of Visual Literacy*, *31*(2), 1–16. doi:10.1080/23796529.2012.11674697

Serna-Bolea, C., Munoz, J., Almeida, J. M., Nhacolo, A., Letang, E., Nhampossa, T., Ferreira, E., Alonso, P., & Naniche, D. (2010). High prevalence of symptomatic acute HIV infection in an outpatient ward in southern Mozambique: Identification and follow-up. *AIDS (London, England)*, *24*(4), 603–608. doi:10.1097/QAD.0b013e328335cda3 PMID:20019574

Sethi, S. (2018). Healthcare Blockchain leads to Transform Healthcare Industry. *International Journal of Advance Research, Ideas and Innovations in Technology*, *4*(1), 607–608. https://www.multichain.com/white-paper/

Shadrick, I. D. (2020). Social and Community Inclusion of People Withwith Blindness, Low Vision, and DeafBlindness. *Journal of Applied Rehabilitation Counseling*, *51*(4), 290–294. doi:10.1891/JARC-D-20-00026

Shamseer, L., Moher, D., Clarke, M., Ghersi, D., Liberati, A., Petticrew, M., Shekelle, P., Stewart, L. A., Altman, D. G., Booth, A., Chan, A. W., Chang, S., Clifford, T., Dickersin, K., Egger, M., Gøtzsche, P. C., Grimshaw, J. M., Groves, T., Helfand, M., … Whitlock, E. (2015). Preferred reporting items for systematic review and meta-analysis protocols (prisma-p) 2015: Elaboration and explanation. *BMJ*, *349*(February), 1–25. . doi:10.1136/bmj.g7647

Sharma, R., Zhang, C., Wingreen, S. C., Kshetri, N., & Zahid, A. (2020). Design of Blockchain-based Precision Health-Care Using Soft Systems Methodology. *Industrial Management & Data Systems*, *120*(3), 608–632. doi:10.1108/IMDS-07-2019-0401

Shaw, N. T. (2002). "CHEATS": A generic information communication technology (ICT) evaluation framework. *Computers in Biology and Medicine*, *32*(3), 209–220. Advance online publication. doi:10.1016/S0010-4825(02)00016-1 PMID:11922936

Shaw, T., McGregor, D., Brunner, M., Keep, M., Janssen, A., & Barnet, S. (2017). What is eHealth (6)? Development of a Conceptual Model for eHealth: Qualitative Study with Key Informants. *Journal of Medical Internet Research, 19*(10), e324. doi:10.2196/jmir.8106 PMID:29066429

Shieshia, M., Noel, M., Andersson, S., Felling, B., Alva, S., Agarwal, S., Lefevre, A., Misomali, A., Chimphanga, B., Nsona, H., & Chandani, Y. (2014). Strengthening community health supply chain performance through an integrated approach: Using mHealth technology and multilevel teams in Malawi. *Journal of Global Health, 4*(2). Advance online publication. doi:10.7189/jogh.04.020406 PMID:25520796

Shiferaw, S., Workneh, A., Yirgu, R., Dinant, G. J., & Spigt, M. (2018). Designing mHealth for maternity services in primary health facilities in a low-income setting–lessons from a partially successful implementation. *BMC Medical Informatics and Decision Making, 18*(1), 1–14. doi:10.118612911-018-0704-9 PMID:29301576

Shuvo, T. A., Islam, R., Hossain, S., Evans, J. L., Khatun, F., Ahmed, T., Gazi, R., & Adams, A. M. (2015). Innovation and Entrepreneurship in Health Dovepress eHealth innovations in LMICs of Africa and Asia: A literature review exploring factors affecting implementation, scale-up, and sustainability. *Innovation and Entrepreneurship in Health, 2*, 95–106. doi:10.2147/IEH.S88809

Sidney, K., Antony, J., Rodrigues, R., Arumugam, K., Krishnamurthy, S., D'souza, G., De Costa, A., & Shet, A. (2011). Supporting patient adherence to antiretrovirals using mobile phone reminders: Patient responses from South India. *AIDS Care, 24*(5), 612–617. doi:10.1080/09540121.2011.630357 PMID:22150088

Silverstone, R. (2005). The sociology of mediation and communication. The SAGE handbook of sociology, 188-207.

Silvestre, E. (2018). *How Electronic Health Records Strengthen the Health Systems of Low- and Middle-Income Countries: Learning from Eswatini and Mexico*. Academic Press.

Skinner, E. A. (1996). A guide to constructs of control. *Journal of Personality and Social Psychology, 71*(3), 549–570. doi:10.1037/0022-3514.71.3.549 PMID:8831161

Smith, R. (2008). The end of disease and the beginning of health. *BMJ Group Blogs 2008*. Retrieved September 10, 2021 from https://blogs.bmj.com/bmj/2008/07/08/richard-smith-the-end-of-disease-and-the-beginning-of-health/

Smith, A. M. (2016). Healthcare Reform Priorities for South Africa: Four Essays on the Financing, Delivery and User Acceptability of Healthcare. *Ph.D.*, (March), 1–244. doi:10.5588/ijtld.15.0312http

Smith, M. K., Rutstein, S. E., Powers, K. A., Fidler, S., Miller, W. C., Eron, J. J. Jr, & Cohen, M. S. (2013). The detection and management of early HIV infection: A clinical and public health emergency.). *Journal of Acquired Immune Deficiency Syndromes, 63*(2), 187–199. doi:10.1097/QAI.0b013e31829871e0 PMID:23764635

Smith, M., & Marx, L. (1994). *Does Technology Drive History?: The Dilemma of Technological Determinism*. MIT Press.

Sockolow, P. S., Bowles, K. H., & Rogers, M. (2015). Health Information Technology Evaluation Framework (HITREF) Comprehensiveness as Assessed in Electronic Point-of-Care Documentation Systems Evaluations. *Studies in Health Technology and Informatics*. Advance online publication. doi:10.3233/978-1-61499-564-7-406 PMID:26262081

Soni, T. C., Ndayizigamiye, P., & Kante, M. (2019). *Determinants of the Adoption of Self-healthcare Monitoring Mobile Applications. Fortieth International Conference on Information Systems (ICIS)*, Munich, Germany.

Stanhope, J., Gregory, M., & Murphy, K. (2014). The current role of orthoptists: A systematic review. *The Internet Journal of Allied Health Sciences and Practice*, *12*(4), 6. doi:10.46743/1540-580X/2014.1501

Stent, A., Syrdal, A., & Mishra, T. (2011). On the intelligibility of fast synthesized speech for individuals with early-onset blindness. In *Proceedings of the 13th international ACM SIGACCESS conference on Computers and accessibility* (pp. 211-218). 10.1145/2049536.2049574

Stephens, A., Lewis, E. D., & Reddy, S. (2018). Towards an inclusive systemic evaluation for the SDGs: Gender equality, environments and marginalized voices (GEMs). *Journals.Sagepub. Com*, *24*(2), 220–236. doi:10.1177/1356389018766093

Stone, D., & Principal, D. (2017). *Blockchain: The challenges and opportunities in healthcare*. www.divurgent.com

Sulaiman, A. (1996). *A Review Of Information Systems Performance Evaluation Measures*. Academic Press.

Suls, J., & Wallston, K. A. (2003). Introduction. In J. Suls & K. A. Wallston (Eds.), *Social psychological foundations of health and illness*. Blackwell Publishing. doi:10.1002/9780470753552

Sumner, A., Hoy, C. & Oritz-Juarez, E. (2020). *Estimates of the impact of COVID-19 on Global Poverty*. World Institute for Development Economics Research (UNU-WIDER) (No. wp-2020-43).

Supriya, S., & Senthilkumar, A. (2009). Electronic braille pad. In 2009 international conference on control, automation, communication, and energy conservation (pp. 1-5). IEEE.

Su, Q., Zhang, R., Xue, R., & Li, P. (2020). Revocable Attribute-Based Signature for Blockchain-Based Healthcare System. *IEEE Access: Practical Innovations, Open Solutions*, *8*, 127884–127896. doi:10.1109/ACCESS.2020.3007691

Taber, K. S. (2018). The Use of Cronbach's Alpha When Developing and Reporting Research Instruments in Science Education. *Research in Science Education*, *48*(6), 1273–1296. doi:10.100711165-016-9602-2

Taddicken, M. (2014). The “Privacy Paradox” in the Social Web: The Impact of Privacy Concerns, Individual Characteristics, and the Perceived Social Relevance on Different Forms of Self-Disclosure1. *Journal of Computer-Mediated Communication, 19*(2), 248–273. Advance online publication. doi:10.1111/jcc4.12052

Tamura, S., Yoshitake, S., Okano, M., Uchikawa, Y., Onitsuka, S., & Kawano, R. (2020). Benefits of consulting a certified orthoptist in a pediatric vision screening program. *Journal of American Association for Pediatric Ophthalmology and Strabismus, 24*(6), 371–374. doi:10.1016/j.jaapos.2020.08.008 PMID:33246111

Tandon, A., Dhir, A., Islam, N., & Mäntymäki, M. (2020). Blockchain in healthcare: A systematic literature review, synthesizing framework and future research agenda. *Computers in Industry, 122*, 103290. Advance online publication. doi:10.1016/j.compind.2020.103290

Tanwar, S., Parekh, K., & Evans, R. (2020a). Blockchain-based electronic healthcare record system for healthcare 4.0 applications. *Journal of Information Security and Applications, 50*, 102407. doi:10.1016/j.jisa.2019.102407

Tapera, J. (2014). The importance of strategic management to business organizations. *Research Journal of Social Sciences and Management*. https://www.academia.edu/download/60296058/THEIMPORTANCEOFSTRATEGICMANAGEMENTTOBUSINESSORGANIZATION20190814-60656-fu9ked.pdf

Taylor, S. (1978). A developing role of social psychology in medicine and medical practice. *Personality and Social Psychology Bulletin, 4*(4), 515–524. doi:10.1177/014616727800400404

The Centre for Health Policy. (2019). *Evaluation of the Phase 1 Implementation of the Interventions in the National Health Insurance Pilot Districts in South Africa*. Author.

The World Bank. (2017). *A wake up call: Nigeria water supply, sanitation, and hygiene poverty diagnostic*. World Bank Publications.

Theodouli, A., Arakliotis, S., Moschou, K., Votis, K., & Tzovaras, D. (2018). On the Design of a Blockchain-Based System to Facilitate Healthcare Data Sharing. *Proceedings - 17th IEEE International Conference on Trust, Security and Privacy in Computing and Communications and 12th IEEE International Conference on Big Data Science and Engineering, Trustcom/BigDataSE 2018*, 1374–1379. 10.1109/TrustCom/BigDataSE.2018.00190

Ting, D. S. W., Carin, L., Dzau, V., & Wong, T. Y. (2020). Digital technology and COVID-19. *Nature Medicine, 26*(4), 459–461. doi:10.103841591-020-0824-5 PMID:32284618

Torraco, R. J. (2016). Writing Integrative Literature Reviews: Using the Past and Present to Explore the Future. In Human Resource Development Review (Vol. 15, Issue 4, pp. 404–428). SAGE Publications Ltd. doi:10.1177/1534484316671606

Training Cognitivo. (2020). *Game Center*. https://www.trainingcognitivo.it/

Trauzettel-Klosinski, S. (2011). Current methods of visual rehabilitation. *Deutsches Ärzteblatt International, 108*(51-52), 871. PMID:22259642

Tripathi, G., Ahad, M. A., & Paiva, S. (2020). S2HS- A blockchain based approach for smart healthcare system. *Health Care*, *8*(1), 100391. Advance online publication. doi:10.1016/j.hjdsi.2019.100391 PMID:31753750

Trzepacz, M., Łagodziński, P., & Grzegorzek, M. (2019). Electrooculography Application in Vision Therapy Using Smart Glasses. In *International Conference on Information Technologies in Biomedicine* (pp. 103-116). Springer. 10.1007/978-3-030-23762-2_10

Tufekci, Z. (2008). Can you see me now? Audience and disclosure regulation in online social network sites. *Bulletin of Science, Technology & Society*, *28*(1), 20–36. doi:10.1177/0270467607311484

UNICEF Malawi. (2020). *Annual Report.* https://www.unicef.org/malawi/media/4981/file/UNICEF%20Malawi%20Annual%20Report%202020.pdf

UNICEF. (2013). *The State of the World's Children 2013.* Available at https://www.unicef.org/sowc2013/files/SWCR2013_ENG_Lo_res_24_Apr_2013.pdf

United Nations Development Programme (UNDP). (2020). http://www.mw.undp.org/

Van Dijk, J. (2020). The network society. *Sage (Atlanta, Ga.).*

Varela-Aldás, J., Buele, J., Ramos Lorente, P., García-Magariño, I., & Palacios-Navarro, G. (2021). A Virtual Reality-Based Cognitive TeleRehabilitation System for Use in the COVID-19 Pandemic. *Sustainability*, *13*(4), 2183. doi:10.3390u13042183

Vélez, O. (2011). *Design and usability testing of an mHealth application for midwives in rural Ghana.* Retrieved October 15 2015 from https://academiccommons.columbia.edu/catalog/ac:137838

Ventegodt, S., Kandel, I., Ervin, D. A., & Merrick, J. (2016). Concepts of holistic care (1935-1941). In *Healthcare for people with Intellectual and developmental disabilities across the Lifespan.* doi:10.1007/978-3-319-18096-0_148

Vis, C., Bührmann, L., Riper, H., & Ossebaard, H. C. (2020). Health technology assessment frameworks for eHealth: A systematic review. *International Journal of Technology Assessment in Health Care Cite This Article*, *36*(3), 204–216. doi:10.1017/S026646232000015X PMID:32297588

Vokinger, K. N., Nittas, V., Witt, C. M., Fabrikant, S. I., & von Wyl, V. (2020). Digital health and the Covid-19 epidemic: An assessment framework for apps from an epidemiological and legal perspective. *Swiss Medical Weekly*, *150*(May), w20282. doi:10.4414mw.2020.20282 PMID:32418194

Vukicevic, M., Koklanis, K., & Giribaldi, M. (2013). Orthoptics: Evolving to meet increasing demand for eye service. Sydney: Insight News.

Wakadha, H., Chandir, S., Were, E. V., Rubin, A., Obor, D., Levine, O. S., Gibson, D. G., Odhiambo, F., Laserson, K. F., & Feikin, D. R. (2013). The feasibility of using mobile-phone based SMS reminders and conditional cash transfers to improve timely immunization in rural Kenya. *Vaccine*, *31*(6), 987–993.

Walker, S. (2019). Effective antimicrobial resistance communication: The role of information design. *Palgrave Communications*, *5*(24), 24. doi:10.105741599-019-0231-z

Wallace, M., & Shelkey, M. (2007). Katz index of independence in activities of daily living (ADL). *Urologic Nursing*, *27*(1), 93–94. PMID:17390935

Walsham, G. (2017). *Research methodologies for information systems in the development context: a tutorial. In The Digital Challenge: Information Technology in the Development Context. Information Technology in the Development context*. Routledge.

Walsham, G. (2020). Health information systems in developing countries: Some reflections on information for action. *Information Technology for Development*, *26*(1), 194–200. doi:10.1080/02681102.2019.1586632

Warren, J. (2017). Communicating Personal Health Information in Virtual Health Communities. *An Integration of Privacy Calculus Model and Affective Commitment.*, *18*(1), 45–81.

Wave, V. (2009). *M-Health for Development: The Opportunity of Mobile Technology for Healthcare in the Developing World*. The United Nations Foundation and Vodafone Foundation Technology Partnership. Available: http://www.globalproblems-globalsolutionsfiles.org/unf_website/assets/publications/technology/mhealth/mHealth_for_Development_full.pdf

Weiss, M., Botha, A., Herselman, M., & Loots, G. (2017, November 8). Blockchain as an enabler for public mHealth solutions in South Africa. *2017 IST-Africa Week Conference*, *2017*, 1–8. Advance online publication. doi:10.23919/ISTAFRICA.2017.8102404

White, J. M., & Bedell, H. E. (1990). The oculomotor reference in humans with bilateral macular disease. *Investigative Ophthalmology & Visual Science*, *31*(6), 1149–1161. PMID:2354915

Whitelaw, S., Mamas, M. A., Topol, E., & Van Spall, H. G. (2020). *Application of digital technology in COVID-19 pandemic planning and response*. The Lancet Digital Health.

WHO. (2020). Contact tracing in the context of Covid-19. In *WHO Guidelines* (Vol. 2019, Issue May 10). https://www.who.int/publications-detail/contact-tracing-in-the-context-of-Covid-19

WHO/UNAIDS. (2007). New Data on Male Circumcision and HIV Prevention: Policy and Programme Implications In WHO/UNAIDS Technical Consultation on Male Circumcision and HIV Prevention: Research Implications for Policy and Programming. Geneva: WHO Press.

WHO/UNAIDS/JHPIEGO. (2009). *Manual for Male Circumcision under Local Anaesthesia*. Retrieved July 8, 2011 from http://www.malecircumcision.org/about/ documents/MC_manual_local_anaesthesia.pdf

Wikipedia. (2020). *Covid 19 stats mali - Google Search*. https://www.google.com/search?client=firefox-b-d&q=covid+19+stats+mali

Wirth, J. (2018). *Dependent Variables in the Privacy-Related Field: A Descriptive Literature Review*. Academic Press.

Wirth, J., Maier, C., & Laumer, S. (2019). *Subjective Norm and the Privacy Calculus: Explaining Self-Disclosure on Social Networking*. Academic Press.

World Economic Outlook. (2018). *Groups and Aggregates Information*. World Economic Outlook. Available at: https://en.wikipedia.org/wiki/Developing_country#cite_note-107

World Health Organization (WHO). (2011). mHealth: New horizons for health through mobile technologies. Global Observatory for eHealth Series, 3.

World Health Organization. (1982). *Medium term program*. World Health Organization.

World Health Organization. (2020). Coronavirus disease (COVID-19): Situation report. WHO.

Wu, A., & Zeng, Z. (2012). Dynamic behaviors of memristor-based recurrent neural networks with time-varying delays. *Neural Networks*, *36*, 1–10. doi:10.1016/j.neunet.2012.08.009 PMID:23037770

Wyscocki, A. (2004). The multiple media of texts: How onscreen and paper texts incorporate words, images, and other media. In C. Bazerman & P. Prior (Eds.), *What writing does and how it does it: An introduction to analyzing texts and textual practices* (pp. 123–163). Lawrence Erlbaum.

Xu, H., Gupta, S., Rosson, M. B., & Carroll, J. M. (2012). *Measuring mobile users' concerns for information privacy*. Academic Press.

Yamuah, L. (2005). *Towards healthy nations with ICT wealth*. Information for Development. Retrieved October 10, 2021, from www.i4d.csdms

Yang, S., Fichman, P., Zhu, X., Sanfilippo, M., Li, S., & Fleischmann, K. R. (2020). The use of ICT during COVID-19. *Proceedings of the Association for Information Science and Technology*, *57*(1), e297. doi:10.1002/pra2.297 PMID:33173819

Yao, M. Z. (2011). Self-Protection of Online Privacy: A Behavioral Approach. In *Privacy Online* (pp. 111–125). Springer Berlin Heidelberg., doi:10.1007/978-3-642-21521-6_9

Yeatman, S. E., Hoffman, R. M., Chilungo, A., Lungu, S. R., Namadingo, H. C., Chimwaza, A. F., & Trinitapoly, J. A. (2015). Brief Report: Health-Seeking Behavior and Symptoms Associated with Early HIV Infection: Results from a Population-Based Cohort in Southern Malawi. *Journal of Acquired Immune Deficiency Syndromes*, *69*(1), 126–130. doi:10.1097/QAI.0000000000000536 PMID:25942464

Yordanova, K., Favela, J., & Marcu, G. (2019). Challenges Providing Ground Truth for Pervasive Healthcare Systems. In IEEE Pervasive Computing (Vol. 18, Issue 2, pp. 100–104). Institute of Electrical and Electronics Engineers Inc. doi:10.1109/MPRV.2019.2912261

Yusof, M. M., & Arifin, A. (2016, November). Towards an evaluation framework for Laboratory Information Systems. *Journal of Infection and Public Health*, *9*(6), 766–773. Advance online publication. doi:10.1016/j.jiph.2016.08.014

Yusof, M. M., Kuljis, J., Papazafeiropoulou, A., & Stergioulas, L. K. (2008). An evaluation framework for Health Information Systems: Human, organization and technology-fit factors (HOT-fit). *International Journal of Medical Informatics*, *77*(6), 386–398. doi:10.1016/j.ijmedinf.2007.08.011 PMID:17964851

Yusof, M. M., Papazafeiropoulou, A., Paul, R. J., & Stergioulas, L. K. (2008, June). Investigating evaluation frameworks for health information systems. *International Journal of Medical Informatics*, *77*(6), 377–385. Advance online publication. doi:10.1016/j.ijmedinf.2007.08.004 PMID:17904898

Zaidi, S. (2017). *E-government services effectiveness evaluation framework (E-GEEF): A case study of Indian e-tax service*. http://repository.londonmet.ac.uk/id/eprint/1254

Zewge, A., & Dittrich, Y. (2017). Systematic mapping study of information technology for development in agriculture (the case of developing countries). *The Electronic Journal on Information Systems in Developing Countries*, *82*(2), 1–25. doi:10.1002/j.1681-4835.2017.tb00602.x

Zhang, P., Schmidt, D. C., White, J., & Lenz, G. (2018). Blockchain Technology Use Cases in Healthcare. In *Advances in Computers* (Vol. 111, pp. 1–41). Elsevier. doi:10.1016/bs.adcom.2018.03.006

Zlatolas, L. N., Welzer, T., Heričko, M., & Hölbl, M. (2015). Privacy antecedents for SNS self-disclosure: The case of Facebook. *Computers in Human Behavior*, *45*, 158–167. Advance online publication. doi:10.1016/j.chb.2014.12.012

Zu, Z. Y., Jiang, M. D., Xu, P. P., Chen, W., Ni, Q. Q., Lu, G. M., & Zhang, L. J. (2020). Coronavirus disease 2019 (COVID-19): A perspective from China. *Radiology*, *296*(2), 200490. doi:10.1148/radiol.2020200490 PMID:32083985

About the Contributors

Patrick Ndayizigamiye obtained his PhD (Information Systems and Technology) from the University of KwaZulu-Natal in South Africa. Patrick is currently employed as a Senior Lecturer at the University of Johannesburg in South Africa and is the ICT4D research cluster leader at the University of Johannesburg. He has more than ten years of experience in teaching information systems modules and has published in international journals and conference proceedings. He has also presented his research outputs at many local and international conferences. He is currently an associate editor for the African Journal of Information Systems and has been a Track Program Committee (TCP) member of many reputable international conferences. Patrick is also a member of the Association for Information systems (AIS) and the South African Institute of Computer Scientists and Information Technologists (SAICSIT). His current research interest is in the design and deployment of ICT-led interventions to provide healthcare services in Resource-Limited Settings. He is also conducting research in ICT4D and Cybersecurity.

* * *

Joel Adépo is a teacher at the Virtual University of Côte d'Ivoire since 2017. He gives lectures on computer networks and security.

Philip Chike Chukwunonso Aghadiuno is a Principal Lecturer in the Department of Library and Information Science, Isa Mustapha Agwai 1 Polytechnic, Lafia, Nasarawa State. He holds a Higher National Diploma from the Federal Polytechnic, Oko, Post-Graduate Diploma in Education from the Benue State University, Makurdi, Master's degree in Library and Information Science from the University of Nigeria, Nsukka, and is currently a Ph.D. student at the University of Nigeria, Nsukka. His major areas of research interests are scholarly communication, information and knowledge management, multimedia, social media, and use of digital technologies in library, information and documentation centres. He is a certified library professional which earned him the Certified Librarian of Nigeria (CLN) awarded by the Librarians Registration Council of Nigeria (LRCN). He holds membership of professional associations, including Nigerian Library Association (NLA), Nigerian Association of Library and Information Science Educators, among others.

Abiodun (Abbey) Alao obtained her Doctor of Philosophy in Information Systems from the University of Cape Town. She has been an active researcher and teaching fellow at various South African Universities. Abiodun is passionate about research and keen to demonstrate her academic capabilities in higher educational institutions using work-integrated learning to equip and prepare young people with the relevant industry skills that will allow them to function in the labour market. She is currently a research fellow at the University of Johannesburg where she derives delight mentoring and working on projects that relate to Human-computer interaction, Organisational digital transformation, Information and Communication Technology for Development (ICT4D), and Sustainable ICTs.

Michel Babri is Professor in Computer Science since 1982. His interest is in network and Data mining.

Chiara Baghino is an orthoptist who obtained her master's degree at University of Genoa. Since the beginning of her career she works with low-vision children, co-operating in a rehabilitation equipe at David Chiossone Istitute (Genoa, Italy) since it is fundamental for the rehabilitation of children with disabilities.

Roelien Brink is a researcher in the Department of Applied Information Systems Management at the University of Johannesburg. She holds a PhD from the University of Johannesburg, South Africa, with a focus on information management for the work-integrated learning process. She is a Vice-Chair in the African region in the International Research Group for World Association for Cooperative Education (WACE). Her research is mainly focused on work-integrated learning. Also, she was part of the international review team for the WACE 2nd International Research Symposium and WACE 20th World Conference. Her research interests focus on work-integrated learning, information systems, information communication and technology for development. She is the cluster leader for the information and communication technology for development (ICT4D) field at the University of Johannesburg and currently supervising postgraduate students in Omni Channels, Cashless Economy and cloud computing and involved in technology projects such as Status of Women in Information Technology (SWIFT) and Sense of Belonging, Social Media and Well-Being: Comparing Co-op and Non-Co-op Student Perceptions and an international experience at the University of Waterloo in Canada.

Elisabetta Capris is an M.D. Opthalmologist, specialized in Low Vision and visual rehabilitation. Director of the childhood unit at David Chiossone Institute (Genoa, Italy). Competences on pediatric visual pathologies and multiple disabilities

Elena Cocchi is the Director of the Visual Rehabilitation Center at David Chiossone Institute (Genoa, Italy).

Silvia Dini, with a degree in Communication, works at David Chiossone Institute for blind, in Genova; She is expert in accessibility and information technology, has been collaborating for years in research projects and publications on innovations and software to improve the quality of life of people with visual disabilities of all ages

Valentina Facchini is an orthoptist, assistant in opthalmology specializing in low vision and in the visual rehabilitation of visually impaired subjects.

Shaivar Girdhari is a very good communicator and finds it easy to relate to other people. He really enjoys learning new things and is constantly seeking out new learning opportunities. His prior experience in customer service has provided him with unique technical skills that he can apply within and around the IT industry. Working at a startup (Launch Code) gave him an opportunity to understand the ins and outs of the industry, and to take on tasks he might not have at a larger company. He is not afraid of failure. In fact, he thinks it is an essential part of the experimental process that gets you to success. When solving problems, he applies both logic and emotional aspects in equal proportion. For instance, he is trained in SEO and understands how to use analytics to ensure a marketing campaign is successful, but he also majored in IS/IT Management and knows how to apply innovative, technological creativity to a project as well. Shaivar is passionate about environmental concerns and technological sustainability. The planet and environment are something that we all share and Green Computing is a gray area in which not many businesses or individuals place enough emphasis. However, the eco-friendly usage of technology could play a prominent role in striving towards a sustainable future alongside safe & environmentally friendly technological devices. Geographical Information Systems (GIS) is a point of peculiar interest for Shaivar. He is very skilled and a quick learner at discerning geographical data and software and most geographical concepts come naturally to him. Shaivar's current endeavors lead him to the forefront of the fourth industrial revolution (4IR), with him specializing in blockchain and its uses/applications towards healthcare within his studies towards a Master's degree. Some of Shaivar's hobbies include fish breeding and caring, learning of astronomical phenomena, hiking, volunteering, and meditation.

Mahamadou Kanté is a public servant of his state and a scientist with research experience in IT, data protection, privacy preservation and related areas. He is currently affiliated with the Virtual University of Ivory Coast working in the area of cyber security and IoT. His papers/chapters have been published in peer-reviewed regional and international journals. He is a reviewer for many journals that include the International Journal of Information Security Science, the African Journal of Social Sciences, and Public Health (board member). He is also a confident teacher able to explain complex information to audiences.

Donald Flywell Malanga is a PhD candidate in Information Systems Program at the University of Cape Town, South Africa. He holds a Master's degree in Library and Information Science from the University of Botswana and a Bachelor's degree in Library and Information Science from Mzuzu University, Malawi. His research focuses on Information and Communication Technology for Development (ICT4D); Health Informatics; Health Information Systems Evaluations; Information Ethics; Open/E-Government; and Digital Information Literacy. He is both a Fellow of Communication Policy Research for the Global South and African School on Internet Governance. He currently works as a Librarian at the University of Livingstonia in Malawi.

Simon Shachia Oryila lectures in the Department of English, Benue State University, Makurdi, Nigeria. He is about completing his Ph.D. in English at the Ahmadu Bello University, Zaria, Nigeria. He holds M.A. in Linguistics (2012), B.A. (Hons.) in English (2005), Diploma in Law (2001) from the Benue State University, Makurdi, and another Diploma in Computer Studies (2007) from the Usmanu Danfodiyo University, Sokoto, Nigeria. He has attended and presented papers at local and international conferences. His major research and teaching interests include: Applied Linguistics; Peace and War Linguistics, Ecolinguistics; Critical Discourse Analysis; Multimodality; Social Semiotics; Stylistics; Pragmatics; Semantics; Digital Media; Editing, Writing, and Publishing. He has written as well as collaborated and authored scholarly works in the fields of Social Sciences, Arts and Humanities, Law, Education, and Library and Information Science, which reflect his multi-disciplinary bent. He is a member of the Association of Nigerian Authors, Society for Research and Academic Excellence, English Scholars' Association of Nigeria (ESAN), among others.

Antonella Panizzi is an orthoptist who completed with laude her master's degree in 2011. Since 2015 she is working at David Chiossone Institute (Genoa, Italy), working about visually impaired children and adults rehabilitation.

Giulia Perasso has a PhD in Psychology, Neuroscience and Data Science obtained at University of Pavia (Italy) in 2021. She is the scientific coordinator of David Chiossone Institute telematic rehabilitation protocol. She is currently adjunct professor of Developmental Psychology at University of Genoa.

Valentina Salvagno is an orthoptist specialised in visual rehabilitation and she is part of the rehabilitation equipe of David Chiossone Institute (Genoa, Italy).

Index

www.ingramcontent.com/pod-product-compliance
Lightning Source LLC
LaVergne TN
LVHW060002031026
849161LV00025B/1310
* 9 7 8 1 7 9 9 8 8 9 1 5 1 *